Clinical Medicine

Clinical Medicine

DAVID RUBENSTEIN

MA BM FRCP (Lond)
Physician
Addenbrooke's Hospital
Cambridge

DAVID WAYNE

MA BM FRCP (Lond & Edin)
Physician
James Paget Hospital
Great Yarmouth

JOHN BRADLEY

B Med Sci, DM, FRCP
Physician
Addenbrooke's Hospital
Cambridge

Fifth edition

**Blackwell
Science**

© 1976, 1980, 1985, 1991, 1997 by
Blackwell Science Ltd
Editorial Offices:
Osney Mead, Oxford OX2 0EL
25 John Street, London WC1N 2BL
23 Ainslie Place, Edinburgh EH3 6AJ
350 Main Street, Malden
  MA 02148 5018, USA
54 University Street, Carlton
  Victoria 3053, Australia
10, rue Casimir Delavigne
  75006 Paris, France

Other Editorial Offices:
Blackwell Wissenschafts-Verlag GmbH
Kurfürstendamm 57
10707 Berlin, Germany

Blackwell Science KK
MG Kodenmacho Building
7–10 Kodenmacho Nihombashi
Chuo-ku, Tokyo 104, Japan

First published 1976
Reprinted 1977, 1978, 1979
Second edition 1980
Reprinted 1981, 1982, 1983, 1984
Third edition 1985
Reprinted 1986, 1987, 1990
Portuguese translation 1981
Spanish translation 1984
German translation 1986
Fourth edition 1991
Reprinted 1992, 1994, 1995, 1996, 1997
Four Dragons edition 1991
Reprinted 1992, 1994, 1996
Fifth edition 1997
Reprinted 2000

A catalogue record for this title
is available from the British Library

ISBN 0-86542-925-1 (BSL)
     0-86542-632-5 (IE)

Library of Congress
Cataloging-in-Publication Data

Rubenstein, David.
    Lecture notes on clinical medicine/
 David Rubenstein, David Wayne,
 John Bradley.—5th ed.
        p.   cm.
    Includes bibliographical references
 and index.
    ISBN 0-86542-925-1
    1. Clinical medicine—Handbooks,
 manuals, etc. 1. Wayne, David.
 II. Bradley, John, MRCP. III. Title.
    [DNLM: 1. Clinical Medicine—
 handbooks.
 WB 39 R895L 1997]
 RC48.R8 1997
 616—dc21
 DNLM/DLC
 for Library of Congress   97-10914
                                  CIP

Set by Excel Typesetters Co., Hong Kong
Printed and bound in Great Britain by
MPG Books Ltd, Bodmin, Cornwall

DISTRIBUTORS

Marston Book Services Ltd
PO Box 269
Abingdon
Oxon OX14 4YN
(Orders: Tel: 01235 465500
              Fax: 01235 465555)

USA
Blackwell Science, Inc.
Commerce Place
350 Main Street
Malden, MA 02148 5018
(Orders: Tel: 800 759 6102
               781 388 8250
         Fax: 781 388 8255)

Canada
Login Brothers Book Company
324 Saulteaux Crescent
Winnipeg, Manitoba R3J 3T2
(Orders: Tel: 204 837-2987)

Australia
Blackwell Science Pty Ltd
54 University Street
Carlton, Victoria 3053
(Orders: Tel: 03 9347 0300
          Fax: 03 9347 5001)

The Blackwell Science logo is a
trade mark of Blackwell Science Ltd,
registered at the United Kingdom
Trade Marks Registry

For further information on
Blackwell Science, visit our website:
www.blackwell-science.com

Contents

other conditions. Valvular heart disease: aortic stenosis, aortic regurgitation, mitral stenosis, mitral regurgitation, tricuspid regurgitation, pulmonary stenosis, atrial myxoma. Congenital heart disease: working classification, atrial septal defect, patent ductus arteriosus, ventricular septal defect, Fallot's tetralogy, pulmonary stenosis, coarctation of the aorta, Eisenmenger's syndrome. Infective endocarditis. Constrictive pericarditis. Acute pericarditis. Syphilitic aortitis and carditis. Cardiomyopathy: hypertrophic cardiomyopathy, dilated (congestive) cardiomyopathy, restrictive cardiomyopathy. Peripheral arterial disease: intermittent claudication, acute obstruction, ischaemic foot, Raynaud's phenomenon.

Preface to the Fifth Edition

In this edition we have included relevant sections on basic physiology, pharmacology and genetics which form a significant number of MCQ questions. We have also highlighted the most important clinical trials. The book has been fully updated, carefully audited and re-engineered to take account of evidence-based practice. As in earlier editions the margin is intentionally wide to allow personal additions. If anything factual needs deleting or altering do please let us know.

David Rubenstein
David Wayne
John Bradley

Preface to the First Edition

This book is intended primarily for the junior hospital doctor in the period between qualification and the examination for Membership of the Royal Colleges of Physicians. We think that it will also be helpful to final-year medical students and to clinicians reading for higher specialist qualifications in surgery and anaesthetics.

The hospital doctor must not only acquire a large amount of factual information but also use it effectively in the clinical situation. The experienced physician has acquired some clinical perspective through practice: we hope that this book imparts some of this to the relatively inexperienced. The format and contents are designed for the examination candidate but the same approach to problems should help the hospital doctor in his everyday work.

The book as a whole is not suitable as a first reader for the undergraduate because it assumes much basic knowledge and considerable detailed information has had to be omitted. It is not intended to be a complete textbook of medicine and the information it contains must be supplemented by further reading. The contents are intended only as lecture notes and the margins of the pages are intentionally large so that the reader may easily add additional material of his own.

The book is divided into two parts: the *clinical approach* and *essential background information*. In the first part we have considered the situation which a candidate meets in the clinical part of an examination or a physician in the clinic. This part of the book thus resembles a manual on techniques of physical examination, though it is more specifically intended to help the candidate carry out an examiner's request to perform a specific examination. It has been our experience in listening to candidates' performances in examinations and hearing the examiner's subsequent assessment, that it is the failure of a candidate to examine cases systematically and his failure to behave as if he were used to doing this every day of his clinical life that leads to adverse comments.

In the second part of the book a summary of basic clinical facts is given in the conventional way. We have included most common diseases but not all, and we have tried to emphasise points which are understressed in many textbooks. Accounts are given of many conditions which are relatively rare. It is necessary for the clinician to know about these and to be on the lookout for them both in the clinic and in examinations. Supplementary reading is essential to understand their basic pathology but the information we give is probably all that need be remembered by the non-specialist reader and will provide adequate working knowledge in a clinical situation. It should not be forgotten that some rare diseases are of

great importance in practice because they are treatable or preventable, e.g. infective endocarditis, hepatolenticular degeneration, attacks of acute porphyria. Some
conditions are important to examination candidates because patients are ambu-
lant and appear commonly in examinations, e.g. neurosyphilis, syringomyelia, atrial
and ventricular septal defects.

We have not attempted to cover the whole of medicine but by cross-
referencing between the two sections of the book and giving information in
summary form we have completely omitted few subjects. Some highly specialised
fields such as the treatment of leukaemia were thought unsuitable for inclusion.

A short account of psychiatry is given in the section on neurology since many
patients with mental illness attend general clinics and it is hoped that readers may
be warned of gaps in their knowledge of this important field. The section on
dermatology is incomplete but should serve for quick revision of common skin
disorders.

Wherever possible we have tried to indicate the relative frequency with which
various conditions are likely to be seen in hospital practice in this country and
have selected those clinical features which in our view are most commonly seen
and where possible have listed them in order of importance. The frequency with
which a disease is encountered by any individual physician will depend upon its
prevalence in the district from which his cases are drawn and also on his known
special interests. Nevertheless, rare conditions are rarely seen; at least in the
clinic. Examinations, however, are a 'special case'.

We have used many generally accepted abbreviations, e.g. ECG, ESR, and have
included them in the index instead of supplying a glossary.

Despite our best efforts, some errors of fact may have been included. As with
every book and authority, question and check everything—and please write to us
if you wish.

We should like to thank all those who helped us with producing this book and
in particular, Sir Edward Wayne and Sir Graham Bull who have kindly allowed us to
benefit from their extensive experience both in medicine and in examining for the
Colleges of Physicians.

David Rubenstein
David Wayne
November 1975

The Clinical Approach

Nervous System

The candidate is usually asked to examine a specific area, e.g. '*Examine the cranial nerves*', '*Examine the lower limbs*', '*Examine the arms*' or '*Examine the eyes*'. By far the commonest neurological disorders suitable for a clinical examination are multiple sclerosis and the results of cerebrovascular disease. Diabetes is a common disorder which fairly frequently gives rise to neurological manifestations. Carcinomatous neuropathy should always be considered when the signs are difficult to synthesize. Parkinsonism is relatively common. Motor neurone disease (MND), myopathies, myasthenia gravis and the neurological manifestations of vitamin B_{12} deficiency are all rare in practice but more frequently seen in examinations. Neurosyphilis is now rarely seen—the patient will belong to the prepenicillin era, i.e. be over 60 years old.

In terms of examination technique the practising physician must examine case after case, both normal and abnormal, in order to develop a system which is rapid, accurate and which becomes second nature. An appearance of professionalism in your neurological examination may encourage the examiner to take a kinder view of minor errors than if you appear hesitant, clumsy or imprecise. Analysis of clinical signs is improved if you can remember some anatomical diagrams (pp. 6, 7 and 24).

3

Cranial nerves

'*Examine the cranial nerves*'
Many abnormalities of the cranial nerves are the results of chronic disease and such patients are commonly seen in examinations.

The commonest disorders in examinations are multiple sclerosis (optic atrophy, nystagmus (often ataxic), cerebellar dysarthria), stroke and Bell's palsy. The manifestation of cerebral tumour, aneurysm, dystrophia myotonica and myasthenia gravis are seen much less frequently. It is useful to memorize diagrams of cross-sections of the brainstem and of the floor of the fourth ventricle (p. 6) since these may greatly improve analysis of a cranial nerve lesion. Do not spend long on the 1st or 2nd cranial nerves unless there is good reason to suspect an abnormality. If the optic fundus is abnormal, the examiner is likely to ask you to look at it specifically. Eye movements must be carefully examined. Do not confuse ptosis (3rd nerve or sympathetic) with paresis of the orbicularis oculi (7th nerve). Make sure you can explain clearly and concisely the difference between an upper and lower motor neuron (UMN and LMN) lesion of the 7th nerve. The corneal reflex is an essential part of the complete examination of the cranial nerves.

The following approach is recommended:

Smell

'*Has there been any recent change in your sense of smell?*' If so, test formally with fresh 'smell bottles' (e.g. freshly ground coffee or instant coffee granules). Colds and sinusitis are the most likely cause.

Eyes

Observe, and test when necessary, for:
- *visual acuity*, either quickly with literature from the bedside locker, or formally with Snellen charts;
- *ptosis*;
    (a) third nerve lesion (complete or partial ptosis);
    (b) sympathetic lesion (partial ptosis) as part of Horner's syndrome. Muscle weakness of myasthenia gravis (and rarely, dystrophia myotonica, facioscapulohumeral dystrophy, congenital and in taboparesis).
NB　Ptosis is not due to a 7th-nerve lesion.
- *pupillary responses* (p. 9)
- *visual fields* to confrontation (2nd nerve; p. 5)
- *external ocular movements* (3rd, 4th and 6th nerve; p. 9) and *nystagmus* (p. 12)
- the *fundi* (2nd nerve; p. 31).

Face (7th nerve)

- '*Screw up your eyes very tightly.*' Compare how deeply the eyelashes are buried on the two sides. Unilateral weakness is invariably due to an LMN lesion.
- '*Grin.*' Compare the nasolabial grooves.

Mouth

- '*Clench your teeth*' (5th nerve, motor). Feel the masseters and test the jaw jerk if indicated. The jaw jerk is obtained from placing one finger horizontally across the front of the jaw and tapping the finger with a tendon hammer with the jaw relaxed and the mouth just open. An increased jaw jerk occurs in UMN lesions of the 5th cranial nerves (pseudobulbar palsy, p. 15).
- '*Open your mouth and keep it open*' (5th nerve, motor: pterygoids). You should not be able to force it closed. With a unilateral lesion, the jaw deviates towards the weaker side (the weak muscle cannot keep it open).
- '*Say aaah*' (9th and 10th nerves: both mixed, but the ninth is mainly sensory for the pharynx and palate, and the 10th for motor). Normally the uvula and soft palate move upwards and remain central and the posterior pharyngeal wall moves a little. With a unilateral lesion the soft palate is pulled away from the weaker side (there may also be 'curtain movement' of the posterior pharyngeal wall away from the weaker side).
- '*Put your tongue out*' (12th nerve). Look for wasting, fasciculation and whether it protrudes to one side (towards the weaker side since the weaker muscle cannot push it out).

Neck (11th nerve)

- '*Lift your head off the pillows*' or '*Put your chin on your right (or left) shoulder*' while you resist the movement. Look at, and palpate the sternomastoids.
- '*Shrug your shoulders*' while you push them down. Look at and palpate the bulk of trapezius.

Ears (8th nerve)

Test hearing by whispering in each ear and perform Weber and Rinne tests (p. 11). You should ask for an auriscope if indicated. The commonest cause of conductive (air conduction) deafness is wax.

Facial sensation (5th nerve)

Test the three divisions on both sides with cotton wool. Check the corneal reflexes (often the first clinical deficit in 5th nerve lesions). Ask the patient if the sensation is equally unpleasant on the two sides.

NB It is frequently helpful to be able to draw cross-sections of the spinal cord and brainstem when considering lesions in those areas (Figs 1.1–1.3).

FIELD DEFECTS

In principle you are comparing the patient's visual fields with your own. When

THE SPINAL CORD

Dorsal columns

Spinocerebellar tracts

Spinothalamic tracts

Pyramidal tract (lateral columns)

Sensory | Motor

Fig. 1.1 Cross-section through the spinal cord.

THE OPEN MEDULLA

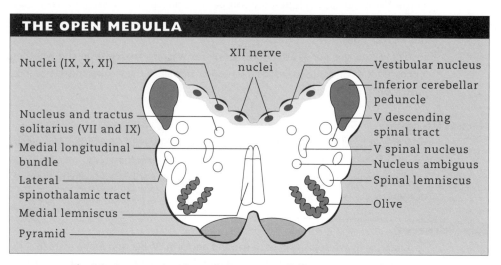

Nuclei (IX, X, XI)

XII nerve nuclei

Vestibular nucleus

Inferior cerebellar peduncle

Nucleus and tractus solitarius (VII and IX)

V descending spinal tract

Medial longitudinal bundle

V spinal nucleus

Nucleus ambiguus

Lateral spinothalamic tract

Spinal lemniscus

Medial lemniscus

Olive

Pyramid

Fig. 1.2 Cross-section through the open medulla.

testing the right eye, the patient should be level with you and look straight into your left eye with the patient's head held at arm's length. '*Keep looking at my eye and tell me when you first see my finger out of the corner of your eye.*' Then bring your finger towards the centre of the field of vision from the four main directions (right, left, up, down). It is preferable to use a white-headed hat pin if you have one.

The nasal and superior fields are limited by the nose and eyebrow respectively but this is not often of clinical importance. Field defects are described by the side of the visual field which is lost, i.e. temporal field loss indicates loss of the tempo-

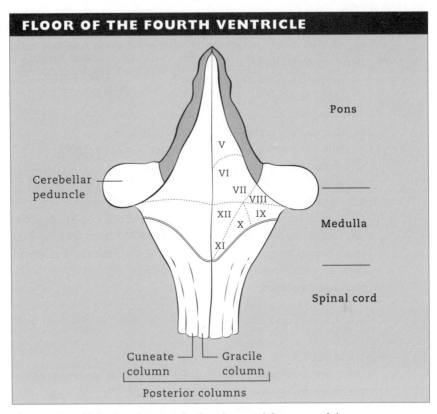

FLOOR OF THE FOURTH VENTRICLE

Pons

Cerebellar peduncle

V
VI
VII
VIII
XII
X
IX
XI

Medulla

Spinal cord

Cuneate column — Gracile column

Posterior columns

Fig. 1.3 Floor of the fourth ventricle showing cranial nerve nuclei.

ral field of vision and denotes damage to the nasal retina or its connections back to the visual cortex. Perimetry will accurately define defects.

• *Temporal hemianopia* in one eye alone or in both eyes (bitemporal hemianopia) suggests a chiasmal compression usually from a pituitary tumour.

• *Homonymous hemianopia* (loss of nasal field in one eye and temporal field in the other). This may occur with any postchiasmal lesion, commonly following a posterior cerebral vascular lesion (usually with macular sparing). The side of the field loss is opposite to the side of the damaged cortex (i.e. a right-sided cerebral lesion produces a left homonymous hemianopia).

• *Upper quadrantic field loss* suggests a temporal lesion of the opposite cortex or optic radiation. It is homonymous.

• *Central scotoma.* Loss of vision in the centre of the visual field is detected by passing a small-diameter white- or red-tipped pin across the front of the eyes which are held looking forward. This occurs in acute retrobulbar neuritis most commonly due to multiple sclerosis.

• Test for visual inattention by presenting the stimulus simultaneously to both eyes.

BLINDNESS

A history of transient blindness, total or partial (with specific field defects usually in one eye) is not uncommon in migraine. Carotid transient ischaemic attacks cause transient unilateral blindness (p. 131).

Sudden blindness also occurs with:

- retinal detachment;
- acute glaucoma;
- vitreous haemorrhage in diabetes;
- temporal arteritis and retinal artery or vein obstruction;
- fractures of the skull; and
- raised intracranial pressure.

NB   The light reflex is absent except in cortical blindness.

Senile changes and *glaucoma* account for about two-thirds of blindness in the UK. Diabetes is the major non-ocular (systemic) cause (7–10%) due chiefly to vitreous haemorrhage, advanced retinopathy and cataract. Trachoma is a common cause on a worldwide basis. *Hysterical blindness* is uncommon and should never be confidently assumed.

The blindness of *temporal arteritis* is preventable if steroid therapy is started in time.

EYE MOVEMENTS

These are controlled by the 3rd, 4th and 6th nerves and conjugate movement integrated by the medial longitudinal bundle. This connects the above nuclei together and to the cerebellum and the vestibular nuclei.

SQUINT (strabismus)

Congenital concomitant squints are present from childhood and are due to a defect of one eye. The angle between the longitudinal axes of the eyes remains constant on testing extraocular movements, and there is no diplopia.

Paralytic squint is acquired and results from paralysis of one or more of the muscles which move the eye, or paralysis from proptosis. On testing external ocular movements, the angle between the eye axes varies and there is diplopia. The following rules should be borne in mind:

1   Diplopia is maximum when looking in the direction of action of the paralysed muscle.

2   The image further from the midline arises from the paralysed eye. This may be determined by covering up each eye in turn and asking which image has disappeared.

NB   It is sometimes easier to test movements in each eye separately.

'Do you see double?'

If so, ask in which direction it is worst. Move your forefinger in that direction and then ask if the two fingers which the patient sees are parallel to each other (lateral rectus palsy: 6th nerve) or at an angle (superior oblique palsy: 4th nerve). If the patient has not noticed diplopia, test the movements formally, right and left, up and down, and note if there is any nystagmus.

Apart from local lesions such as pressure from tumour or aneurysm, isolated external ocular palsies may result from diabetes mellitus (ischaemia), multiple sclerosis, migraine, raised intracranial pressure, mononeuritis multiplex (e.g. polyarteritis), and rarely from sarcoidosis, syphilis (ischaemia) and meningitis (usually tuberculosis or pneumococcal).

Lateral rectus palsy (6th nerve)

This produces failure of lateral movement with convergent strabismus. It is the commonest external ocular palsy. The diplopia is maximal on looking to the affected side. The images are parallel and separated horizontally. The outermost image comes from the affected eye and disappears when that eye is covered. The palsy is produced as a false localizing sign in raised intracranial pressure or by direct involvement with tumour, aneurysm, or rarely with acoustic neuroma (p. 150).

Superior oblique palsy (4th nerve)

This type is rare. Palsy produces diplopia which is maximal on downward gaze. The two images are then at an angle to each other when the palsied eye is abducted and one above the other when the eye is adducted. The diplopia is therefore noticed most on reading or descending stairs.

Third nerve palsy

It may not present with diplopia because there may be complete ptosis. When the lid is lifted the eye is seen to be 'down and out' (divergent strabismus) and there is severe (angulated) diplopia. The pupil may be dilated. It occurs with space-occupying lesions, brainstem vascular lesions (Weber's syndrome) after surgery (e.g. for pituitary lesions) and aneurysm of the posterior communicating artery (painful).

The muscles themselves are involved in myasthenia gravis (p. 168) and in the ophthalmoplegia of thyrotoxicosis (particularly looking up and out) (p. 204).

PUPILLARY REFLEXES

The balance between parasympathetic (constrictor) and sympathetic (dilator) tone controls pupil size.

Constriction of the pupil in response to light. This is relayed via the optic nerve, optic tract, lateral geniculate nuclei, the Edinger–Westphal nucleus of the 3rd nerve and the ciliary ganglion. The cortex is not involved.

Constriction of the pupil with accommodation. Convergence originates within the cortex and is relayed to the pupil via the 3rd nerve nuclei. The optic nerve and tract and the lateral geniculate nucleus are not involved.

Therefore:

• if the direct light reflex is absent and the convergence reflex is present, a local lesion in the brainstem or ciliary ganglion is implied, possibly due to degeneration in the ciliary ganglia, e.g. the Argyll Robertson pupil of syphilis;

• if the convergence reflex is absent and the light reflex is present, a lesion of the cerebral cortex is implied, e.g. cortical blindness.

Examination of the pupillary reflexes should be performed in subdued light. The pupil should be positively inspected for irregularity. A torch is flashed twice at each eye (once for direct and once for consensual responses), preferably from the side so that the patient does not focus on it (and hence have an accommodation–convergence reflex).

If the pupil is constricted consider: Horner's syndrome (below); morphine; pilocarpine; pontine haemorrhage; Argyll Robertson pupil (must be irregular and have no light reflex). It also occurs in normal old age.

If the pupil is dilated consider: mydriatics (e.g. homatropine, tropicamide or cyclopentolate); a 3rd-nerve lesion; the Holmes–Adie syndrome (pupils constrict sluggishly to light, e.g. in half an hour in a bright room, and absent tendon reflexes); and congenital (ask the patient). In the unconscious patient a fixed dilated pupil (3rd-nerve lesion) may indicate temporal lobe herniation (from raised intracranial pressure) on the same side, intracranial bleeding, tumour or abscess.

HORNER'S SYNDROME

This is rare in practice but common in examinations. The syndrome comprises unilateral:

• ptosis (partial, i.e. sympathetic)
• miosis (constricted pupil) with normal reactions
• anhidrosis (decreased sweating over face)
• enophthalmos (indrawing of orbital contents), i.e. everything gets smaller or contracts.

The syndrome results from lesions of the sympathetic nerves to the eye, anywhere from the hypothalamus downwards through the sympathetic nucleus of the brainstem and during their passage through the cervical and upper thoracic cord, the anterior spinal first thoracic root, the sympathetic chain, stellate ganglion and carotid sympathetic plexus. It is essential to look for evidence of a T1 lesion (p. 26) and to palpate the neck and supraclavicular fossae for malignant glands.

Aetiology

• Carcinoma of the bronchus (T1, Pancoast tumour)
• Cervical node secondary deposits

- Cervical sympathectomy (look for the scar)
- Brainstem vascular disease (lateral medullary syndrome, p. 128) and demyelinating disease
- Local neoplasms and trauma in the neck
- Rarely, carotid or aortic aneurysms
- Very rarely, syringomyelia and intrinsic cervical cord disease (vascular and neoplastic).

HEARING

Roughly assess auditory acuity in each ear in succession, by blocking the sound in the other ear with a restless finger tip, and then whisper at arm's length. Compare the ears. A clockwork watch, if available, is a suitable alternative.

Weber test

A vibrating tuning fork is held in the middle of the forehead. In the absence of nerve deafness, the sound is louder in the ear where air conduction is impaired, e.g. wax or otitis media. (This can easily be checked by placing a vibrating tuning fork on one's own forehead and putting a finger in one ear.)

Rinne test

Air conduction is normally better than bone conduction. The vibrating tuning fork is first placed behind the ear on the mastoid process and then rapidly held with its prongs in line with the external meatus. The patient is asked: 'Is it louder behind (with the tuning fork on the mastoid) or in front (with the tuning fork in line with the external meatus)?' Normally it is louder in front — this is termed Rinne-positive. Negative is abnormal and implies conductive (air) deafness in that ear — usually wax.

DIZZINESS AND GIDDINESS

Dizziness and giddiness are very common neurological presenting features.

The important clinical observation is to determine whether there is true vertigo or not (see below). If this is present, it strongly suggests a disorder of the brainstem (vascular or demyelinating) or its vestibular connections, e.g. labyrinthitis, Menière's disease (see below). Dizziness or unsteadiness without vertigo, particularly if intermittent, may suggest postural hypotension, which is relatively common in the elderly, in those on overenthusiastic hypotensive regimes and in those who stand stationary too long, particularly in warm weather. It may also suggest a cardiovascular disorder such as a transient cardiac arrhythmia including heart block, or, less commonly, aortic stenosis or emboli, e.g. from carotid artery stenosis. Transient dizzy sensations may very rarely be a feature of temporal lobe epilepsy (p. 136). Usually no organic cause is found and the complaint may be a marker of emotional distress.

NB   'Something wrong with the brain, think of the heart.'

VERTIGO

Vertigo refers to unsteadiness with a subjective sensation of rotation of the patient or of the environment around. Vertigo results from disease of the inner ear, 8th cranial nerve or its connections in the brainstem.

Labyrinthine. Menière's disease, acute labyrinthitis.

Eighth nerve. Acoustic neuroma and other posterior fossa tumours, aminoglycosides (streptomycin and gentamicin).

Brainstem. Neoplasm, vascular disease (vertebrobasilar ischaemia, lateral medullary syndrome), demyelination (multiple sclerosis), migraine, aneurysms, degeneration (syringobulbia).

MENIÈRE'S DISEASE

The onset is usually in people over 40 years old with progressive deafness and tinnitus usually only in one ear. There are attacks of vertigo, nausea and vomiting. Attacks cease when deafness is complete. Progression can be so slow that this may never occur. Examination shows a defect of 8th nerve conduction and abnormal results to caloric tests of vestibular function. Nystagmus is present during attacks of vertigo.

Treatment

Phenothiazines (e.g. prochlorperazine) and some antihistamines (e.g. promethazine) act as sedatives and against nausea during acute episodes. They may reduce the incidence and severity of attacks. Betahistine, a histamine analogue, may specifically help in this condition by reducing endolymph pressure. If very severe, ultrasonic destruction of the labyrinth should be considered, though it results in total deafness on that side.

NYSTAGMUS

Nystagmus may result from any disturbance of either the 8th nerve and its connections in the brainstem or the cerebellum, and in phenytoin intoxication. Its direction is named after the quick phase (of 'saw-tooth' nystagmus). Nystagmus is usually more pronounced when the patient looks in the direction of the quick phase. Nystagmoid jerks may be produced in normal eyes by errors of examination technique—either holding the object too close to the patient or too far to one side.

Horizontal nystagmus

Vestibular nystagmus occurs following damage to the inner ear, 8th nerve or to its brainstem connections and is present only in the first few weeks after the damage because central compensation occurs. It is greater on looking *away* from the side of a destructive lesion. It may be caused by acute viral labyrinthitis, acute alcoholism, Menière's disease, middle-ear disease and surgery. It is usually associated with vertigo and often with vomiting, deafness and tinnitus. Multiple sclerosis, basilar artery ischaemia and syringobulbia cause less constitutional upset.

Cerebellar nystagmus occurs usually with lateral lobe lesions: even central (vermis) lesions causing severe truncal ataxia may cause no nystagmus. Since cerebellar disease is frequently bilateral, nystagmus may occur to both sides. If it is unilateral it is greater *towards* the side of the *destructive* lesion.

Cerebellar lesions occur in multiple sclerosis, hereditary ataxias and vascular disease.

Nystagmus is often seen in patients who have taken high doses (though sometimes within the therapeutic range) of sedative drugs, especially phenytoin and barbiturates.

Ataxic nystagmus. The degree of nystagmus in the abducting eye is greater than in the adducting eye, which may fail to adduct completely. This is virtually pathognomonic of multiple sclerosis and is due to damage to the medial longitudinal bundle.

Vertical nystagmus

The direction of jerks is vertical. Vertical gaze usually makes it more pronounced. It may be produced by sedative drugs (especially phenytoin) but otherwise localizes disease to the brainstem (although brainstem disorders more commonly produce horizontal nystagmus).

Pendular and rotary nystagmus

Unlike all the above, the phases of the nystagmus are equal in duration. It is secondary to an inability to fix objects and focus with one or both eyes due to partial blindness, e.g. albinism.

FACIAL PALSY

In unilateral UMN lesions (e.g. stroke) movements of the upper face are retained because it is represented on both sides of the cerebral cortex. A flattened forehead and sagging lower eyelid are seen in complete LMN lesions (e.g. Bell's palsy and middle-ear surgery). Taste sensation from the tongue in the chorda tympani leaves the facial nerve in the middle ear, and therefore loss of taste over the anterior two-thirds of the tongue means that a facial nerve paresis must be due to a lesion above this level, e.g. herpes zoster of the geniculate ganglion—the Ramsay Hunt syndrome. Lesions caused by tumours of the parotid gland do not give these signs. Facial palsy is a very late sign of acoustic neuroma. It may occur in an unusually extensive lateral medullary syndrome (p. 128).

AETIOLOGY OF CRANIAL NERVE PALSIES

The causes of single-nerve palsies include cerebral aneurysm, diabetes mellitus, trauma, surgery, cerebral tumour and multiple sclerosis. The various eponymous vascular lesions of the brainstem need not be separately remembered, but you should be able to discuss the localization of such lesions with the help of diagrams: they are relatively common causes of cranial nerve palsy. Polyarteritis nodosa, sarcoidosis, meningitis, and Wernicke's encephalopathy are less common causes.

SPEECH DISORDERS

'Would you like to ask this patient some questions?'
It is likely that the patient has a speech disorder, but there may be some degree of dementia (p. 171).

- Ask name, age, occupation and address.
- Test orientation in time (date, season) and place, for dementia.
- If indicated, test memory and intellectual capacity.
- Test ability to name familiar objects (pen, coins, watch)—nominal dysphasia.
- Test articulation, e.g. 'baby hippopotamus', 'West Register Street'.
- If dysarthria is present, look in the mouth for local lesions and test the lower cranial nerves.

Dysphasia (or aphasia)

This is a disorder of the symbolic aspects of language both written and spoken. In right-handed people and 50% of left-handed people, the left hemisphere is dominant in this respect. It usually follows cerebrovascular accidents and hence is common. Before assessing dysphasia it is important to exclude a dysarthria due to a neuromuscular lesion affecting the muscles of speech. Depression and parkinsonism may cause slow responses but not a dysphasia.

Pure expressive (motor) dysphasia tends to result from lesions in the postero-inferior part of the frontal lobe (Broca's area, see Fig. 11.3 p. 123). Receptive (sensory) dysphasia is a specific failure to understand the meaning of words and results from lesions of the temporo-parietal lobes (Wernicke's area, see Fig. 11.3).

A form of expressive dysphasia where patients cannot name objects whilst knowing what they are is called 'nominal dysphasia' (e.g. Ask when holding up a pen, 'What is this?' Pause. 'Is it a watch?' 'No.' 'Is it a key?' 'No.' 'Is it a pen?' 'Yes').

Dysarthria

Inability to articulate properly due to local lesions in the mouth or disorders of the muscles of speech or their connections. There is no disorder of the content of speech.

- Paralysis of cranial nerves, e.g. Bell's palsy (7th), 9th, 10th or 12th nerves.
- Cerebellar disease—'scanning' speech or staccato, seen in multiple sclerosis.
- Parkinson's disease: speech is slow, quiet, slurred and monotonous.
- Pseudobulbar palsy (spastic dysarthria): monotonous, high-pitched 'hot potato' speech (rare).
- Progressive bulbar palsy (rare).

BULBAR AND PSEUDOBULBAR PALSIES

	Pseudobulbar (UMN lesion)	Bulbar (LMN lesion)
Emotions	Labile	Normal
Dysarthria	Donald Duck speech	Nasal
Tongue	Spastic, small for mouth	Flaccid, fasciculating
Jaw jerk	Increased	Normal or absent
Associated findings	Bilateral UMN lesions of limbs	Sometimes other evidence of MND, e.g. fasciculation in limbs

UMN, Upper motor neuron; LMN, lower motor neuron; MND, motor neurone disease.

Table 1.1 Clinical signs of bulbar and pseudobulbar palsies.

- General paralysis of the insane (very rare nowadays).
- Stutter (usually physiological).

BULBAR AND PSEUDOBULBAR PALSIES (Table 1.1)

Both forms are rare. The symptoms of dysarthria, dysphagia and nasal regurgitation result from paralysis of the 9th, 10th and 12th cranial nerves.

Pseudobulbar (UMN) palsy is commoner than bulbar palsy and is due to bilateral lesions of the internal capsule, most often the result of cerebrovascular accidents affecting both sides, usually sequentially. It can also occur in multiple sclerosis (p. 140). Bulbar (LMN) palsy is rare because MND, and the infective causes (poliomyelitis, Guillain–Barré), are rare.

Tests of higher cerebral functions

'Would you like to have a few words with this patient?' or *'Assess the higher cerebral functions'* or *'Assess this patient's personality/mental state/intellectual function'*
This usually implies dysphasia (p. 14), dysarthria (p. 14) or dementia (p. 171). You should have some all-purpose questions to ask such as 'What is your name?' 'Where do you live?' or 'What is your job?' The answers to these questions may give you some indication of the best lines for further questioning.

Orientation. Orientation in time and space is assessed by asking the patient his or her name, the date and the place of the interview.

Motivation. Non-dominant lesions may cause loss of motivation.

Personality and mood. Subtle personality changes are best obtained from the relatives' history. Recent personality changes are common in depression, with feelings of exhaustion, guilt and self-deprecation and a tendency to cry when asked 'Are you depressed?' (see Depression, p. 177).

In dementia, the common personality changes are lack of social awareness, e.g. a previously religious person blaspheming in front of the vicar; lack of love for close and previously loved relatives and lack of interest in dress and appearance. In disseminated sclerosis, patients frequently appear happy despite serious disability. (This is also seen in lesions of the frontal lobes.) Labile emotional expression with alternate laughing and crying for no obvious cause, and often without appropriate mood, is a feature of pseudobulbar palsy (p. 15).

Intellectual function. Intellectual function tests must be related to the patient's previous abilities.

Loss of memory for recent events more than for distant events is a feature of organic cerebral disease and an early feature of dementia. Commonly used tests of intellectual function are:

1   Naming the monarch, prime minister, members of favourite sports teams, famous places and capitals.
2   Serial 7s: the patient is asked to subtract successive 7s from 100.
3   Ability to remember numbers forward and backward. Most people can remember five or more forward and four or more backward.
4   Repetition of complex sentences, e.g. the Babcock sentence: 'The one thing a nation requires to be rich and famous is a large secure supply of wood'.
5   Interpretation of proverbs, e.g. 'People who live in glass houses should not throw stones.'

Dyslexia (difficulty in reading), dysgraphia (difficulty in writing) and dyscalculia (difficulty in calculating) are features of lesions in the posterior parietal lobe.

Agnosia is inability to understand or recognize objects and forms in the presence of normal peripheral sensation. Tactile agnosia is most common and tested by asking the patient to recognize and distinguish objects placed in the hand (astereognosis) or figures drawn on the palm with the eyes closed (dysgraphaesthesia).

Agnosia denotes damage to the contralateral sensory cortex. Inability to recognize objects when viewed (visual agnosia) denotes a lesion of the occipital cortex.

Apraxia is the inability to perform complex and sequential actions to command in the presence of normal coordination, sensation and motor power. It occurs with lesions of the parietal cortices connected by the corpus callosum, e.g. inability to light a match (given the closed box); difficulty dressing (dressing dyspraxia) and inability to copy designs (constructional dyspraxia — most often seen in patients with hepatocellular failure).

Arms

'*Examine this patient's arms (neurologically)*'

You may be asked to look at a patient whose neurological syndrome involving the arm is part of a more central lesion such as a stroke or cerebral tumour (perhaps producing cortical sensory or motor loss), a cerebellar lesion, brainstem involvement or cervical cord disease (e.g. vascular disease, tumour, syringomyelia). Peripheral neuropathies affecting the hands are uncommon (cf. isolated peripheral nerve lesions).

Amongst the commonest neurological lesions of the arms are:
• *Carpal tunnel syndrome* (median nerve palsy).
• *Ulnar nerve palsy* (usually involved in the ulnar groove at the elbow — by osteoarthritis or trauma).
• *Cervical spondylosis* (usually of roots C5 and C6 but occasionally lower).

All three syndromes may present with motor and/or sensory signs and symptoms.

A mononeuropathy is usually due to a mechanical cause or old injury and is only rarely due to polyarteritis, diabetes mellitus, sarcoidosis or underlying carcinoma. Leprosy is very rare in the UK.

An examiner may indicate that neurological examination is required. If not, it is important to ensure that there are no obvious bone, soft-tissue or joint abnormalities. Quickly look at the face for parkinsonism or signs of a stroke. (Ask 'Are the arms or joints painful?') Then try to identify the problem more precisely by asking the patient 'Have you any loss of strength in your arms or hands?' and 'Have you had any numbness or tingling in your hands?' If you suspect a specific lesion, demonstrate the complete syndrome. If not, perform a methodical examination. The following scheme is recommended.

MOTOR SYSTEM

'*Examine the motor system*' (p. 20).

Look for obvious muscle wasting and test the strength of the appropriate muscle if it is present. If there is wasting of the small hand muscles, note whether it is generalized (ulnar) or thenar (median). Note any fasciculation or tremor (p. 29).

Test muscle tone — easiest at the elbow, though cogwheel rigidity may be more obvious at the wrist.

Test muscle power in groups (Table 1.2). 'I am going to test the strength of some of your muscles.'
• *Shoulder: C5.* 'Hold both arms out in front of you and close your eyes.' Look for drifting of one arm. This test checks not only weakness of the muscles at the shoulder but also for loss of position sense (when there is no evidence of weakness) and for lesions of the cerebral cortex (when the patient will not be aware of

MOTOR ROOT VALUES

Joint	Movement	Roots	Muscles	Reflex
Shoulder	Abduction	C4, 5, 6	Supraspinatus, deltoid	
	External rotation	C4, 5, 6	Infraspinatus	
	Adduction	C6, 7, 8	Pectorals	+
Elbow	Flexion	C5, 6	Biceps	+
	Extension	C7, 8	Triceps	+
	Pronation	C6, 7		
	Supination	C5, 6	Biceps	+
Wrist	Flexion (palmar): radial	C6, 7		
	ulnar	C8		
	Extension (dorsiflexion)	C6, 7		
Fingers (long)	Flexion	C8		+
and thumb	Extension	C7		
Fingers (short)	Flexion	T1		
Hips	Flexion	L1, 2, 3	Iliopsoas	
	Extension	L5	Glutei	
		S1, 2		
	Adduction	L2, 3, 4	Adductors	+
	Abduction	L1, 4, 5	Glutei and tensor	
		S1	fascia lata	
Knee	Flexion	L5	Hamstrings	
		S1, 2		
	Extension	L3, 4	Quadriceps	+
Ankle	Dorsiflexion	L4, 5	Anterior tibial	
	Plantar flexion	S1, 2	Calf	+
	Eversion	L5	Peronei	
		S1		
	Inversion	L4	Anterior and posterior tibial	
Toes	Flexion	S1, 2		
	Extension	L5		
		S1		
Anus		S2, 3, 4, 5		+
Cremaster		L1, 2		+

Notes

1 A simple *aide-mémoire* for reflexes and controlling muscle groups is:

Ankle jerk   S1, 2
Knee jerk   L3, 4
Biceps jerk   C5, 6
Triceps jerk   C7, 8

2 All muscles on the back of the upper limb (triceps, wrist extensors and finger extensors) are innervated by C7.

3 T1 innervates the small muscles of the hand.

Table 1.2 Motor root values (including reflexes).

the drift, sometimes even with open eyes). You should also notice any winging of the scapula (nerve to seratus anterior, C5, 6, 7).

- *Elbow flexion*: C5, 6, 7: biceps. 'Bend your elbow up; don't let me straighten it.'
- *Elbow extension*: C7: triceps. 'Now straighten your elbows and push me away.'
- *Wrist and finger extension*: C7. 'Keep your wrist and fingers straight, don't let me bend them.'
- *Hand grip: C8, T1.* 'Squeeze my fingers hard and stop me pulling them out.'

Only allow the patient two of your fingers or they may be crushed.

Ulnar nerve tests (fingers)

Abduction of fingers ('Spread your fingers apart'). Try to squash them together and note how much effort this requires. Note also the bulk of the first dorsal interosseous muscle.

Adduction of fingers. Hold a piece of paper between straight fingers ('Don't let me pull it out').

Median nerve tests (thumb)

Abduction of thumb. The patient places the hand down flat with the palm upwards and the thumb overlying the forefinger. Ask the patient to lift the thumb vertically against resistance.

Opposition of thumb. 'Put your thumb and little finger together and stop me pulling them apart with your forefinger'.

NB   Thenar adduction is ulnar.

REFLEXES
Examination

See Table 1.2, p. 18.

SENSORY SYSTEM
Screening

For light touch (cotton wool) and pain (disposable pin; see Fig. 1.4, p. 24). As a minimum, you should test once each on the front and back of the upper and lower arms and on each digit. Check vibration and position senses on a finger.

COORDINATION

See p. 27.

Legs

'*Examine this patient's legs (neurologically)*'
The commonest neurological lesions affecting chiefly the legs are:
- *Peripheral neuropathy* (particularly diabetes mellitus).

- *Lumbar root lesions* (prolapsed intervertebral disc).
- *Lateral popliteal (common peroneal) nerve palsy.* Local pressure at the head of the fibula causes paralysis of the peroneal muscles and foot-drop. There may be sensory loss.
- *Spastic paraparesis.*

  Try to identify the problem more precisely by asking the patient about any motor or sensory deficit. If no obvious lesion or syndrome is noted, perform systematic examination. The following scheme is recommended.

MOTOR SYSTEM
Examination (p. 25)

Look for obvious muscle wasting and test the strength of the appropriate muscles if it is present. Note any fasciculation or tremor.

Test muscle tone. Lift the knee off the bed briskly while the patient is relaxed and see if the heel is lifted. Let it drop: observe how stiffly it falls. Then roll the leg to and fro, and see if the foot is rigid at the ankle or normally loose. Alternatively, bend the knee to and fro with an irregular rhythm (so that the patient cannot consistently resist the movement) or briskly abduct one leg to observe whether bilateral adductor spasm makes the other leg follow.

Test muscle power in groups. 'I am going to test the strength of some of your muscles.'
- *Hip flexion: L1, 2: iliopsoas.* 'Lift your leg up straight.' Push down on the patient's knee.
- *Hip extension: L5, S1: glutei.* 'Lift your leg up straight: push my hand down to the bed.' Push up to resist this.
- *Knee flexion: L5, S1, 2: hamstrings.* 'Bend your knee: don't let me straighten it.' Keep one hand above the patient's patella and pull up on the ankle.
- *Knee extension: L3, 4: quadriceps* (femoral nerve). 'Keep your knee straight: don't let me bend it.' Put your forearm behind the patient's knee and push down on the ankle.
- *Ankle plantar flexion: S1.* 'Push your foot down: don't let me push it up'.
- *Ankle dorsiflexion: L4, 5* (common peroneal nerve). 'Pull your foot up towards you and don't let me pull it down'.

KNEE AND ANKLE REFLEXES
Also examine ankle and patella clonus if these are brisk. Practise the technique.

PLANTAR RESPONSE
Gently but firmly draw a key or orange stick up the outer border of the sole and across the heads of the metatarsals.

SENSORY SYSTEM (p. 22)

Light touch and pinprick:

- once each on the medial and lateral sides of thigh and calf; and
- on the dorsum of the foot, tip of the big toe and lateral border of the foot.

Vibration sense at the medial malleolus and, if it is absent there, progress to the knee and hip.

Position sense. Test position sense at the big toes. If absent, check it at progressively more proximal joints.

Reduction or absence of vibration and position senses suggests not only dorsal column loss (now usually due to B_{12} deficiency) but also may be part of a peripheral neuropathy (now usually diabetic). However, in peripheral neuropathy you expect the other modalities to be reduced (pin and touch).

COORDINATION (p. 27)

Heel–shin test. 'Put your heel (touching the patient's heel) on your knee (touching the patient's knee) and slide it down your leg (sliding your finger down the patient's shin).' This is primarily a test for intention tremor. If present, you should look for other signs of cerebellar disorders (arms, eyes, speech). Then ask the patient to stand and stand nearby (to assist if the patient stumbles). Look for:

- *Rombergism* (more unsteady with the eyes closed than with them open), which indicates loss of position sense (posterior column lesion);
- *Truncal ataxia* while standing with feet together (cerebellar lesion);
- *Ataxic gait* on walking heel to toe—note direction of fall (ipsilateral cerebellar lesion); and
- *Abnormalities of gait* on normal walking (including turning).

Abnormality of gait (excluding orthopaedic disorders)

'*Watch this patient walk*'

HEMIPLEGIA

The leg is rigid and describes a semicircle with the toe scraping the floor (circumduction).
Aetiology: almost invariably a stroke.

PARAPLEGIA

Scissors or 'wading through mud' gait.
Aetiology: multiple sclerosis, cord compression; rarely congenital spastic diplegia.

FESTINANT GAIT OF PARKINSONISM

The patient is rigid, stooped and the gait shuffling. The arms tend to be held flexed and characteristically do not swing. The patient appears to be continually about to fall forwards and may show propulsion or retropulsion. Turning is poor. There may be 'freezing' in doorways.

CEREBELLAR GAIT

The patient walks on a wide base with the arms held wide. He or she is ataxic, veering and staggering towards the side of the disease.

Aetiology: usually multiple sclerosis. Cerebellar tumour (primary or secondary), the cerebellar syndrome of carcinoma (non-metastatic) and familial degenerations should be remembered.

SENSORY (DORSAL COLUMN) ATAXIA

A stepping and stamping gait. The patient walks on a wide base and looks at the ground. The patient tends to fall if he or she closes the eyes (rombergism).

Aetiology: diabetic pseudotabes, subacute combined degeneration of the cord, Friedreich's ataxia, tabes dorsalis. Ataxia in multiple sclerosis may very rarely be of this kind (it is usually cerebellar).

STEPPAGE (DROP-FOOT) GAIT

There is no dorsiflexion of the foot as it leaves the ground and the affected legs (or leg) are lifted high to avoid scraping the toe.

Aetiology: usually lateral popliteal nerve palsy (mechanical or diabetic). Less commonly poliomyelitis or peroneal muscular atrophy. Very rarely, heavy metal (lead, arsenic) poisoning.

WADDLING GAIT

The pelvis drops on each side as the leg leaves the ground.

Aetiology: wasting disorders of the muscles of the pelvic girdle and proximal lower limb muscles (p. 25) and osteomalacia.

Notes

SENSORY TESTING (vibration and position, touch, pain, temperature)

It is important that the patient understands what sensations you are testing and what is an appropriate response. Two of the stimuli conventionally used (vibration and position senses) are strange ones and the patient needs quickly to be taught about them. If you already have a good and professional system the following suggested scheme will be unnecessary.

Vibration sense

Ensure that the patient can recognize vibration by placing the vibrating tuning fork on the patient's sternum. 'Now with your eyes closed tell me if you can feel the vibration.' Start at the big toes and work proximally to the medial malleoli, patellae and anterior superior iliac spines, comparing right with left (and with yourself if necessary).

Position sense

With the patient looking, hold a big toe or a finger by its sides (holding the top and bottom introduces light touch sensation). Move the toe away from the patient— 'this is down'—and then towards the patient—'this is up. Now with your eyes closed tell me whether I move the toe (finger) up or down.'

Light touch (cotton wool) and pinprick

These stimuli should be familiar to the patient. Appropriate instructions might be: 'Say *now* every time I touch you', and/or 'Say *pin* when you feel a pinprick'. No person is entirely consistent in sensory testing and a few discrepant responses are to be expected and ignored. Increasingly inconsistent responses are often due to wandering attention. Areas of anaesthesia are easily produced by suggestion. The pin should be safely discarded after use on one patient because of the risks of transmission of infection, especially human immunodeficiency virus (HIV) and hepatitis B.

Ask the patient to outline for you the extent of any numbness or tingling: you may then confirm and define the extent of sensory loss with the cotton wool or a pin.

You must have an approximate idea of the dermatomes (Fig. 1.4). The following points may be found useful:

• *C4* and *T2* are the neighbouring dermatomes over the front of the chest at the level of the first and second ribs;
• *C5, 6, 7, 8, T1* supply the upper limb;
• *C7* supplies the middle finger front and back;
• *T7* supplies the lower ribs;
• *T10* supplies the umbilical region;
• *T12* is the lowest nerve of the anterior abdominal wall;
• *L1* supplies the inguinal region;
• *L2, 3* supply the anterior thigh (lateral and medial);
• *L4, 5* supply the anterior shin (medial and lateral); and
• *S1* supplies the lateral border of the foot and sole, and the back of the calf up to the knee.

PATTERNS OF SENSORY LOSS IN LIMBS
Peripheral sensory neuropathy (p. 151)

All modalities tend to be lost symmetrically starting distally. The loss is more marked in the lower limbs than in the upper. This pattern is seen in diabetes mellitus, carcinomatous neuropathy, vitamin B_{12} deficiency, and with some drugs or chemicals.

NB 'Glove-and-stocking' anaesthesia, with a very well-demarcated upper border, may occur in hysteria and in malingerers.

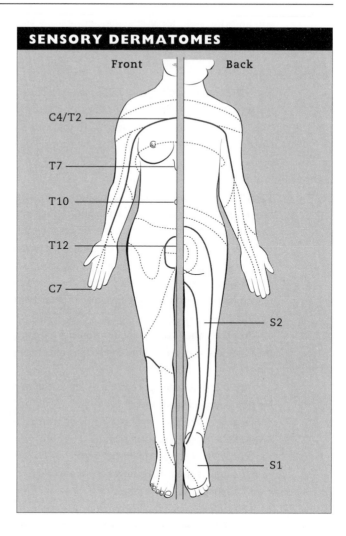

Fig. 1.4 Sensory dermatomes with the key points to remember.

Spinal cord lesions (Fig. 1.1)

Dissociated sensory loss is a feature of spinal cord lesions. Classically, vibration and position sense are carried in the dorsal columns which decussate in the medulla.

All other sensations are carried in the lateral spinothalamic tracts which decussate at the level of the origin in the cord, or just above it.

NB   Do not confuse them with the lateral columns, which are the pyramidal tracts.

Dorsal column loss without spinothalamic loss occurs in both legs in vitamin B_{12} deficiency. (It also occurs in the ipsilateral leg in hemisection of the cord—Brown-Séquard syndrome.)

Spinothalamic loss without dorsal column loss (dissociated anaesthesia) occurs in syringomyelia, usually in the arms. (It also occurs in the contralateral leg in hemisection of the cord.)

Cerebral cortical lesions

Astereognosis and dysgraphaesthesia are used to determine parietal sensory loss. They are tested by asking the patient to recognize, with the eyes closed, respectively objects placed in the hands, or numbers drawn on the palm. Two-point discrimination is also a sensitive test of parietal cortical function.

MOTOR TESTING (involuntary movement, tone, power, wasting, coordination)

First look for *involuntary movements* at rest — fasciculation, tremor or choreoathetosis (p. 30).

Then test *muscle tone* (before testing for power, since this may leave the patient tense). Engage the patient in conversation so that he or she is relaxed. Tone is most easily assessed at the elbow (though cogwheel rigidity may be more obvious at the wrist) and at the knee. Move the joint to and fro with an irregular rhythm so that the patient cannot consistently resist the movement.

Ask the patient which movements were weak and then try to confirm these observations and look for related deficiencies.

Test *muscle power* in groups. Make your instructions slow and precise. Look at and feel the bulk of the muscles as you test their strength. You must have an approximate idea of the root values of at least certain movements so that you can perform a rapid 'motor root' screen (upper limb, p. 17; lower limb, p. 20).

You must know the root values of the common reflexes (Table 1.2, p. 18).

PATTERNS OF MOTOR LOSS IN LIMBS
Lower motor neuron lesion

There is reduced or absent power with marked muscle wasting in the established lesion. The muscles are flaccid and the reflexes absent. In the foot there is no plantar response. The lesion affects the motor distribution of the spinal root or peripheral nerve.

Upper motor neuron lesion

There is reduced or absent power with relatively little wasting. The muscle tone and reflexes are increased and clonus is often present. In the foot the plantar response is upgoing. There tends to be a characteristic distribution of weakness. Thus in the arms weakness is more marked in elbow extension than flexion and wrist dorsiflexion than palmar flexion. In the legs it is more marked in hip flexion, knee flexion and ankle dorsiflexion than in their antagonist movements. This is most easily remembered by recalling the posture of the limbs in the hemiplegic patient when walking.

Proximal myopathy

Proximal muscle wasting and weakness also occur in polymyositis, carcinomatous neuromyopathy, hereditary muscular dystrophies, Cushing's syndrome usually from steroid therapy, thyrotoxicosis, osteomalacia and diabetes (amyotrophy; p. 224). *Trichinella spiralis* infection of muscles may produce acute myositis.

ISOLATED PERIPHERAL NERVE LESIONS

Median nerve lesion (carpal tunnel syndrome)

These patients, often middle-aged and female, may complain of tingling and numbness of the fingers and/or weakness of the thumb, which is at its worst on walking. It is often unilateral at the time of presentation and remains so if idiopathic. Pain at the flexor aspect of the wrist may occasionally radiate up to the elbow and exceptionally as far as the shoulder. You should examine for:

• motor loss: thenar wasting and weakness of thumb abduction and opposition;

• sensory loss, palmar surface only, on the thumb and two and a half fingers (i.e. to the middle of the ring finger);

• Tinel's sign. Percuss over the flexor retinaculum to elicit tingling in the same area; and

• evidence of pregnancy (or ask if the patient is on the pill), myxoedema, rheumatoid arthritis and acromegaly. It is commonest in overweight middle-aged women with none of these.

NB   Bilateral carpal tunnel syndrome is commonly due to rheumatoid arthritis and also occurs in chronic renal dialysis patients (amyloid deposits of β_2-microglobulin). In the examination also consider cervical spondylosis (T1 lesion), MND and syringomyelia if you are in doubt about the diagnosis.

Ulnar nerve lesion

The ulnar nerve supplies all the small muscles of the hand except the thenar eminence (but including adductor pollicis). It may be compressed in the ulnar tunnel at the wrist or in the ulnar groove at the elbow (e.g. if the arm has been incorrectly positioned in general anaesthesia). These patients may complain of tingling or deadness and/or weakness of the ring and little fingers. You should examine for:

• motor loss with flattening of the contours of the hand due to muscle wasting. The ring and little fingers are held slightly flexed, and there is loss of power in abduction and adduction of the fingers (claw hand);

• sensory loss, back and front, over the one and a half ulnar fingers (i.e. little finger and half the ring finger); and

• 'filling in' of the ulnar groove at the elbow and limitation of movement at the elbow. X-rays of the elbow may show osteoarthritis or local fracture.

NB   If you are in doubt about the diagnosis consider a lesion in the neck and look for restricted movements of the cervical spine (T1 lesion).

Radial nerve lesion

These are rare and result from local pressure (e.g. an arm over the back of the chair) which causes wrist-drop. Sensory loss may be very limited because the median and ulnar nerve territories overlap the radial territory.

Lateral cutaneous nerve of the thigh

Compression causes meralgia paraesthetica, a syndrome characterized by hyperalgesia, burning pain and numbness in the lateral aspect of the thigh and is associated with tight jeans or obesity.

Lateral popliteal palsy

The lateral popliteal (common peroneal) nerve supplies the peroneal muscles which dorsiflex and evert the foot. The nerve may be damaged as it passes over the head of the fibula, resulting in foot-drop. There may be sensory loss over the outer aspect of the leg and foot.

Wasting of the small hand muscles

These are innervated by the T1 root. Wasting of the muscles in both hands occurs with:
- old age and cachexia;
- rheumatoid arthritis;
- bilateral cervical ribs;
- MND;
- syringomyelia; and
- bilateral median and ulnar nerve lesions.

If present in one hand only, the following should also be considered:
- cervical cord lesions, including tumours;
- brachial plexus trauma; and
- a Pancoast tumour.

Proximal myopathy

This characteristically produces difficulty in standing from the sitting position and difficulty in raising the arms above the head. It occurs (often slight) in thyrotoxicosis, diabetes mellitus, polymyositis, carcinomatous neuromyopathy, osteomalacia, Cushing's syndrome (usually iatrogenic) and in the hereditary muscular dystrophies.

Mixed motor and sensory neuropathy

See peripheral neuropathy (p. 151) and mononeuritis multiplex (p. 152).

INCOORDINATION

There are two chief patterns of incoordination, one dominated by a failure in controlling accurate limb movements (cerebellar) and the other dominated by an ignorance of limb position when visual and cutaneous clues are excluded (proprioceptive).

Cerebellar incoordination

'*Demonstrate some cerebellar signs.*' The signs are ipsilateral to a destructive lesion.

Finger–nose test. The intention tremor is more marked when the patient has to stretch to reach your finger. If you keep your finger still and then ask the patient to repeat the test with the eyes closed, you may bring out past-pointing — deviation of the patient's finger consistently to one side of your own (the same side as the cerebellar lesion). The tremor is not altered by closing the eyes. The heel–shin test has similar significance. Remember that muscular weakness alone may make the patient unsteady in these tests, and that this may resemble an intention tremor.

Dysdiadochokinesia. ('Tap rapidly on the back of your hand like this . . . and now the other side'). The test is more sensitive if the patient taps alternately with the front and backs of his fingers, i.e. pronates and supinates. Rapid repetitive alternating movements of the wrists are irregular in both force and rate in cerebellar disease. There also tends to be abnormal movement at elbow and shoulder. Supination/pronation tests are more sensitive than flexion/extension ones.

Nystagmus (p. 12), typically horizontal, is more marked on looking towards the side of the lesion. Do not get the patient to focus on an object too far laterally or too near the eyes.

Dysarthria. Slurred and explosive, sometimes as if drunk.

Truncal ataxia. The gait is reeling and staggering as if drunk with a tendency to fall to the side of the lesion. Heel–toe walking may accentuate the sign. It may be the sole cerebellar sign in midline (vermis) cerebellar lesions.

Causes of cerebellar signs
- Multiple sclerosis.
- Brainstem vascular disease.
- Anticonvulsant therapy may produce gross nystagmus.
- Rarely, brainstem tumours, posterior fossa tumours (especially acoustic neuroma), degenerative disorders (e.g. alcoholism and hereditary ataxias), the cerebellar syndrome of bronchial carcinoma and (very rarely) hypothyroidism.

Proprioceptive incoordination (dorsal column loss)

The signs are ipsilateral to the lesion. When there is loss of proprioception, the patient can still place the limbs accurately by looking at them. Incoordination is therefore only obviously present when the eyes are closed. Tests are performed with the eyes open and the eyes closed. When the patient's coordination is worse with the eyes closed than with them open, he or she is said to have loss of position sense (i.e. dorsal column loss or proprioceptive loss). If there is dorsal column loss (vibration and position senses) but no spinothalamic loss (pain and temperature senses), there is said to be a dissociated sensory loss. (This term also describes the rarer reverse situation of spinothalamic loss without dorsal column loss.) Dissociated sensory loss is evidence of spinal cord disease.

Finger–nose test and heel–shin test are normal when the patient can see but incoordinate when he or she cannot. Rombergism is present when the patient, standing with the feet together, is more unsteady with the eyes closed than when they are open. The gait is ataxic and the patient walks on a wide base with high steps. Muscle tone and the tendon reflexes may be diminished (or increased in B_{12} myelopathy).

Causes of dorsal (posterior) column loss

Subacute combined degeneration of the cord. This may progress sufficiently to give dorsal column loss—peripheral neuropathy is the earliest manifestation. It is very rare in the clinic but patients treated with vitamin B_{12} may be seen in examinations (when the peripheral neuropathy may be considerably recovered, though the spinal cord lesions are not).

Tabes dorsalis. This is now very rare, though a few cases in older individuals may appear in the examinations.

Hemisection of the cord (Fig. 1.1, p. 6).

TREMOR

'*Look at this patient's tremor*'
There are four common tremors.
1 The resting tremor of parkinsonism, maximal at rest and with emotion and inhibited by movement (4–6 Hz). It is best demonstrated by passive, slow flexion–extension movements at the wrist. It is mainly distal and asymmetrical.
2 Essential tremor (5–8 Hz). This is an accentuation of physiological tremor present at rest and brought out by placing a sheet of paper on the outstretched fingers. It increases with age. It is faster (8–12 Hz) when associated with β_2-adrenergic stimulation (bronchodilators), caffeine, anxiety, after exercise and hypoglycaemia. In thyrotoxicosis it is associated with warm moist palms, tachycardia and eye signs of Graves' disease. It is occasionally familial. In alcoholics, the tremor is often reduced by ethanol and exacerbated by its withdrawal. It may improve with β-blockade.
3 The intention tremor of cerebellar disease (finger–nose test; 3 Hz). It is reduced or absent at rest and associated with past-pointing, nystagmus, dysarthria and ataxia, including truncal ataxia. It is rare except in multiple sclerosis.

4 Flapping tremor occurs in hepatic precoma and in the carbon dioxide retention of respiratory failure.

Athetosis refers to slow sinuous, writhing movements of the face and limbs, especially the distal parts. In torsion spasm (dystonia) the movements are similar but
slower and affect the proximal parts of the limbs. The movements are purpose-
less. Both occur in lesions of the extrapyramidal system. They are rare.

Choreiform movements are non-repetitive, involuntary abrupt jerky movements of
face, tongue and limbs. They may be localized or generalized (both are rare). They
occur in lesions of the extrapyramidal system and with phenothiazine toxicity and
occasionally in pregnancy or those taking an oral contraceptive. Rheumatic
chorea (Sydenham's chorea; p. 148) is now very rare. Huntington's chorea is
an inherited triplet repeat disease (p. 148).

Eyes

'Look at these eyes'
'Unless specifically instructed (i.e. *'Look at the pupils'* or *'Look at the fundi'*), a complete examination is required. There may be obvious exophthalmos (p. 204) or squint (p. 8): otherwise follow the scheme in Table 2.1.

Optic fundus

First check that the ophthalmoscope is adjusted to suit your own eyes (usually no lens) and that the light beam is circular and bright by shining it on your other hand. It is useful to start by observing the patient's eye through the ophthalmoscope from about 2 feet to see if there is any loss of the red light reflex (indicating opacities is the translucent media which may cause difficulty when trying to inspect the retina). You should interpret the fundal findings in the light of the patient's refractive errors (you may discover this from a quick look at the patient's glasses) and you should use a similar lens in the ophthalmoscope. Short-sighted (myopic) patients have a negative (concave) lens in their glasses (objects look smaller through them) and tend to have a deep optic cup and some temporal pallor of the disc. Long-sighted patients (hypermetropic) have a positive lens in their glasses (convex, magnifying) and their optic disc tends to look small and have ill-defined margins. You should be able to recognize and comment on the following.

MYELINATED NERVE FIBRES

A normal variant in which there are bright white streaky irregular patches, usually adjacent to the disc margin and radiating from it.

DIABETIC FUNDUS

This is characterized by:
• Background retinopathy (capillary leak of proteins, lipids, red cells); microaneurysms (dots), most frequent temporal to the macula; retinal haemorrhages (blots); hard exudates.

EYE EXAMINATION

Observe	For	Clinical association
Eyes and eyelids (from in front)	Squint (congenital or acquired) Xanthelasma	Diabetes, atheroma, myxoedema, primary biliary cirrhosis (p. 298)
	Ptosis (partial, i.e. 3rd nerve or sympathetic, or complete, i.e. 3rd nerve)	(p. 4) If bilateral: myasthenia dystrophia myotonica
Cornea	Corneal arcus Calcification Kayser–Fleischer rings	Age and hyperlipidaemias Hypercalcaemia (rare) Wilson's disease (very rare)
Visual acuity (Snellen chart)		May pick up early change in diabetes
Visual fields to confrontation (p. 5)		
Eye movements (p. 8)	Failure of lateral movements Failure of down and in movement Failure of other movements (with ptosis and fixed dilatation of pupil) Failure of all movements Nystagmus (p. 12)	6th nerve palsy 4th nerve palsy 3rd nerve palsy Usually myasthenia, glass eye Cerebellar, vestibular or brainstem lesion
Pupils	Dilatation Constriction	Homatropine or part of 3rd-nerve lesion, Holmes–Adie syndrome Horner's syndrome, Argyll Robertson pupil Morphine Pilocarpine
NB *Check light and accommodation reflexes (p. 9) (Glass eyes have neither).*		
Iris (with ophthalmoscope)	Iritis (p. 34)	
Lens	Lens opacities or cataract (shine light obliquely across lens); this is often missed and may make examination of the fundus difficult or impossible	Senility, diabetes, trauma Rare causes include congenital rubella syndrome, parathyroidism, dystrophia myotonica and drugs (chloroquine, amiodarone and steroids)
Fundus (p. 31)		

Table 2.1 Examination of the eyes.

• Maculopathy: oedema and/or background changes at the macula, associated with reduced visual acuity.
• Preproliferative (secondary to retinal hypoxia): soft exudates (cotton-wool spots) of retinal oedema; venous beading and reduplication.
• Proliferative (response to retinal hypoxia): new vessel formation; haemorrhage (vitreous, obscuring the retina and preretinal).
• Advanced (secondary to fibrosis): fibrous proliferation; traction retinal detachment.
• Results of treatment (photocoagulation): spots of retinal burns.
NB Glaucoma and cataract are commoner in diabetes than in the general population.

HYPERTENSIVE FUNDUS

There are usually the changes of arteriosclerosis (grades 1 and 2, including tortuosity, arterial nipping, silver wiring, varying vessel calibre). Hypertension produces haemorrhages and exudates (grade 3) and more severe disease in addition produces papilloedema (grade 4, malignant hypertension). Note that the subhyaloid haemorrhage sometimes seen in subarachnoid haemorrhage may indicate underlying hypertension.

PAPILLOEDEMA

The earliest findings are redness of the disc and blurring of the nasal margin. Small vessels may appear to dip over the swollen edge, and the optic cup disappears. Later small haemorrhages appear. The blind spot may enlarge. The main causes are:
• raised intracranial pressure (tumour, abscess, meningitis, and the rare benign intracranial hypertension found chiefly in young overweight women);
• malignant hypertension; and
• rarely, optic retrobulbar neuritis, venous obstruction and the hypercapnia of respiratory failure.
NB Papillitis should be distinguished from papilloedema. It is usually due to multiple sclerosis. There may be impaired colour vision and acuity, a central scotoma and pain. The disc is red and swollen with a blurred margin, exudates and haemorrhages.

OPTIC ATROPHY

• Glaucoma.
• Secondary to papilloedema (disc edge blurred)—rare.
• Primary (disc margin sharp with cup and cribriform plate well-defined) occurs after papillitis (almost invariably multiple sclerosis), from optic nerve pressure and in retinal artery thrombosis. Rarely, methanol abuse, B_{12} deficiency and the hereditary ataxias.

CAUSES OF IRITIS AND CHOROIDITIS	
Iritis	**Choroiditis**
Diabetes	Idiopathic (i.e. unexplained), the most
Sarcoid	frequent in the UK
Ankylosing spondylitis	Toxoplasmosis (invariably acquired)
Reiter's syndrome	Diabetes
Ulcerative colitis and	Sarcoid
Crohn's disease	(Rare causes include *Toxocara*, tuberculosis,
Still's disease	syphilis)
(Rare causes include gonorrhoea,	
Toxoplasma, *Brucella*,	
tuberculosis, syphilis)	

Table 2.2 Causes of iritis and choroiditis.

EXUDATES AND HAEMORRHAGES

Chiefly in hypertension and diabetes mellitus but also in uraemia, acute leukaemia, raised intracranial pressure, severe anaemia and carbon dioxide retention.

Uveitis, iritis and choroiditis

The uveal tract comprises the choroid (posterior uvea), the ciliary body and the iris (anterior uvea). Uveitis occurs alone or as part of other generalized diseases, some of which tend to involve either the iris (iritis, or anterior uveitis) or the choroid (choroiditis or posterior uveitis), although virtually all may involve both. Iritis is recognized by ocular pain and blurring of vision with vascularization around the corneal limbus and a 'muddy' iris. It is usually unilateral. The causes are listed in Table 2.2.

Limbs (joints and peripheral vascular disease)

Legs

In the legs the usual abnormalities are neurological or vascular. Diabetes mellitus is very common and may cause both, and you may be presented with a 'diabetic foot' (ischaemia, peripheral sensory neuropathy with ulceration and deformity). The skin and joints should also be considered. Many neurological diseases such as multiple sclerosis and strokes are chronic and appear in examinations. Paget's disease commonly shows as an enlarged, hot, bowed tibia. Erythema nodosum occasionally appears in examinations because, although it is short-lived, it is fairly common. Pretibial myxoedema is occasionally shown. Relatively rare cases include the results of spinal injury or prolapsed intervertebral discs (cervical or lumbar), peripheral nerve damage and subacute combined degeneration. Even patients with motor neurone disease or a carcinomatous neuropathy may be well enough to be included. Syringomyelia and the myopathies are rare but these patients have a better prognosis and are often available for examinations.

'Look at these legs'
Unless attention is directed towards a particular part of the legs such as the feet or knees, the following scheme is recommended.

1   Look for obvious *joint deformity*. Also note *bone deformity*, leg shortening and external rotation of fractured neck of femur, Paget's disease, previous rickets (rare except in the elderly), the results of previous poliomyelitis, and Charcot's joints of diabetes and very rarely, syphilis. Note if *oedema* is present.

2   Look at the *skin* (purpura, rash, ulcer) and note cyanosed or necrotic toes.

3   Examine abnormal joints.

4   *Peripheral vasculature*. Compare and assess the temperature of the dorsa of both feet, noting asymmetry and any interdigital infection and loss of hair. If the feet are cold, feel the dorsalis pedis and posterior tibial pulses, and if these are absent, proceed to feel for the popliteal and femoral pulses, and listen for arterial bruits. Ask the patient about a history of intermittent claudication. If there are ulcers, ask the patient if they are painful. If not, there is a neuropathy, most frequently diabetic.

5   Then examine the legs neurologically (p. 19).

Arms

In the arms the usual abnormalities seen are of the joints or the nervous system. The commonest neurological conditions in the upper limbs are the results of multiple sclerosis, stroke or peripheral nerve compression. Rarer conditions which may be seen in examinations are the results of pressure on the cord or brachial plexus (remember cervical spondylosis and cervical rib), motor neurone disease, syringomyelia and dystrophia myotonica.

'Look at the arms' (upper limb, hands)
This may mean primarily the hand, which should always be inspected first, or the joints (including elbow or wrist). Usually it means a neurological examination (wasting, nerve palsies, root lesions) but:
• observe any tremor at rest (parkinsonism);
• observe the skin for purpura (p. 102) and signs of liver disease (liver palms, spider naevi) and Dupuytren's contracture;
• look at the fingers and nails for clubbing (p. 58), cyanosis, nicotine staining, anaemia and the splinter haemorrhages and Osler's nodes of subacute bacterial endocarditis (Splinter haemorrhages are often occupational and not diagnostic, and Osler's nodes very rare.);
• glance at the patient's face as this may provide a further clue, e.g. pallor, exophthalmos, parkinsonian facies, acromegaly, spider naevi, and tophi on the ears in gout; and
• note any joint swelling (ask if the joints are painful before touching them) and any associated muscle wasting (often marked in rheumatoid arthritis).

Notes

If there is evidence of joint disease, look for the conditions listed below.

RHEUMATOID ARTHRITIS (p. 188)

This is usually symmetrical, with ulnar deviation at the metacarpophalangeal joints, spindling of the fingers, nail fold infarcts, muscle wasting and swelling of the joints, except the terminal interphalangeal joints. Look for the changes of psoriatic arthritis, including pitting of the nails and onycholysis with involvement of the terminal interphalangeal joints, psoriasis at the elbows and for the skin changes of steroid therapy. Rheumatoid arthritis may produce gross deformity. Nodules (20%) may be present at the elbow and down the radial border of the forearm. Note characteristic proximal interphalangeal deformities: boutonnière (flexion) and swan-neck (hyperextension).

OSTEOARTHRITIS (osteoarthrosis; p. 199)

Asymmetrical and most frequently seen in old people as Heberden's nodes — osteophytes around the terminal interphalangeal joints. Any joint of the hand may be involved, but it involves especially the terminal interphalangeal and first carpo-metacarpal joints.

GOUT (p. 256)

May attack any joint of the body. It may be monarticular or polyarticular. Usually the metatarsophalangeal joint of the big toe is involved first. It becomes red, hot, shiny and tender. There is often marked soft-tissue swelling and there may be superficial tophi over joints and in the cartilage of the ear. Ask about thiazide diuretics and note any polycythaemia.

NB   Osteo-, rheumatoid and gouty arthritis may mimic each other but rheumatoid is usually symmetrical.

Monarticular arthritis may well be purulent: joint aspiration and blood culture are essential.

If a rapid examination as above reveals no abnormality, proceed to examine the upper limbs neurologically (p. 17).

Head and Neck

Head

'Look at this patient's face'

This somewhat unsatisfactory request usually implies either that the patient has an abnormal facies (or neck), or that he or she has abnormal facial movements, or poverty of movement (parkinsonism and myxoedema). If the abnormality is not immediately obvious, the following checklist of the systems which may be involved might be found useful.

ENDOCRINE AND METABOLIC

- Cushing's, usually iatrogenic otherwise rare.
- Myxoedema; thyrotoxicosis.
- Acromegaly.
- Pagetic skull.

NEUROLOGICAL

- Facial palsy from stroke or Bell's palsy.
- Ptosis and ocular palsies (3rd nerve, sympathetic in Horner's syndrome and myasthenia gravis).
- Parkinsonism.
- Myopathy (including dystrophia myotonica with cataract and baldness).
- Ophthalmic herpes (zoster), including the conjunctiva.

CARDIORESPIRATORY

- Cyanosis of lips (look at the tongue) of chronic obstructive airway (note pursing lips on expiration, and poor expansion), or cardiac failure.
- Elevated jugular venous pressure of heart failure (or fluid overload). Kussmaul's sign may be present with cardiac tamponade, and there will be no pulse wave in the extremely elevated pressure due to mediastinal obstruction.

Obstructive airways disease gives elevation of the jugular venous pressure during expiration (in proportion to the obstruction).

GASTROINTESTINAL

- Jaundice and spider naevi.
- Peutz–Jeghers syndrome (p. 315).
- Hereditary haemorrhagic telangiectasia.
- Anaemia (white hair, glossitis and lemon-yellow skin of pernicious anaemia).
- Angular cheilitis is usually caused by over-closure from aged dentures and mandibular resorption rather than anaemia.

COLLAGEN DISEASE

- Systemic lupus erythematosus (butterfly rash).
- Scleroderma (tight mouth and shiny tight skin of fingers).
- Dermatomyositis (periorbital rash).

SKIN DISEASES

- Acne vulgaris.
- Rosacea.
- Psoriasis.
- Port wine stain (of Sturge–Weber syndrome).

Neck

'Examine the neck'
This usually means that there is enlargement of the lymph glands, or that a goitre is present, or that the jugular venous pressure is raised (see Table 7.2, p. 66).

CERVICAL LYMPHADENOPATHY (p. 107)

This is often easier to feel from behind.

Do not forget the occipital group. If lymphadenopathy is present, check for local infection or neoplasm over the whole head and neck. Remember to look into the mouth and pharynx. Check the nose for blood, discharge and patency.

Glands in the root of the neck may be symptomatic of pulmonary, abdominal (including the testes) or breast malignancy.

Cervical glands may be the presenting symptom of a generalized lymphadenopathy. Further examination should include all lymph gland groups and palpation for enlargement of the liver and spleen. Consider secondary carcinoma, the reticuloses, leukaemia, local sepsis and the granulomatous disorders, including tuberculosis, sarcoid, *Brucella* and infectious mononucleosis. Look for primary ear, nose and throat carcinoma and do not forget the testes.

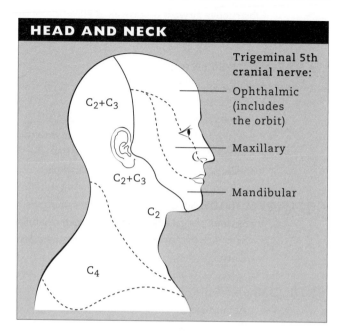

HEAD AND NECK

C$_2$+C$_3$

Trigeminal 5th cranial nerve:

Ophthalmic (includes the orbit)

Maxillary

C$_2$+C$_3$

Mandibular

C$_2$

C$_4$

Fig. 4.1 Sensory dermatomes—head and neck.

NB   'Lump in the neck: look in the mouth.'

ENLARGED THYROID

'Look at this patient's thyroid gland'

This means the patient has a goitre. It is unlikely that the patient is hyperthyroid but this must first be excluded by looking for the evidence, such as fine finger tremor, hyperkinesia, eye signs of Graves' disease (lid lag, lid retraction, exophthalmos), tachycardia or fast atrial fibrillation and hot, sweaty hands. Similarly, check for the characteristic facies, slow movements, dry thick skin, hair changes and croaking voice of hypothyroidism and proceed to test the ankle jerks if indicated.

Look at the patient's neck and ask him or her to swallow. Palpate the gland first from behind and then from the front. The patient's chin should be flexed to relax the tissues (untrained patients invariably extend the neck). If the patient has to swallow more than two or three times, give a glass of water. Pay special attention to the following.

• *Character.* Diffuse of multinodular. The gland is diffusely enlarged in Graves' disease, Hashimoto's thyroiditis, iodine deficiency and dyshormonogenesis. Patients with multinodular goitres are usually non-toxic (euthyroid). The usual clinical problem is their bulk, which may produce compression (of trachea, oesophagus or laryngeal nerve) and cause distress from their appearance. Single nodules should be regarded as malignant (though most are not), and removed or biopsied.

• *Tenderness.* This is unusual except in viral thyroiditis (very rare) and occasionally in autoimmune thyroiditis and carcinoma.

- *Mobility.* Attachment to surrounding tissues suggests carcinoma.
- *Retrosternal extension.* Feel in the suprasternal notch and percuss the upper sternum for dullness.
- *Lymph glands.* An enlarged chain of lymph glands suggests papillary thyroid carcinoma.
- *Trachea* central or displaced.
- *Thyroidectomy scar.* If present, you should suspect hypothyroidism or hypoparathyroidism. Elicit Chvostek's sign (may be present in normal people) and perform Trousseau's test (p. 255).
- Auscultate over the gland for a systolic bruit. Look for vitiligo, acropachy and pretibial myxoedema if autoimmune thyroid disease is suspected.

You should ask about pressure symptoms of dyspnoea, any drugs (especially medicines containing iodine) and take a family history for inborn enzyme deficiency (dyshormonogenesis). If you are asked to suggest investigations you should consider:

- Thyroid function tests. These should include as appropriate (and available) serum free thyroxine, free triiodothyronine and thyroid-stimulating (thyrotrophic) hormone.
- Tests for thyroid microsomal autoantibodies.
- X-rays for tracheal deviation or compression.
- Laryngoscopy to observe vocal cords if the voice has changed.
- Radioiodine scan (for cold nodules) and ultrasound (to distinguish solid from cystic masses) are not sufficiently reliable and therefore perform needle biopsy of isolated nodules for cytology, or total removal.

NB   The observed incidence of simple goitre, autoimmune thyroiditis and carcinoma in one series was 89%, 10% and 1% respectively. Carcinoma is suggested by a hard fixed gland, lymph gland enlargement, pressure symptoms, vocal cord paralysis, rapid increase in size and evidence of metastasis to bone (p. 207).

Abdomen

Examination

'Examine this patient's abdomen'

The most usual abnormality seen in examinations is a palpable mass or the presence of free fluid, or both. These are relatively rare in the clinic, where the clinician more commonly elicits only areas of maximum tenderness. The commonest conditions suitable for examination purposes are diseases which are chronic and produce enlargement of the spleen or liver, such as the chronic leukaemias, myelofibrosis or chronic liver disorders. Other palpable masses include renal swellings, especially polycystic kidneys. Neoplastic or inflammatory swellings may be present and it is usually not possible to distinguish between these on physical examination alone. Patients with acute abdominal disease virtually never appear in clinical examinations. Remember always to look before palpation, to have warm hands and to palpate gently so as to gain the patient's confidence and to avoid hurting him or her. You should ask the patient to let you know if you are hurting and look at the patient's face periodically during palpation, especially if you elicit guarding or rebound tenderness.

A complete examination of the alimentary system involves inspection of the tongue, mouth, teeth and throat but this is rarely required in examinations. Loss of weight, clubbing, jaundice, anaemia and spider naevi should always be looked for. Hence:
- Look at the hands especially for clubbing leukonychia, tobacco staining, liver palms, spider naevi and Dupuytren's contracture.
- Palpate the neck, supraclavicular fossae, axillae and groins for lymph nodes (the testes drain to the para-aortic and cervical glands).
- Inspect the eyes and conjunctivae for anaemia and jaundice.
- Lie the patient flat (one pillow) with arms by the sides.
- Observe the abdomen for:
  - (a) general selling with eversion of the umbilicus in ascites and visible enlarge-

ment of internal organs (liver, spleen, kidneys, gall bladder, stomach (in pyloric stenosis), urinary bladder and pelvic organs);

(b) abnormal veins or abnormally distended veins usually in cirrhosis with the direction of flow away from the umbilicus (portal hypertension). The flow is upwards from the groin in inferior vena cava obstruction;

(c) scars of previous operations, striae, skin rashes and purpura;

(d) pigmentation localized or generalized; and

(e) visible peristalsis suggests obstruction except in very thin patients.

• Palpate for internal organs and masses. It is often of value to percuss the liver and spleen areas initially to avoid missing the lower border of a very large liver or spleen. It is essential to start palpation in the right iliac fossa and work upwards towards the hepatic and splenic areas, first superficially and then deeper. Ascites may obscure a liver edge, but firm 'dipping' on to an enlarged liver should always be attempted unless it causes pain.

The 'scratch test' can often help *roughly* to define the extent of hepatomegaly. Place the stethoscope firmly just below the xiphisternal cartilage, which is a surface relation of liver in normal people. Sound is conducted through solid objects, so firm stroking of the skin progressing from the right costal margin downwards will be audible until the liver edge is reached.

Liver

The upper border is in the fourth to fifth space on percussion. It moves down on inspiration. If enlarged, the edge may be tender, regular or irregular, hard, firm or soft. Note if it is pulsatile (tricuspid incompetence). The liver may be of normal size but low because of hyperinflated lungs in chronic obstructive airway disease.

Spleen

Smooth rounded swelling in left subcostal region, usually with a distinct lower edge (as compared with the kidney). It enlarges diagonally downward and across the abdomen in line with the ninth rib. The examining hand cannot get above the swelling. Percussion over it is dull. There is a notch on the swelling. It may occasionally be more easily palpated with the patient lying on the right side.

Kidneys

They are palpated in the loin bimanually, i.e. most easily felt by pushing the kidney forwards from behind on to the anterior palpating hand. They move slightly downwards on inspiration. Percussion is resonant over the kidney. The examining hand can easily get between the swelling and the costal margin. The lower pole of the right kidney can often be felt in thin normal persons.

Abnormal masses

Palpate for abnormal masses particularly in the epigastrium (gastric carcinoma) and suprapubically (an overfilled bladder and ovarian and uterine masses are often missed) and note colonic swellings. The descending colon is commonly palpable in the left iliac fossa (faeces may be indented). The abdominal aorta, which is pulsatile and bifurcates at the level of the umbilicus (L4), is easily palpable in thin and lordotic patients. This is very seldom the only evidence of aortic aneurysm.

If general swelling is present, suspect ascites and examine for shifting dullness and ballottment of the liver (dipping). A fluid thrill may be demonstrable in large, tense effusions.

Complete the examination by feeling for inguinal and (if relevant) cervical glands (the drainage from the testes is to the para-aortic and cervical glands), the femoral pulses, checking for leg oedema, and listening for renal bruits and bowel sounds. Do not forget the hernial orifices—inguinal and femoral—and check for a cough impulse.

External genitalia

It is essential to examine them in practice but rarely required in examinations. Seminoma is a treatable and curable disease of the relatively young and very rarely left-sided varicocoele may suggest a left renal carcinoma.

Rectal examination

Essential in practice as rectal carcinoma is common but should not be performed in examinations unless suggested by the examiner. Some examiners will expect the candidates to comment on its desirability, particularly in the presence of gastrointestinal disease.

NOTES
Splenomegaly

There are two common causes of a very large spleen:
- chronic myeloid leukaemia; and
- myelofibrosis.

NB   Other causes, rare in the UK but very common on a worldwide basis, are malaria and kala-azar.

There are two additional causes of a moderately enlarged spleen (4–8 cm):
- reticuloendothelial disease, e.g. Hodgkin's disease and chronic lymphatic leukaemia; and
- cirrhosis with portal hypertension.

But there are many causes of a slightly enlarged spleen:
- any of the above;
- glandular fever, *Brucella* and infectious hepatitis (unlikely in the examination); and
- subacute septicaemia, including subacute bacterial endocarditis and in many infections.

Other rare causes include amyloid (rheumatoid arthritis the commonest cause; chronic sepsis is less common), Felty's syndrome, multiple myeloma, sarcoid, collagen disease and storage diseases. Other blood disorders which can give splenic enlargement are idiopathic thrombocytopenia, pernicious anaemia, congenital spherocytosis and polycythaemia rubra vera.

Hepatomegaly

There are three common causes:
- congestive cardiac failure;
- secondary carcinomatous deposits; and
- cirrhosis (usually alcoholic).

Other causes include:
- infections—glandular fever, infectious hepatitis;
- leukaemia and reticuloendothelial disorders;
- tumours (primary hepatoma, amoebic and hydatid cysts);
- amyloid, sarcoid and storage diseases;
- primary biliary cirrhosis (large regular liver in women with jaundice and xanthelasmata); and
- haemochromatosis (look for pigmentation).

Hepatosplenomegaly

The list is much the same as for splenomegaly alone since the commonest causes are chronic leukaemia, cirrhosis with portal hypertension, reticuloendothelial disease and myelofibrosis but each of these is usually associated with other clinical signs.

Palpable kidneys

The left kidney is nearly always impalpable but the lower pole of a normal right kidney may be felt in thin people. *Unilateral enlargement* may result from a local lesion, e.g. carcinoma, hydronephrosis, cysts or from hypertrophy of a single functioning kidney. *Bilateral enlargement*, usually gross, occurs in polycystic disease (the liver may also be enlarged) and very rarely in bilateral hydronephrosis and amyloidosis. Following *renal transplantation* a kidney may be palpable in the iliac fossa, and the patient may be cushingoid in appearance due to steroid therapy. Look for scars of previous renal surgery and arteriovenous shunts.

Mass in right subcostal region

It may be difficult to decide the nature of a mass in this region which may be derived from the liver (including Riedel's lobe), colon, kidney or occasionally gall bladder. If you are uncertain, say so, giving the most likely possibilities and the reasons for your conclusions. This will determine the approach to further investigation, which should start with simple studies:
- Urine for haematuria and proteinuria;
- Stool for occult bleeding; and
- Ultrasound for solid or cystic masses.

Then proceed as indicated by clinical suspicion and the results of simple studies of one or more of the following:

- Liver—liver function tests, ultrasound scan and biopsy;
- Kidney — ultrasound, computed tomography (CT) scan or intravenous urogram;
- Colon—sigmoidoscopy, barium enema and colonoscopy;
- Gall bladder—ultrasound;
- CT scan may be helpful for masses which remain obscure and which arise from the pelvis; and
- Laparotomy.

Ascites

The clinical features are abdominal distension, dullness to percussion in the flanks, shifting dullness and a fluid thrill.

The common causes are:
- intra-abdominal neoplasms (remember gynaecological lesions);
- hepatic cirrhosis with portal hypertension (relatively late in the disease; p. 300);
- congestive cardiac failure and, rarely, constrictive pericarditis;
- nephrotic syndrome (and other low albumin states); and
- tuberculous peritonitis (rare in this country, but should be suspected in Asian and Irish patients).

Paracentesis of a few millilitres of fluid for diagnosis is simple. The specimen should be examined for:
- protein content (>30 g/l suggests an exudate; less, a transudate);
- microscopy and bacterial culture (including tuberculosis); and
- cytology for malignant cells.

Paracentesis may occasionally be required for the relief of severe symptoms but not otherwise because the fluid tends to reaccumulate, and repeated paracentesis leads to excessive protein loss.

The suprapubic region is often neglected by physicians examining the abdomen. The commoner causes of a suprapubic mass are the distended bladder (retention from prostatic hypertrophy, tricyclic antidepressants), pregnancy, uterine and ovarian tumours (ovarian fibroids, ovarian cysts, carcinoma).
NB   See p. 301 for management.

Jaundice

Yellow coloration of the skin and sclerae is usually only apparent when the serum bilirubin is over 35 μmol/l. Keep in mind the three basic causes of jaundice (haemolytic, hepatocellular and obstructive) but remember that most cases are due to:
- Acute viral hepatitis (p. 293): most of these patients are not admitted to hospital unless they are very ill, recovery is unduly prolonged, or intrahepatic cholestasis persists;

- Bile duct obstruction from gallstones or carcinoma of the head of the pancreas;
- Drugs (p. 303);
- Multiple secondary deposits of carcinoma in the liver (clinical jaundice is not common when the patient presents but the bilirubin is frequently slightly raised);
- Intrahepatic cholestasis (durgs, viral hepatitis, ascending cholangitis and primary biliary cirrhosis);
- Infectious mononucleosis;
- Gilbert's syndrome (p. 51) is intermittent and harmless; and
- Less common causes include: haemolytic anaemia, congenital hyperbilirubinaemia, stricture or carcinoma of the major bile ducts or ampulla.

'Would you like to ask this (jaundiced) patient some questions?'

Ask about

- *Age.* As a cause of jaundice, carcinoma becomes commoner and hepatitis less common the older the patient.
- *Injections or transfusions* in the last 6 months (virus hepatitis), including drug addicts. Look for evidence of injections.
- *Contacts* with jaundice and residence abroad.
- *Occupation.* Farm and sewage workers are at risk for leptospirosis.
- *Presence of dark urine and pale stools* of biliary obstruction.
- *Recent drug therapy,* especially phenothiazines and the 'pill'.
- *Period of onset* from first symptoms to jaundice. In general, hepatitis A is short (1–3 weeks), carcinoma is medium (1–2 months) and cirrhosis is long. Hepatitis B is from 6 weeks to 6 months.
- *Alcohol consumption.*
- *Recent abdominal pain,* or a history of chronic dyspepsia may suggest cholecystitis, cholangitis, gallstones or pancreatic carcinoma.
- *Recent surgery,* anaesthesia (halothane).
- *Family history* if Gilbert's syndrome is suspected.

'Would you like to examine this (jaundiced) patient?'

Examine

Skin of the face and abdomen and assess the degree of jaundice—deep green suggests long-standing obstruction and pale lemon suggests haemolysis. The sclerae often show minor degrees of jaundice not evident elsewhere.

Face, upper chest and hands for spider naevi and the hands for Dupuytren's contracture, liver palms and clubbing. Note that xanthelasmata with deep jaundice in a middle-aged woman probably indicate primary biliary cirrhosis.

Neck for lymph node enlargement due to secondary spread of abdominal carcinoma.

Abdomen for:
• recent operation scars which suggest cholecystectomy or surgery for intra-abdominal carcinoma;
• hepatomegaly. Irregular when infiltrated with carcinoma, tender in infectious and acute alcoholic hepatitis (and when enlarged in congestive heart failure) and sometimes with carcinoma;
• splenomegaly in portal hypertension (and spherocytosis and infectious mononucleosis);
• palpable enlarged gall bladder suggesting bile duct obstruction due to carcinoma of the pancreas (rather than gallstones); and
• ascites (which is probably more often due to gynaecological malignancy than to the portal hypertension of cirrhosis, where it occurs late).

Urine if available (see below).
In obstructive jaundice the difficulty is usually to distinguish between benign causes (gallstone obstruction) and malignant causes (carcinoma of the head of the pancreas). Remember that hepatitis A and B, which usually occur in younger patients, and drug jaundice, often present with the typical clinical picture of obstructive jaundice from intrahepatic cholestasis and that this may occasionally be persistent.
    Drug jaundice should always be reconsidered.

'What investigations would you perform?'
The aims of investigation are:
• to discover the site of any obstruction to the outflow of bile and to determine whether operative interference is necessary;
• to determine the degree of impairment of liver cell function and its cause, and to observe its course; and
• to eliminate rare causes such as haemolysis.

HAEMATOLOGY

Including a reticulocyte count and Coombs test, which may give evidence of haemolytic anaemia. A normal reticulocyte count virtually excludes haemolytic jaundice. Leukocytosis may indicate infection (cholangitis) or carcinoma. Abnormal mononuclear cells suggest infectious mononucleosis (Paul–Bunnell) or, possibly, viral hepatitis.

URINE ANALYSIS

Conjugated bilirubin renders the urine yellow.

Urobilinogen is colourless but on standing the urine turns brown as urobilinogen is converted to urobilin by oxidation.

Haemolytic jaundice is acholuric (no bilirubin in the urine) but the urine contains excess urobilinogen because excess bilirubin reaches the intestine and is re-excreted as urobilinogen.

Obstructive jaundice gives urine coloured dark brown with excess bilirubin but a reduction of urinary urobilinogen, because little or no bilirubin reaches the gut due to the obstruction and therefore cannot be reabsorbed and re-excreted. In the early stages of hepatocelluar jaundice in acute viral hepatitis, excess urobilinogen may sometimes be present before clinical jaundice becomes apparent. This is due to failure of the liver to take up the excess urobilinogen absorbed from the gut. With increasing severity, biliary obstruction develops and as bilirubin (conjugated) appears in the urine, it disappears from the gut and therefore urobilinogen disappears from the urine. The reciprocal effect also occurs during recovery.

LIVER FUNCTION TESTS
Protein synthesis
Serum albumin and prothrombin concentrations are reduced in long-standing liver disease. The latter is usually partially responsive to vitamin K.

Alkaline phosphatase
Serum alkaline phosphatase is characteristically greatly elevated in obstructive jaundice and less so in hepatocellular jaundice. A raised level in the absence of other signs of liver disease or abnormal LFTs suggests the presence of malignant secondary deposits in the liver (or bone) or Paget's disease. It is very seldom raised in myeloma. The normal range is higher in growing adolescents and in pregnancy.

Bilirubin metabolism
Serum bilirubin is predominantly unconjugated in haemolytic jaundice and the other liver function tests are usually normal. It is mainly conjugated in obstructive jaundice.

Hepatocellular damage
Shown by raised serum level of aminotransferases (transaminases). Very high values suggest viral hepatitis or toxic damage. Slight elevation is consistent with obstructive jaundice. γ-Glutamyl transferase, an inducible microsomal enzyme, is probably the most sensitive index of alcohol ingestion, but it is raised in most forms of liver disease including acute and chronic hepatitis and cirrhosis (or large bile ducts in obstruction) and drugs which induce microsomal enzymes, e.g. phenytoin.

SEROLOGY

Always check hepatitis antibody serology in jaundice cases of unknown cause. Anti-mitochondrial antibodies are detected in 90% of cases of primary biliary cirrhosis. Antinuclear factor and smooth-muscle antibodies are detected in over 50% of cases of chronic active hepatitis. Anti-mitochondrial antibodies may also be positive.

X-RAY AND ULTRASOUND OF ABDOMEN

May show gallstones and will put on record the size of the liver and spleen. *Barium swallow* and meal may show oesophageal varices or a distorted duodenal loop from pancreatic carcinoma. *Isotopic liver scans* may demonstrate 'holes' due to carcinomatous secondaries (or large bile ducts in obstruction). *Ultrasound* and *CT scan* may show secondary tumour, stones in the gall bladder and dilated ducts in obstruction (not always shown when the obstruction is due to stones).

NEEDLE LIVER BIOPSY

Biliary obstruction is a relative contraindication because of the potential danger of causing biliary peritonitis. Biopsy may provide the histological diagnosis sometimes even in focal lesions. In experienced hands it is a safe procedure provided the prothrombin concentration and platelet counts are normal. Fresh frozen plasma will quickly reverse the prothrombin time for the duration of the procedure.

Other investigation procedures which may be helpful.

- For hepatoma: α-fetoprotein and selenomethionine scan.
- For carcinoma of the pancreatic head: CT scan.
- For obstructive jaundice: endoscopic retrograde cholangiopancreatography (ERCP) is valuable to define obstruction of the pancreaticoduodenal tree for sphincterotomy, to release stones and to relieve obstruction by insertion of a stent.
- *Percutaneous cholangiography.* This may be valuable in clinical obstructive jaundice where the cause is in doubt after initial investigations and ultrasound is inconclusive. The needle is inserted and contrast medium injected if a dilated bile duct is entered. If not, a liver biopsy is taken.

NB   In obstructive jaundice if the cause is not clinically obvious:

- retake the drug history;
- perform blood and urine tests as above;
- perform ultrasound, or abdominal CT scan for large ducts, pancreatic carcinoma, stones, secondary carcinoma;
- liver biopsy if the ducts are not enlarged on ultrasound or CT;
- ERCP if ducts are enlarged.

Congenital non-haemolytic hyperbilirubinaemias

These may explain persistent jaundice in the young after viral hepatitis or slight jaundice in the healthy.

Gilbert's syndrome (autosomal dominant)

• This is the only common congenital hyperbilirubinaemia (1–2% of the population). There is impaired glucuronidation of bilirubin (reduced uridine diphosphate glucuronyl transferase (UDPGT)) resulting in a raised unconjugated plasma bilirubin and acholuria. About 40% have a reduced red cell survival with a consequent increase in bilirubin production.

• The plasma bilirubin is usually <35 μmol/l.

• Diagnosis is by exclusion: there is no haemolysis and the other liver function tests are normal. Fasting and intravenous nicotinic acid produce a rise in plasma bilirubin.

• Liver biopsy is very rarely indicated (unless the diagnosis is uncertain) and the liver is histologically normal.

• The prognosis is excellent and treatment unnecessary. It is important because it should not be confused with serious liver disease.

Dubin–Johnson (autosomal recessive)

A rare benign disorder, usually in adolescents, of failure to excrete conjugated bilirubin. The plasma bilirubin is conjugated. The liver is stained black by centrilobular melanin and there is a late rise in the Bromsulphalein (BSP) elimination curve at 90 min.

Rotor syndrome

A benign disorder with conjugated hyperbilirubinaemia. It is distinguished from the Dubin–Johnson syndrome by a normal liver biopsy.

Crigler–Najjar (autosomal recessive)

It is exceedingly rare and presents in neonates with kernicterus and unconjugated hyperbilirubinaemia (due to absence of UDPGT). Type I with complete deficiency is fatal in the first year of life, but type II with partial deficiency is not.

Uraemia

'This patient is uraemic. Would you ask him some questions and examine him?'

Ask about

• Symptoms of renal failure—thirst, polyuria and nocturia, anorexia, nausea and vomiting, fatigue and itching.

• Symptoms of urinary tract infection (dysuria), prostatism (poor stream), renal stone, acute nephritis (haematuria) and nephrotic syndrome (ankle oedema).

- Drug therapy, analgesics.
- Past history: nephritis, diabetes and, in women, pelvic surgery (ureteric obstruction), hypertension and pre-eclamptic toxaemia.
- Family history: hypertension, polycystic kidneys and gout.

Examine for
- Brownish pallor of uraemia and the brown line near the ends of the finger nails.
- Bruising.
- Hypertension and its consequences, especially cardiac enlargement or failure.
- Hypotension (especially postural) and reduced tissue turgor from dehydration.
- Hyperventilation from acidosis (Kussmaul's respiration).
- Palpable bladder in outflow obstruction.
- Palpable kidneys (polycystic disease and hydronephrosis).
- Ankle (or sacral) oedema of nephrotic syndrome or congestive failure.
- Signs of dialysis (abdominal scars, arteriovenous fistula).
- Peripheral neuropathy.
- Pericarditis is a late event in uraemia.
- Muscular twitching, hiccup, fall in blood pressure and uraemic frost are rare terminal manifestations.
- Rectal examination for prostatic hypertrophy or carcinoma must be performed in practice.

Investigate initially
- Urine for microscopy, protein and glucose.
- Blood for urea, creatinine, potassium and bicarbonate.
- Ultrasound for pelvic dilatation of outflow obstruction and for renal size.

Dysphagia

'This patient complains of dysphagia; please question and examine him'
This term includes both difficulty with swallowing and pain on swallowing. The former symptom is more prominent in obstruction and the latter with inflammatory lesions.

The history should be taken of the commoner causes, remembering that previous reflux oesophagitis suggests peptic stricture and that recurrent chest infections occur with achalasia, bronchial carcinoma or pharyngeal pouches.

Examine the mouth and pharynx (pallor, carcinoma, neurological abnormalities), neck (goitre, and glands from carcinoma) and abdomen (carcinoma) with an initial glance at the hands for koilonychia.

Commonest causes
Carcinoma of the oesophagus and gastric fundus usually gives a history of increasing painless difficulty with swallowing foods for the previous 2–3 months. The

patient is frequently reduced to taking only soups and drinks by the time of presentation.

Peptic oesophagitis (with pain) proceeds to stricture with difficulty in swallowing.

Rarer causes

• Achalasia of the cardia, mainly in the relatively young. Food 'sticks' and is regurgitated unchanged a short while later (without acid); 25% present with recurrent pulmonary infection.

• External pressure. Since the oesophagus is slippery, symptoms of pressure from outside masses (especially carcinoma of the bronchus) are very seldom presenting ones. A retrosternal goitre large enough to produce dysphagia is usually obvious.

• The elderly may develop a dysmotility syndrome which may spontaneously resolve.

Very rare causes

Neurological disease: myasthenia gravis (p. 168) and bulbar palsies (p. 15).

Plummer–Vinson syndrome (Paterson–Kelly–Brown). Sideropenic dysphagia usually occurs in middle-aged women who have iron-deficiency anaemia, koilonychia and glossitis. It may be associated with a postcricoid web which is precancerous.

NB   Globus hystericus is diagnosed only after full investigation and when positive evidence of psychological stress exists.

Investigation

If you are asked to discuss investigation, suggest:

• Haemoglobin, serum iron and ferritin;

• Endoscopy (May differentiate between benign peptic stricture and carcinoma.); and

• Barium swallow.

NB   The postcricoid web occurs in the anterior oesophageal wall and appears on barium swallow as an anterior indentation at the top of the oesophagus at the level of the cricoid cartilage.

Diarrhoea

Acute gastroenteritis with diarrhoea and vomiting is the second most common group of disorders affecting the community (second only to acute respiratory infections).

Aetiology

Infectious diarrhoea

Usually *acute*, e.g. winter vomiting disease and travellers' diarrhoea. The aetiology of these syndromes remains unknown, with the exception of some outbreaks of diarrhoea due to specific serotypes of *Escherichia coli* to which the local population may be immune. They may be caused by viruses but none of the common enteroviruses (Coxsackie, polio, echoviruses) can be confidently incriminated. Infant diarrhoea is usually caused by a rotavirus. The vast majority of patients are successfully treated symptomatically.

Food poisoning. *Salmonella typhimurium* is responsible for 75% of bacterial food poisoning. *S. enteritidis* infection from eggs and poultry is common. Staphylococcal food poisoning results from eating precooked meats and dairy foods, and is produced by the bacteria toxin.

Enteric fevers. Typhoid and paratyphoid must also be considered in patients returning from endemic areas.

Dysentery (p. 443). Results from ingestion of organisms of the genus *Shigella* (bacillary dysentery). Amoebic dysentry and giardiasis should also be considered in patients recently returned from the tropics.

Campylobacter infection may cause bloody diarrhoea.

Clostridium difficile infection (pseudomembranous colitis) usually follows antibiotic therapy.

Cryptosporidium can cause persistent, severe and intractable diarrhoea in acquired immunodeficiency syndrome (AIDS).

Non-infectious diarrhoea
The following conditions must be considered:
* Drugs, including purgatives (common);
* Diverticulitis (common);
* Colonic carcinoma, sometimes with spurious diarrhoea secondary to partial obstruction (usually alternates with spells of constipation);
* Irritable bowel syndrome (p. 321) 'nervous diarrhoea' (common);
* Ulcerative colitis and Crohn's disease;
* Malabsorption syndromes;
* Diabetes, thyrotoxicosis (rare); and
* Post-vagotomy.

'This patient has developed diarrhoea. Would you question and examine him?'
In hospital, the acute diarrhoeas are seen less frequently than in general practice. It is important to determine whether the recent attack is an isolated one or part of a chronic or recurrent history. If it is isolated and acute, ask about travel and residence abroad, contact history, previous antibiotic therapy and, if food poison-

ing is suspected, the time relationship to previous food and its effect on other eaters. If the diarrhoea is recurrent or chronic, ask about appetite, weight loss, abdominal pain, blood or mucus in the stools, drug ingestion including purgatives and operations.

Examination

In practice a complete medical examination is required. In examinations, note particularly weight loss, anaemia and clubbing (Crohn's disease). Look for abnormal abdominal masses (usually carcinoma, but Crohn's disease should be suspected in young patients). Rectal examination and sigmoidoscopy should invariably be performed in chronic and recurrent diarrhoeas but these should not be attempted in examinations (though the examiner should be told of their necessity).

Investigation

'How would you investigate this patient?'

If it is a single episode of acute diarrhoea and has not settled within 5–7 days or if the patient is ill, perform:

- Full blood count for anaemia and blood cultures for *Salmonella typhi, S. paratyphi* and *S. enteritidis*, particularly in travellers from abroad.
- Stool to laboratory for examination for cysts, ova and parasites (amoeba, *Giardia*) and for culture (typhoid and paratyphoid, *Campylobacter, Clostridium difficile*).
- Sigmoidoscopy, particularly in suspected ulcerative colitis or carcinoma (or amoebic colitis). Biopsy and histology may be diagnostic.

If acute diarrhoea remains undiagnosed or fails to respond to simple symptomatic remedies within 1–2 weeks or in chronic diarrhoea, it is usually necessary (if not previously indicated) to proceed to further investigation, including sigmoidoscopy with biopsy followed after a few days (to allow healing) by barium enema. If the history suggests malabsorption (p. 316), perform endoscopic duodenal biopsy and if Crohn's disease is suspected, obtain small-bowel barium studies.

Bloody diarrhoea suggests:

- colonic carcinoma;
- diverticular disease;
- ulcerative colitis;
- dysentery;
- ischaemic colitis; and
- *Campylobacter* enteritis

but the most common cause of rectal bleeding is haemorrhoids and fissures. If the cause is not obvious, rectal bleeding needs full investigation with sigmoidoscopy and barium enema, proceeding to colonoscopy if necessary.

NB   Dysentery (bacillary and amoebic), typhoid and paratyphoid, and cholera are notifiable to the public health authorities.

Respiratory System

The most usual types of clinical case seen in examinations are those secondary to carcinoma of the bronchus or due to long-standing chronic disease. Asthma and chronic bronchitis are very common chronic disabilities. Bronchiectasis is still sufficiently common to appear in examinations. Pleural effusions are usually secondary to underlying carcinoma (primary or secondary) or to infection. There are still some patients with long-standing healed tuberculous fibrosis (mainly of the upper lobes) with mediastinal shift.

Examination

'Examine the chest' or *'Examine the lungs'*
This means *'Examine the respiratory system'* unless otherwise specified.

If allowed to question the patient, enquire about smoking, occupation, dyspnoea, chest pain, cough, sputum and haemoptysis, allergy, family history of allergy and past history of asbestosis or mining. The diagnosis of chronic bronchitis is made on the history of 3 months' productive cough in 2 consecutive years.

Observation

1   On approaching the patient note dyspnoea and cyanosis and any evidence of loss of weight.

2   Examine the hands for clubbing, tobacco-staining and feel for the bounding pulse of carbon dioxide retention if you suspect respiratory failure. Ask the patient's age and occupation (for occupational lung diseases) and assess hoarseness.

3   Quickly check the height of the jugular venous pressure, and the tongue for cyanosis.

4   Remove all patient's clothes above the waist and observe the shape of the chest and spine, any scars and the movements for symmetry and expansion (subtle differences are best seen from the end of the bed), and the use of accessory muscles in the neck and shoulders.

5 Count the respiratory rate.

Palpation

Palpate for chest expansion, comparing movements on both sides. *Diminished movement means pathology on that side.*

Palpate the trachea in the suprasternal notch (easier with the head partially extended). Deviation denotes fibrosis or collapse of the upper lobe or whole lung in the direction of deviation, or pneumothorax (or very rarely a large pleural effusion) on the other side.

NB Local causes may produce deviation in the absence of lung disease, e.g. goitre and spinal asymmetry. The position of the apex beat is of no help in assessing lung disease except if there is marked mediastinal shift.

Palpate for cervical lymphadenopathy.

Percussion

Percuss by moving down the chest comparing both sides. Stony dullness in

PHYSICAL SIGNS

	Movements on side of lesion	Trachea	Percussion	Breath sounds	Tactile fremitus and vocal resonance
Pleural effusion	Diminished	Usually central May be deviated away from lesion if very large	Dull (stony)	Diminished, often with bronchial breathing at top of effusion	Diminished
Pneumothorax	Diminished	Usually central May be deviated away if very large	Hyperresonant	Diminished	Diminished
Consolidation (pneumonia)	Diminished	Central or deviated towards side of lesion if associated with collapse	Dull	Bronchial (tubular) if airway open Absent if airway obstructed, e.g. carcinoma	Increased if airway open Diminished if airway obstructed
Fibrosis	Diminished	Deviated towards fibrosis if upper lobe affected	Dull	Bronchial	Increased
Chronic obstructive pulmonary disease		Central, possibly with tug	Normal or hyperresonant	Scattered added sounds	Normal

NB All the abnormal signs—bronchial breathing, increased vocal resonance, increased tactile fremitus, whispering pectoriloquy—occur in consolidation.

Table 6.1 Physical signs in lung disease.

the axilla usually indicates pleural effusion. Pleural thickening and collapse, consolidation or fibrosis of the lung also gives dullness.

NB   Upper-lobe fibrosis in an otherwise fit elderly patient is probably due to old tuberculosis.

Diminished movement with resonance on one side usually means pneumo-thorax (or occasionally a large bulla).

Auscultation

Bronchial breathing occurs in consolidation, including that at the top of effusions. Diminished breath sounds occur overlying an effusion, pleural thickening, pneu-mothorax and, in the obese, due to interposition of abnormal features between the lung surface and the stethoscope. Diminished breath sounds also occur with obstructed airways.

Added sounds are either wheezes (*rhonchi*) or crackles (*crepitations* — sounds like rubbing strands of hair between finger and thumb behind the ear, rales). Wheezing is common in asthma and bronchitis but sometimes occurs in left ven-tricular failure ('cardiac asthma'). Crackles are fine in pulmonary congestion and fibrosing alveolitis and coarse in the presence of excess bronchial secretions. *Vocal resonance* is increased over areas of consolidation. Friction rubs occur with pleurisy.

Whispering pectoriloquy occurs in association with consolidation. The patient is asked to whisper (not phonate) '1–2–3–4' and this is heard by the exploring stethoscope on the chest wall overlying the consolidation. (It can be imitated by whispering with both ears blocked with index fingers.)

Notes

CLUBBING

Associated with diseases in the lungs, heart and abdomen:
- Carcinoma of bronchus (the only common cause);
- Pus in the pleura (empyema), lung (abscess) or bronchi (bronchiectasis, cystic fibrosis);
- Fibrosing alveolitis;
- Cyanotic congenital heart disease;
- Subacute bacterial endocarditis;
- Crohn's disease (less commonly, ulcerative colitis and cirrhosis).

HAEMOPTYSIS
Aetiology
Common
- Bronchial carcinoma (or, rarely, other vascular tumours).
- Tuberculosis (active or healed). NB Aspergilloma in healed cavity.
- Pulmonary embolism with infarction.
- Infection (pneumococcal pneumonia, lung abscess and *Klebsiella pneumoniae*).

The presence of chronic bronchitis, a common cause of slight haemoptysis, does not exclude any of the above.

Uncommon
- Bronchiectatic cavities or chronic bronchitis.
- Mitral stenosis.
- Foreign body—history of general anaesthetic, visit to dentist or inhalation of food, especially peanuts.
- Coagulation disorders.

Very rare
- Wegener's granulomatosis (a generalized vasculitis which may present with rhinitis and round lung shadows with or without ear, nose and throat masses and/or renal failure).
- Goodpasture's syndrome (glomerulonephritis with haemoptysis).

Investigation
The usual clinical problem is to exclude carcinoma and tuberculosis. A full history and clinical examination will usually identify pulmonary infarction, foreign body, bronchiectasis, mitral stenosis and pulmonary oedema.

Chest X-ray
- *Sputum for culture*, including tuberculosis and cytology for malignant cells.
- *Bronchoscopy* with biopsy for cytology and culture. Visible lesions are biopsied —this is essential in all patients suspected of early bronchial carcinoma, which is amenable to surgery only if diagnosed early.
- *Isotope (V/Q) lung scan* for suspected pulmonary embolism.
- *CT or MRI scan.*

NB About 40% of patients with haemoptysis have no demonstrable cause. Patients who have had a single small haemoptysis, no other symptoms and a normal chest X-ray (posteroanterior and lateral) probably do not require further investigation, but a follow-up appointment with a chest X-ray is advisable after 1–2 months. Patients who have more than one small haemoptysis should be regarded as having carcinoma or tuberculosis until proved otherwise, and be submitted to bronchoscopy.

PLEURAL EFFUSION
Aetiology
- Carcinoma: primary bronchus (the effusion implies pleural involvement) or secondary (commonly breast).
- Cardiac failure.
- Pulmonary embolus and infarction.
- Tuberculosis.
- Other infections (pneumonia).

- Rarely, lymphomas, systemic lupus erythematosus, rheumatoid arthritis and transdiaphragmatic spread of ascites including peritoneal dialysis and Meigs' syndrome (usually a right-sided transudate from benign ovarian fibroma).

NB   Aspiration of the fluid is usually necessary both for treatment and to assist diagnosis. A pleural biopsy should be performed at the same time. Specimens are sent to the laboratory for:

- microscopy;
- bacterial culture, including tuberculosis;
- histology;
- cytology for malignant cells; and
- protein content: 30 g/l approximately divides exudates from transudates.

CYANOSIS

'Cyanosis' is a clinical description and refers to the blue colour of a patient's lips, tongue (central) or fingers (peripheral). Central cyanosis is almost always due to the presence of an excess of reduced haemoglobin in the capillaries. Over 3 g/100 ml is usually present before cyanosis is apparent. Thus, in anaemia, severe hypoxaemia may be present without cyanosis.

'Look at this (cyanosed) patient'
It is often difficult to tell whether cyanosis is present or not. Comparison of the colour of the patient's tongue or nail beds with your own nail beds (presumed to be normal) may help if both hands are warm.

Look at the patient's tongue. If it is cyanosed, the cyanosis is central in origin and secondary to:

- chronic bronchitis and emphysema, often with cor pulmonale;
- congenital heart disease (cyanosis may be present only after exercise);
- polycythaemia; and
- massive pulmonary embolism.

In central cyanosis there is always cyanosis at the periphery.

If the tongue is not cyanosed but the fingers, toes or ear lobes are, the cyanosis is peripheral:

- physiological due to cold; and
- pathological in peripheral vascular disease (the cyanosed parts feel cold)

NB   Left ventricular failure may produce cyanosis which is partly central (pulmonary) and partly peripheral (poor peripheral circulation).

A rare cause of cyanosis, which is not due to increased circulating reduced haemoglobin, is the presence of methaemoglobin (and/or sulphaemoglobin). The patients are relatively well and not necessarily dyspnoeic. *Methaemoglobinaemia* is usually the result of taking certain drugs, e.g. sulphonamides, primaquine (an 8-amino quinoline) or nitrites.

Cyanosis is an unreliable guide to the degree of hypoxaemia.

Blood gases

'Comment on these blood gases'
The normal arterial values are:

Po_2	12–14 kPa
Pco_2	4.7–6.0 kPa
pH	7.37–7.42
Standard HCO_3^-	23–27 mmol/l

Look at the pH to diagnose an acidosis or alkalosis.

Look at the Pco_2. If it is raised this may account for an acidosis of respiratory origin (respiratory failure). If it is reduced this may account for an alkalosis due to hyperventilation (pain, stiff lungs, anxiety and hysterical hyperventilation or artificial ventilation).

Look at 'standard HCO_3^-' (measured at a normal Pco_2, i.e. with simulated normal ventilation). If it is raised this accounts for a metabolic alkalosis. If it is reduced it accounts for a metabolic acidosis (usually renal or ketotic).

Look at Po_2. If it is high, the patient is on added oxygen. If low, the patient has either lung disease (the Pco_2 is usually high) or a right-to-left shunt.

INTERPRETATION

- Pco_2 reflects alveolar ventilation.
- Po_2 reflects ventilation/perfusion imbalance, gas transfer or venous to arterial shunts.

Arterial gas patterns

High Pco_2, low Po_2. Respiratory failure due to chronic obstructive pulmonary disease, asthma or chest wall disease (e.g. ankylosing spondylitis or neuromuscular disorders).

Normal or low Pco_2, low Po_2. Hypoxia due to parenchymal lung disease with normal airways. These patients hyperventilate and hence lower the Pco_2 because of hypoxia (and 'stiff lungs'), e.g. pulmonary embolism, fibrosing alveolitis. Another cause is venous admixture from right-to-left shunts (e.g. Fallot).

Low Pco_2, normal Po_2. A common pattern usually seen after painful arterial puncture (causing hyperventilation), and in hysterical hyperventilation.

Causes of hypoxaemia

- Low inspired oxygen concentration due to altitude or faulty apparatus.
- Hypoventilation due to sedative drugs, central nervous system disease, neuromuscular disease, crushed chest/or obstructive sleep apnoea. The arterial Pco_2 is characteristically high.
- Ventilation/perfusion imbalance. Hyperventilation of some alveoli cannot

compensate for the hypoxaemia which results from the hypoventilation of other alveoli. This is the usual cause of a reduced transfer factor.

• Physiological shunt (venous admixture) when deoxygenated blood passes straight to the left heart without perfusing ventilated alveoli. This occurs in cyanotic congenital heart disease. The arterial Po_2 is not significantly improved by the administration of 2 litres of oxygen/min.

Type 1 respiratory failure refers to patients with lung disease which produces hyperventilation as well as hypoxaemia such as pulmonary oedema, pneumonia, asthma, pulmonary fibrosis and pulmonary thromboembolism.

Type 2 respiratory failure with a high Pco_2 (and hypoxaemia) implies a defect in ventilation with obstructed airways, reduced chest wall compliance, or central nervous system disease because otherwise the excess carbon dioxide would be blown off.

Ventilatory function tests

The simplest tests of lung function are spirometric. If a patient exhales as fast and as long as possible from full inspiration into a spirometer, the volume expired in the first second is the forced expiratory volume in 1 s (FEV_1) and the total expired is the forced vital capacity (FVC). Relaxed (slow) vital capacity may provide a better measure of trapped gas volume in chronic airways obstruction and is as easy to measure as these other values. Constriction of the major airways (e.g. asthma) reduces the FEV_1 more than the FVC. Restriction of the lungs (e.g. by fibrosis) reduces the FVC and, to a lesser degree, the FEV_1. The ratio of FEV_1 to FVC (FEV%) thus tends to be low in obstructive airways disease (e.g. chronic bronchitis and asthma) and normal or high in fibrosing alveolitis (p. 355). It is best to see the shape of the actual curve as well as the figures derived from it (Fig. 6.1). Spirometry is often performed before and after bronchodilation.

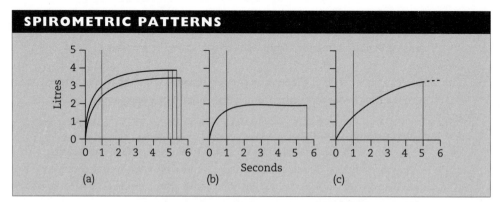

SPIROMETRIC PATTERNS

Fig. 6.1 Spirometric patterns. (a) Normal (elderly man) forced expiratory volume/forced vital capacity (FEV/FVC) = 3.0/4.0 = 75%; (b) restrictive, FEV/FVC = 1.8/2.0 = 90%; and (c) obstructive, FEV/FVC = 1.4/3.5 = 40%.

The peak expiratory flow rate (PEFR) measures the rate of flow of exhaled air at the start of a forced expiration. It gives similar information to the FEV_1.

Normal values for all these tests vary with age, sex, size and race, and suitable nomograms should be consulted unless the changes observed are gross.

TRANSFER FACTOR

The patient must have a vital capacity of over 1 litre and be able to hold the breath for 15 s. This test measures the transfer of a small concentration of carbon monoxide in the inspired air on to haemoglobin. It is reduced in diseases which reduce ventilation or perfusion or alters the balance between them, and increased in pulmonary haemorrhage. Correction must be made for haemoglobin concentration, because the transfer factor varies directly with haemoglobin. Its chief value is for monitoring progression in interstitial disease, including fibrosing alveolitis and confirming a diagnosis of pulmonary haemorrhage.

Cardiovascular System

There is no shortage of patients with cardiovascular disease who are suitable for inclusion in examinations. Patients with ischaemic heart disease have few physical signs and the diagnosis of angina of effort will be made on symptoms alone. Valvular disease, whether acquired or congenital, and septal defects often give rise to murmurs which may be diagnostic. The penalties for failing to elicit and describe and interpret these correctly are often disproportionate to their real importance in diagnosis and treatment. A cardiologist rarely reaches a final decision on physical signs alone unsupported by an electrocardiogram, chest X-ray and echocardiogram. Patients with congestive heart failure and cases of myocardial infarction are very common in hospital and during the recovery phase may be sufficiently well to be included in an examination list.

Arterial pulse

'Examine the (arterial) pulse'
If you are asked this, there is frequently an arrhythmia (often atrial fibrillation or multiple ectopic beats). Less commonly, you may feel the very slow pulse of complete heart block or there may be a tachycardia such as that associated with thyrotoxicosis, the clinical features of which you may notice on approaching the patient (though not so obvious in the elderly).

Do not attempt to estimate the blood pressure from the pulse.

Examine a carotid, brachial or radial pulse, whichever you are familiar with assessing. Describe as follows:

SPECIAL PULSES

Type	Character	Seen in
Plateau	Low amplitude, slow rise, slow fall	Aortic valve stenosis
Collapsing (water hammer)	Large amplitude, rapid rise, rapid fall	Aortic regurgitation. Also severe anaemia, hyperthyroidism Arteriovenous shunt, heart block, patent ductus arteriosus
Small volume	Thready	Low cardiac output due to obstruction: valve stenosis (tricuspid, pulmonary, mitral, aortic) or pulmonary hypertension Shock
Alternans	Alternate large- and small-amplitude beats rarely noted in pulse; usually on taking blood pressure (note doubling in rate as mercury falls)	Left ventricular failure
Bisferiens	Double-topped	Aortic stenosis with aortic regurgitation
Paradoxus	Pulse volume decreases excessively with inspiration (of little diagnostic value)	Cardiac tamponade, constrictive pericarditis, severe inspiratory airways obstruction (chronic bronchitis and asthma)
Absent radial		Congenital anomaly (check brachials and blood pressure) Tied off at surgery or catheterization Arterial embolism (usually atrial fibrillation)

Notes
1 The state of one vessel wall does not necessarily correlate with the state of the arteries elsewhere.
2 It takes little time to check if the other radial (or brachial) pulse is present.
3 If you think the patient may have hypertension, you should look for radial femoral delay (aortic coarctation).
4 If the character of the pulse is abnormal you should ask whether you may take the blood pressure, to estimate the pulse pressure (and to check alternans).

Table 7.1 Abnormalities of the arterial pulse.

Approximate rate

Glance at the jugular venous pressure whilst counting, since this may give valuable additional information about cardiac rhythm and failure (see below).

Rhythm

Regular, basically regular with extra or dropped beats, or completely irregular. If it is clinically atrial fibrillation, remember that the pulse rate is different from the heart rate; also listen at the apex.

VOLUME AND CHARACTER (Table 7.1)

These abnormalities fall into three categories:
• Useful to confirm or assess other findings in the cardiovascular system (plateau, collapsing, small volume);
• Rare and/or difficult (alternans, bisferiens and paradoxus); and
• Examination 'catch' (absent radial).

NB The rate and rhythm are relatively easy to assess but the character of the pulse is extremely difficult to evaluate.

Neck veins

'Look at the veins of the neck' ('Examine the jugular venous pressure')

RAISED JUGULAR VENOUS PRESSURE (Table 7.2)

You should comment on the *vertical* height of the top of the column of blood above the sternal angle. The patient will usually be lying at 45° and the neck should be relaxed. The sternal angle is about 5 cm above the left atrium when the patient

RAISED JVP		
Character	**Compression of neck and abdomen**	**Conclusion**
Non-pulsatile	No change in jugular venous pressure	Superior mediastinal obstruction (usually carcinoma of bronchus), platysmal compression or large goitre
Pulsatile	Jugular vein fills and empties	Right heart failure (p. 70) Expiratory airways obstruction (asthma and bronchitis) Fluid overload Cardiac tamponade (very rare)

Note
There is no 'a' wave in atrial fibrillation.

Table 7.2 Raised jugular venous pressure (JVP).

is lying at 45°. The normal central venous pressure (CVP) is <7 cm and therefore the jugular vein is normally just visible. The deep venous pulse is seen welling up between the heads of sternomastoid in the front of the neck on expiration, and is a better guide to right atrial pressure than the superficial venous pulse which may rarely be obstructed by the soft tissues of the neck. If you can find neither:

- Look at the other side of the neck.
- Suspect a low level and press on the abdomen firmly (unless the liver is tender) in order to raise the column. A positive reflux may have no pathophysiological significance and the sole purpose of this manoeuvre is to demonstrate the vein and to show that it can be filled (i.e. the pressure is not high).
- Suspect a high level with distension of the veins (not easily seen) with the top of the column above the neck. Check if the ear lobes move with the cardiac cycle and sit the patient vertical to get a greater length of visible jugular vein above the right atrium. The venous pressure can sometimes be demonstrated in dilated veins of an arm or hand held at a suitable height above the right atrium. The level at which pulsation occurs should be determined.

If the jugular venous pressure is raised (especially if >10 cm):
- A large 'a' wave (corresponds with atrial systole) occurs in tricuspid stenosis, pulmonary hypertension, pulmonary stenosis and mitral stenosis. A cannon wave is a massive 'a' wave occurring in complete heart block when the right atrium contracts against a closed tricuspid valve.
- Look for a large 'v' wave (corresponds with ventricular systole) indicating tricuspid regurgitation (usually secondary to heart failure): a murmur may be audible on auscultation of the heart.
- Examine the abdomen for an enlarged tender pulsatile liver.
- Check the ankles for oedema and then sit the patient up and examine the back of the chest for crepitations and for pleural effusions (unilateral or bilateral) and for sacral oedema. These should be done even if the jugular venous pressure is not raised since oedema of cardiac failure may persist after jugular venous pressure has been reduced by treatment.
- Examine for the underlying cause, e.g. heart valve lesion or fluid overload.

Heart

'Examine the heart'
Most heart cases in an examination have a murmur. Such patients make it easy for an examiner to assess the candidate's ability to elicit and describe accurately the physical signs which are present. You may be watched throughout your examination and you must therefore have devised a system of examination which is second nature to you even in this stressful situation.

A full examination of the heart is not advisable without examining the arterial and venous pulses and this is usually done first. It is important to know not only the auscultatory features of the various heart abnormalities but also to know which of them are found in association with each other and to examine for these with particular care. Thus a patient in whom you have diagnosed mitral stenosis should be examined with special attention to the aortic valve.

Chronic rheumatic heart disease is still the commonest type of heart case in examinations, though most have had cardiac surgery. It is becoming progressively less common in clinical practice because rheumatic fever is now a rare disorder. You may see patients with ventricular septal defects; the smaller lesions may not require surgery and often produce loud murmurs (*maladie de Roger*). For similar reasons you may be shown a patient with an atrial septal defect (ASD)—often not diagnosed until middle age—but the auscultatory findings may be difficult to elicit. Beware of coarctation of the aorta where loud murmurs may originate in collateral vessels over the chest wall.

On approaching the patient note any cyanosis, dyspnoea or malar flush.
- Examine the arterial pulses and look for clubbing (p. 58).
- Examine the jugular venous pulse.
- Examine the front of the chest. First look for the scars of previous surgery and then for the localized thrusting apex beat of left ventricular hypertrophy and the parasternal lift of right ventricular hypertrophy. Then palpate for these phenomena and for thrills (palpable murmurs). Note that a tapping apex is thought to be an accentuated mitral first sound and in subsequent examination you will be trying to substantiate a diagnosis of mitral stenosis. Finally listen to the heart, starting at the apex. It may be difficult to establish which are the first and second sounds, but an experienced clinician recognizes them by their quality. A thumb on the right carotid artery can help to time the first sound.
- Examine each part of the cardiac cycle for murmurs. (Remember to listen for a friction rub of pericarditis and a triple rhythm of cardiac failure. These are easily missed.) There is no alternative to experience for this and it is essential to know the character of the murmurs of the commoner cardiac lesions. Their description is formalized and stereotyped so that if you say there is a rumbling diastolic murmur at the apex, you have diagnosed mitral stenosis. You should attempt to make whatever you hear fit one of the known patterns (Table 7.3).
- Listen to the lungs, especially at the bases posteriorly for fine crepitations. Look for sacral and ankle oedema. Establish the blood pressure.

DIFFICULT SYSTOLIC MURMURS

It may be impossible to define the valve lesion causing an apical systolic murmur on auscultation without echocardiography. The possibilities include:
- mitral regurgitation (papillary muscle dysfunction, floppy valve, ruptured chordae tendineae);
- aortic ejection murmur (siderosis especially in old women and stenosis); and
- ventricular septal defect (VSD) (very occasionally).

CHARACTERISTICS OF MURMURS

Lesion	Murmur and position	Radiation and notes
Aortic stenosis (often with aortic incompetence)	Basal mid systolic, often loud and with a thrill. Possible ejection click	Maximal in second RICS and radiating into neck. Also at apex
Pulmonary stenosis (may be part of Fallot's tetralogy)	Basal mid systolic with click if stenosis is valvar	Maximal in second LICS. Increase on inspiration (with increased blood flow) Pulmonary component of second sound is quiet and delayed
Aortic regurgitation (often accompanying mitral stenosis in the UK because syphilis is now rare)	Early immediate blowing diastolic murmur	Usually maximal in third LICS or, less often, in second RICS. Radiation between right carotid and cardiac apex. Look for Argyll Robertson pupils, etc.
Pulmonary regurgitation very rare	Early immediate blowing diastolic murmur	Maximal in second and third LICS
Mitral stenosis	Mid or late rumbling diastolic murmur at apex	Loud mitral first sound. Opening snap. Turn patient on left side (and exercise) to accentuate murmur. Presystolic accentuation if in sinus rhythm
Mitral regurgitation (often mitral stenosis is present as well)	Pansystolic at apex	Radiation to axilla (but often heard parasternally)
Tricuspid regurgitation	Pansystolic and lower sternum	'v' wave in neck and pulsatile liver
Ventricular septal defect (small ones are common, severe are rare)	Rough, loud and pansystolic. Maximal at third to fourth LICS parasternally	
Atrial septal defect	Pulmonary systolic murmur with fixed split second sound (no murmur from blood flow through the defect)	Possible diastolic murmur from tricuspid valve if atrial septal defect flow is large
Patent ductus arteriosus	Machinery murmur, maximal in late systole and extending into diastole. Maximal in second to third LICS in mid clavicular line	Also audible posteriorly
Coarctation	Loud rough murmur in systole, maximum over apex of left lung both posteriorly and anteriorly	Murmurs of scapular and internal mammary shunt collaterals. Radial femoral delay. Hypertension in arms
Friction rub	Scratchy noise, usually systole and diastole	Varies with posture and breathing

Notes: 1 'Base' denotes the first and second intercostal spaces. **2** RICS and LICS refer to right and left intercostal spaces.

Table 7.3 Characteristics of murmurs.

CONTINUOUS MURMURS

These are murmurs maximal in systole and pass through the second sound into diastole.

They are caused by:

- patent ductus arteriosus (best heard in second left intercostal space);
- aortic stenosis with regurgitation;
- arteriovenous malformation in the lung;
- coronary arteriovenous fistula; and
- ruptured sinus of Valsalva (the pockets behind each leaflet of the aortic valve) —a high-pitched murmur because of high pressure.

NB   The unsatisfactory question, '*listen here or listen at this point*': usually the apex or aortic area is used to ensure that the candidate roll the patient on to the left side for mitral stenotic murmurs, or sits the patient forward and asks him or her to exhale fully for aortic regurgitation.

HEART FAILURE (p. 365)

The signs of left ventricular failure are tachycardia, triple rhythm, fine basal crepitations of pulmonary oedema and pleural effusion usually associated with signs of right ventricular failure, i.e. raised jugular venous pressure, hepatomegaly, ankle and sacral oedema.

If right ventricular failure is secondary to lung disease (cor pulmonale), there is usually clinical evidence to suggest chronic obstructure pulmonary disease (p. 328) or, less commonly, pulmonary embolism (p. 351). Other rare causes include bronchiectasis, fibrosing alveolitis, cystic fibrosis and primary pulmonary hypertension. Treatment is discussed on p. 372.

Hypertension

'*This person has hypertension—please examine him to demonstrate the key signs*'

If you are allowed to question the patient, ask about anginal chest pain, intermittent claudication, headaches, visual changes, family history, salt intake, breathlessness and drugs taken (especially the contraceptive pill, cold cures containing sympathomimetic drugs and monoamine oxidase inhibitors).

Slight or moderate hypertension usually gives no abnormalities detectable on physical examination. In long-standing or severe hypertension there will usually be left ventricular hypertrophy and a loud aortic second sound. The other consequences of sustained hypertension should be looked for — hypertensive retinopathy, heart failure, renal failure, cerebrovascular disease. It is essential to think of the less common causes of hypertension and therefore to consider the following:

- Observe the face for evidence of Cushing's syndrome—usually due to steroids.
- Feel both radial arteries and take the blood pressure in both arms for coarctation.
- Examine for aortic coarctation (radial–femoral delay, weak femoral pulses and

the bruits of the coarctation and of the scapular anastomoses and visible pulsation of the anastomoses).
- A renal artery bruit may be present in the epigastrium in renal artery stenosis.
- The kidneys are palpable in polycystic disease.
- Think also of the chronic renal diseases (test the urine), of phaeochromocytoma (rare) and of primary hyperaldosteronism (very rare).

Myocardial infarction

'This patient has had a myocardial infarction: would you ask him some questions?'
The patient will be in the recovery stage. The history is more important than the physical signs. Symptoms (pain or fatigue) are often present in the preceding weeks.

Ask about
- *Pain.* Onset (rest or exercise), quality (compressing), distribution (including radiation), duration (usually over half an hour). Tearing interscapular pain suggests dissecting aneurysm.
NB   Intensity is no guide to the extent of the infarct, especially in the elderly where pain may be absent.
- *Breathlessness.* About a quarter of all cases describe an acute attack of dyspnoea as a feature of the attack and in the elderly it may be the only feature.
- *Cold sweat.* Also common, and often associated with nausea and vomiting.
- *Pallor.* Normally reported by witnesses.
- *Previous attacks of angina.* If they have had a previous infarct or angina their new pain will usually resemble that which they have had previously.
- *Past history* of hypertension, strokes, symptoms of peripheral vascular disease and, in young women, whether they have diabetes mellitus or are on the contraceptive pill.
- *Family history* of heart attacks, especially if young; diabetes; hypertension; raised cholesterol; gout.
- *Other risk factors*, e.g. smoking, occupation.

Examination
'Would you like to examine him?'
- Evidence of a low cardiac output (hypotension and small-volume rapid pulse).
- Signs of cardiac failure, including crepitations at the lung bases.
- Arrhythmias, tachycardia, bradycardia.
- Pericardial friction (immediate and post-infarction Dressler's syndrome).
- Evidence of mitral regurgitation (papillary muscle dysfunction).
- Evidence of a cardiac aneurysm (double impulse)—rare.
- Evidence of septal perforation (acquired VSD)—rare and acute.
- Deep venous thrombosis—a complication of immobilization.

- Evidence of hyperlipidaemia, especially xanthelasmata and tendon xanthomata.
- Evidence of associated diseases: hypothyroidism, diabetes mellitus, gout, cigarette smoking (smell and finger-staining).
- Evidence of the relevant alternatives in the differential diagnosis, especially pulmonary embolism, pericarditis, dissecting aneurysm, pleurisy, cholecystitis, reflux oesophagitis, radicular pain.

CARDIAC ARRHYTHMIAS

Rhythm	Rate Atrial	Ventricular	Diagnosis	Underlying diseases	Therapy (treat underlying disease; pp. 364–368)
Regular	90+	90+	Sinus tachycardia	Anxiety, cardiac failure, thyrotoxicosis, fever, anaemia	Treat underlying disease
	120–200	120–200	Supraventricular tachycardia	None (60%), thyrotoxicosis, digitalis, tobacco, caffeine, Wolff–Parkinson–White syndrome	Vagal stimulation (pressure on the carotid sinus), β-blocker or verapamil or digoxin
	200–400	100–200	Atrial flutter with block	Ischaemic heart disease, thyrotoxicosis (digitalis)	Digoxin, DC cardioversion, verapamil
	80+	30–45	Complete heart block with cannon 'a' waves in jugular vein pulse, variable intensity first sound, wide pulse pressure	Post-infarction, idiopathic, digitalis, cardiomyopathy	Nil if asymptomatic Atropine, isoprenaline or cardiac pacemaker after myocardial infarction
	40–50	40–50	Sinus bradycardia	Athletes, myocardial infarction, myxoedema, hypothermia, sinoatrial disease	As heart block if following infarction
Irregular			Multiple ectopics (including coupled beats) ECG basically regular	Ischaemia, digitalis, thyrotoxicosis, cardiomyopathy	Stop digitalis and give potassium if necessary. Lignocaine, disopyramide or mexiletine, β-blocker if due to digitalis
		60–100 treated 100+ untreated	Atrial flutter with varying block Atrial fibrillation (apex rate is only guide to true heart rate. ECG essential)	Ischaemia, rheumatic heart disease (MS), thyrotoxicosis. Rarely pulmonary embolism, constructive pericarditis, cardiomyopathy or bronchial carcinoma	Digoxin, or DC cardioversion following myocardial infarction and following treated mitral stenosis and thyrotoxicosis
Cardiac arrest	120–200		Ventricular tachycardia	Myocardial infarction and ischaemia (p. 360)	
		No peripheral pulse	Ventricular fibrillation and sometimes ventricular tachycardia Ventricular asystole		

ECG, Electrocardiogram; MS, mitral stenosis; DC, direct current.

Table 7.4 Cardiac arrhythmias.

Investigation

'What investigations would you perform?'

Ask for an ECG series and a cardiac enzyme series, e.g. hydroxybutyrate dehydro-genase, aspartate transferase or MB isoenzyme (see p. 362) of creatine phosphok-inase. You may note rises in the white cell count, erythrocyte sedimentation rate and temperature. A chest X-ray is necessary in all cardiac investigations.

Management

'Discuss the management'

The following aspects should be considered (p. 363):

• Aspirin;
• Bed rest;
• Analgesia and sedation;
• Oxygen therapy;
• Anticoagulants;
• Beta blockade;
• Complications (cardiac failure and shock, arrhythmias, rupture of septum, papillary muscle dysfunction and cardiac aneurysm);
• Thrombolytic therapy (p. 363);
• Smoking;
• Obesity;
• Hyperlipidaemia (p. 231); and
• Advice on discharge from hospital, i.e. work, driving, sexual activities (p. 368).

Arrhythmias

SUPRAVENTRICULAR TACHYCARDIAS

Supraventricular tachycardias arise from the atria or atrioventricular junction. QRS complex is normal unless there is also bundle branch block.

SINUS TACHYCARDIA

Sinus rhythm, rate >100 beats/min. An underlying cause (anxiety, exercise, fever, anaemia, heart failure, thyrotoxicosis) can usually be identified.

ATRIAL FIBRILLATION

Atrial fibrillation (AF) is predominantly a disease of the elderly, occurring in 0.2% of men aged 47–56 and 3% of those aged 77–86 (Framingham study, 1949).

Rheumatic AF occurs in association with rheumatic valve disease, whereas in non-rheumatic AF there is an underlying metabolic disorder or other form of cardiac disease.

Lone AF occurs in the absence of valvular, myocardial or other identifiable disease.

The common causes are:

• ischaemic heart disease;

- cardiomyopathy;
- valvular disease; and
- thyrotoxicosis.

Management

The aims are to restore sinus rhythm or control the ventricular rate and minimize the risk of embolization.

Direct current (DC) cardioversion establishes sinus rhythm in 90% of patients, but relapse is common. Long-term amiodarone reduces the frequency of relapse, although side effects can limit its use.

NB   Side effects of amiodarone are reversible corneal microdeposits, photosensitivity, skin discoloration, hypothyroidism, hyperthyroidism, diffuse pulmonary alveolitis and fibrosis, peripheral neuropathy and myopathy.

Medical therapy

Quinine, flecainide and amiodarone have all been used to restore and maintain sinus rhythm.

Digoxin does not restore sinus rhythm, but is effective in controlling the ventricular rate, either alone or in combination with β-blockers.

The incidence of ischaemic stroke (embolic or thrombotic) is increased in patients with non-rheumatic AF. Five prospective trials have shown that using warfarin is effective in reducing the risk of stroke. Aspirin is effective when warfarin is contraindicated.

ATRIAL FLUTTER

The atria discharge at around 300/min, giving the characteristic saw-tooth baseline on ECG (see Fig. 7.14). There is usually atrioventricular block, leading to a ventricular rate of 150/min (2:1) or 100/min (3:1).

The causes are similar to AF, although atrial flutter is less common.

Management

Drugs such as sotalol, flecainide, disopyramide and amiodarone are often effective in restoring sinus rhythm. DC cardioversion can also be used to terminate atrial flutter.

ATRIAL TACHYCARDIA

The atrial rate is slower than in atrial flutter, being between 120 and 200/min. The ECG shows abnormally shaped P waves (see Fig. 7.15). There is often a degree of atrioventricular (AV) block.

Management

Atrial tachycardia is commonly due to digoxin toxicity, which should be stopped. If not, digoxin, verapamil or β-blockers may be used to control the ventricular rate. Sinus rhythm may be restored by DC cardioversion.

TRIALS

AFASAK (Atrial Fibrillation Aspirin Anticoagulation) studied 1007 patients with chronic non-rheumatic AF. A total of 335 patients received warfarin openly (INR 2.8–4.2), and in a double-blind study 336 received aspirin 75 mg daily or placebo. The incidence of thromboembolic complications and vascular mortality was significantly lower in the warfarin group than in the aspirin or placebo groups, which did not differ significantly. *Lancet* 1989; **i**: 175–179.

BAATAF (Boston Area Anticoagulation Trial for Atrial Fibrillation) compared warfarin (INR 1.5–2.7) with placebo in 420 patients. Warfarin reduced the risk of stroke by 14%. *N Engl J Med* 1990; **323**: 1505–1511.

SPAF (Stroke Prevention in Atrial Fibrillation) studied 1330 patients with constant or intermittent AF. Systemic embolization was reduced by 42% in patients receiving aspirin, and 67% in a subgroup of patients eligible to receive warfarin (INR 1.3–1.8). *Circulation* 1991; **84**: 527–539.

The **SPAF** (Stroke Prevention in Atrial Fibrillation) **III study** compared low-dose warfarin (initial INR 1.2–1.5) plus aspirin with adjusted-dose warfarin (INR 2.0–3.0) in 1044 patients with AF and other risk factors for thromboembolism (LV dysfunction, hypertension, previous thromboembolism). Dose-adjusted warfarin was significantly better at preventing stroke. *Lancet* 1996; **348**: 633–638.

CAFA (Canadian Atrial Fibrillation Anticoagulation) compared warfarin (INR 2–3) and placebo in 378 patients. Warfarin reduced the risk of stroke by 79%. *J Am Coll Cardiol* 1991; **18**: 349–355.

VASP (Veterans Affairs Stroke Prevention in non-rheumatic AF) compared warfarin (INR 1.2–1.5) and placebo in 571 men with chronic AF. Warfarin reduced the risk of stroke by 79%. *N Engl J Med* 1992; **327**: 1406–1412.

EAFT (European Atrial Fibrillation Trial) compared warfarin and placebo in patients with non-rheumatic AF and a history of minor ischaemic stroke or TIA within the previous 3 months. Warfarin reduced the risk of subsequent stroke by 67%. *N Engl J Med* 1995; **333**: 5–10.

AF, Atrial fibrillation; INR, international normalized ratio; LV, left ventricular; TIA, transient ischaemic attack.

PRE-EXCITATION SYNDROMES

In addition to the AV node, an additional connection (accessory pathway) between the atria and ventricles allows atrial impulse to be transmitted more quickly to the ventricles — hence the term pre-excitation syndrome. The main types are Wolff–Parkinson–White and Lown–Ganong–Levine syndromes.

Wolff–Parkinson–White syndrome is caused by an accessory pathway (bundle of Kent) which bypasses the AV junction. It is characterized by a short PR interval and a widened QRS complex due to the presence of a δ wave (see Fig. 7.6). In type A the ventricular complex is positive in lead V1; in type B it is negative.

Two main arrhythmias occur:

• In *re-entrant tachycardia* the normal (AV node) conduction pathway and the accessory pathway form a circuit through which impulses repeatedly circulate. The δ wave is lost. Drugs which block the AV node (e.g. adenosine, verapamil) usually restore sinus rhythm.

• In *atrial fibrillation* most ventricular complexes are broad due to the presence of large δ waves. AV nodal blocking drugs may increase the ventricular rate and should be avoided. DC cardioversion usually terminates AF. Amiodarone may be used to slow conduction in the accessory pathway.

Lown–Ganong–Levine is characterized by a short PR interval, normal QRS and paroxysmal tachycardia.

VENTRICULAR TACHYCARDIA

The ventricular rate is usually 120–200/min. It usually reflects serious underlying myocardial disease. It is often self-limiting, but if sustained may cause hypotension and shock. The ECG shows a broad-complex tachycardia, and P waves dissociated from the ventricular activity may be seen (see Fig. 7.16). The axis is often bizarre.

Management

Lignocaine may terminate ventricular tachycardia (p. 365). Amiodarone can be used if lignocaine fails, but DC cardioversion should be performed if there is shock.

In *torsade de pointes* the QRS axis progressively changes so that the complexes appear to twist continuously. There is QT prolongation in sinus rhythm. Underlying causes should be identified and treated (antiarrhythmic drugs, hypokalaemia, hypomagnesaemia, tricyclic antidepressants). Antiarrhythmic agents may aggravate the condition. DC cardioversion or pacing is often effective in terminating attacks.

VENTRICULAR FIBRILLATION

See cardiac arrest (p. 77).

HEART BLOCK

In *first-degree block* the PR interval is prolonged (see Fig. 7.4).

In *second-degree block* the normal 1 : 1 ratio of P : QRS complexes is lost but a relationship between P waves and QRS complexes still exists. The relationship may be either progressive lengthening of the PR interval until one QRS complex is dropped (Mobitz type I or Wenckebach) or dropped QRS complexes without a change in the PR interval (see Fig. 7.4).

If there is complete dissociation between P waves and QRS complexes *third-degree heart block* (see Fig. 7.5) exists. The QRS complex rate (and hence ventricular rate) is usually slow (15–50/min) and regular. Cardiac pacing is often required.

CARDIORESPIRATORY ARREST

Clinical features

- Sudden loss of consciousness
- Absent carotid and femoral pulses
- Respiratory arrest follows shortly after.

Aetiology

- Almost invariably cardiac arrhythmia (ventricular fibrillation (VF), ventricular tachycardia (VT) or asystole)
- Rarely, the primary event is respiratory arrest (e.g. severe asthmatic attack).

Management

- Watch patient for 1–2 s to ensure correct diagnosis (observe for fluttering and opening of eyelids or return of consciousness).
- Recheck carotid pulse.
- If absent, call cardiac arrest team and strike sternum hard.
- Carry out external cardiac massage and ventilation through Brooke's airway.
- Establish intravenous line.
- Defibrillate as soon as machine arrives with 200 J (ensure everyone is away from the bed or trolley).
- Continue until the cardiac arrest team arrives, then:
- Intubate and ventilate.
- Check rhythm on ECG monitor.
- Treat according to Fig. 7.1.

ELECTROCARDIOGRAMS

Hints and facts (Fig. 7.2)

- 1 little square is 0.04 s; 1 big square is 0.2 s.
- 1 little square vertically is 1 mV.
- Normal PR interval is 0.12–0.2 s (three small squares to one big square).
- Normal QRS duration is up to 0.12 s (three small squares).

The QT interval varies with rate. Upper limits of normal are approximately:

- rate 60/min QT 0.43 s
- rate 75/min QT 0.39 s
- rate 100/min QT 0.34 s.

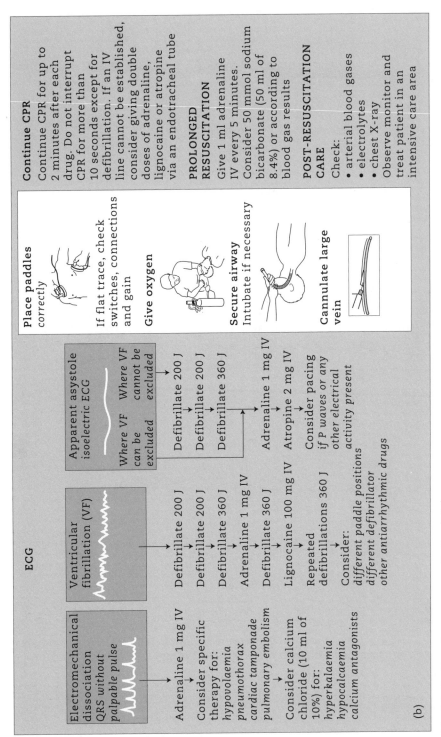

ECG

Ventricular fibrillation (VF)

Defibrillate 200 J
↓
Defibrillate 200 J
↓
Defibrillate 360 J
↓
Adrenaline 1 mg IV
↓
Defibrillate 360 J
↓
Lignocaine 100 mg IV
↓
Repeated defibrillations 360 J
↓
Consider:
different paddle positions
different defibrillator
other antiarrhythmic drugs

Apparent asystole isoelectric ECG

Where VF can be excluded / Where VF cannot be excluded

Defibrillate 200 J
↓
Defibrillate 200 J
↓
Defibrillate 360 J

Adrenaline 1 mg IV
↓
Atropine 2 mg IV
↓
Consider pacing if P waves or any other electrical activity present

Electromechanical dissociation QRS without palpable pulse

Adrenaline 1 mg IV
↓
Consider specific therapy for:
hypovolaemia
pneumothorax
cardiac tamponade
pulmonary embolism
↓
Consider calcium chloride (10 ml of 10%) for:
hyperkalaemia
hypocalcaemia
calcium antagonists

Place paddles correctly

If flat trace, check switches, connections and gain

Give oxygen

Secure airway
Intubate if necessary

Cannulate large vein

Continue CPR

Continue CPR for up to 2 minutes after each drug. Do not interrupt CPR for more than 10 seconds except for defibrillation. If an IV line cannot be established, consider giving double doses of adrenaline, lignocaine or atropine via an endotracheal tube

PROLONGED RESUSCITATION

Give 1 ml adrenaline IV every 5 minutes.
Consider 50 mmol sodium bicarbonate (50 ml of 8.4%) or according to blood gas results

POST-RESUSCITATION CARE

Check:
• arterial blood gases
• electrolytes
• chest X-ray
Observe monitor and treat patient in an intensive care area

(b)

Fig. 7.1 Cardiopulmonary resuscitation (CPR).

(a)

(b)

Fig. 7.2 (a) Normal 12-lead electrocardiogram (ECG). AVF, augmented voltage F; AVL, augmented voltage L; AVR, augmented voltage R. (b) Waves of the normal ECG.

When presented with an ECG, check that it is labelled correctly (patient's name, date, leads for each group of complexes) and then assess the rate and rhythm.

Rate

Assess the rate by counting the large squares between two QRS complexes and dividing into 300 (i.e. if two squares, the rate is 150/min; three squares: 100/min; four squares: 75/min; five squares: 60/min). If the rate is less than 60/min the patient has a bradycardia; if greater than 100/min, a tachycardia.

Regularity

Use the edge of a piece of paper to mark off a series of R waves, and then shift the paper along one or more complexes. The marks on the paper will still correspond with the R waves if the rhythm is regular. Total irregularity is almost always due to AF. Proceed as always, quickly and methodically to:

Check the mean frontal QRS axis

Use the limb leads, and remember the angles at which these leads 'see' the heart (lead I = 0°; Fig. 7.3). To gain a rough idea of the axis, find the lead with the maximum positive deflection (sum of the positive R wave and negative Q and S waves) — the axis lies close to this. Then calculate the total deflection (R wave minus Q and S waves) in leads I and AVF which are perpendicular to each other (at 0 and 90° respectively). Add these together as vectors (use the squares on the ECG paper) — the net vector is the axis. (For examples see Fig. 7.3.)

The normal range is 0–90°.

Causes of axis deviation

Left — left ventricular strain or hypertrophy (e.g. hypertension, aortic stenosis), ostium primum atrial septal defect.

Right — right ventricular strain or hypertrophy (e.g. pulmonary embolus, chronic lung disease, pulmonary valve stenosis), ostium secundum, atrial septal defect (ASD).

Check individual waves

Do this in order (i.e. P wave, PR interval, QRS complex, ST segment, QT interval, T wave) for their presence, shape and duration. This always needs to be performed for each lead in turn, although you will come to recognize certain patterns (e.g. bundle branch block, myocardial infarction). It is usually safe to ignore augmented voltage R (AVR).

P wave (atrial depolarization). Most easily seen in V1 and V2. It is peaked in right atrial hypertrophy, and bifid in left atrial hypertrophy (left atrial depolarization occurs slightly later than right, giving a second peak). It may be 'lost' (in the QRS complex) in nodal rhythm (originates from the AV node).

Fig. 7.3 (a) Position of the limb leads; (b) calculation of the cardiac axis.

PR interval

If the PR interval is longer than 0.2 s (one large square), first-degree heart block is present (Fig. 7.4).

If the normal 1 : 1 ratio of P : QRS complexes is lost but a relationship between P waves and QRS complexes still exists, second-degree heart block is present. The relationship may be either progressive lengthening of the PR interval until one QRS complex is dropped (Mobitz type I or Wenckebach) or dropped QRS complexes without a change in the PR interval (Fig. 7.4).

If there is complete dissociation between P waves and QRS complexes, third-degree heart block (Fig. 7.5) exists. The QRS complex rate (and hence ventricular rate) is usually slow (15–50/min) and regular. Cardiac pacing is often required.

(a)

(b)

(c)

Fig. 7.4 (a) First-degree heart block. PR interval 0.30 s. (b) Second-degree heart block (Wenckebach or Mobitz type I). (c) Third-degree heart block (complete). Atrioventricular dissociation.

Fig. 7.5 Third-degree heart block (complete). Atrioventricular dissociation.

A short PR interval occurs in the Wolff–Parkinson–White syndrome in which an abnormal AV conduction pathway (bundle of Kent) predisposes to arrhythmias. The PR interval is short and the QRS complex slurred by a δ wave at the beginning (Fig. 7.6).

QRS complex

If the QRS complex is longer than 0.12 s (three small squares), bundle branch block exists. In left bundle branch block the complex is negative (V- or W-shaped) in V1 (Fig. 7.7). In right bundle branch block the complex is positive (M-shaped) in V1 (Fig. 7.8).

Pathological (broad, deep) Q waves are greater than 0.04 s (1 small square) wide and greater than 0.2 mV (two small squares deep). They may be normal in AVR or V1. In the absence of bundle branch block, ventricular rhythms and the Wolff–Parkinson–White syndrome they indicate myocardial infarction. The site of such pathological Q waves indicates the site of the myocardial infarction—

Fig. 7.6 Wolff–Parkinson–White (WPW) syndrome. Short PR interval and δ waves. Lown–Ganong–Levine (LGL) has no δ wave but is otherwise identical.

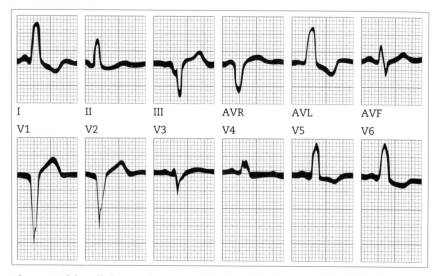

| I | II | III | AVR | AVL | AVF |
| V1 | V2 | V3 | V4 | V5 | V6 |

Fig. 7.7 Left bundle branch block. RSR (M-shaped QRS complex) is visible in some of the left ventricular leads, I, AVL, and V4–6, and notched QS complexes in the right ventricular lead, V1–2.

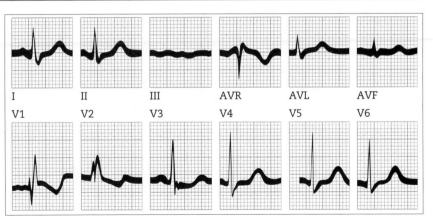

Fig. 7.8 Right bundle branch block. RSR in the right ventricular leads V1–2 and slurred S waves in the left ventricular leads I, AVL and V4–6.

inferior if in AVF, III (the inferior leads—Fig. 7.9), anterior if in the chest leads (Fig. 7.10).

ST segment
The ST segment is depressed in myocardial ischaemia (Fig. 7.11), digoxin therapy and left ventricular hypertrophy.

It is raised in myocardial infarction (convex or domed; Figs 7.9 and 7.10) and pericarditis (concave; Fig. 7.12).

T wave
The T wave is peaked in hyperkalaemia (see below) and sometimes acutely in myocardial infarction.

It is inverted in ventricular strain or hypertrophy, myocardial ischaemia and infarction (as with myocardial infarction, the leads indicate the site), bundle branch block, digoxin therapy and cardiomyopathies (abnormalities of cardiac muscle which may be ischaemic, drug or alcohol, familial or idiopathic in origin).

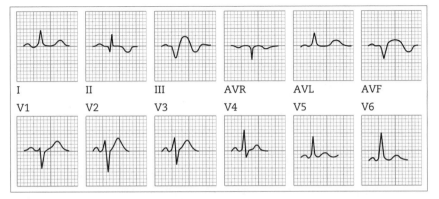

Fig. 7.9 Inferior myocardial infarction.

Fig. 7.10 Anterior myocardial infarction.

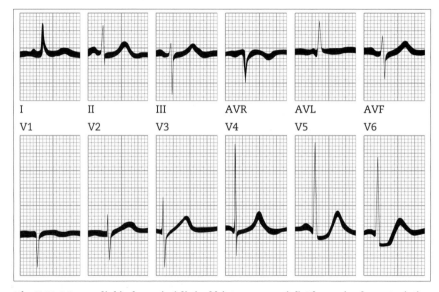

Fig. 7.11 Myocardial ischaemia (clinical history essential). The main characteristic is a depressed ST segment in leads standard II and V. Also not inverted U waves in II, II AVF and V4–6.

U wave
Follows the T wave and can be present normally. It is increased in hypokalaemia (see below).

COMMON ABNORMALITIES
Rhythm
Causes of bradycardia
- Sinus (originating from sinoatrial node; normal P waves) — physiological (e.g. athletes), β-blockers, hypothyroidism, hypothermia.
- Complete heart block.

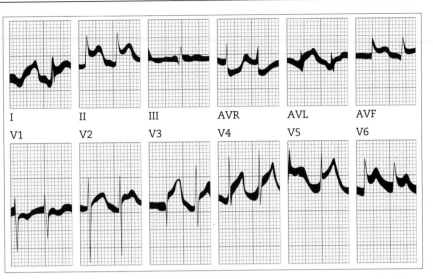

Fig. 7.12 Acute pericarditis. Raised concave-upwards ST segments in most leads, maximal in leads II and V5–6.

Causes of tachycardia

Possibilities

Narrow-complex tachycardia. Normal duration of QRS complex, i.e. depolarization starts in or above the AV node.

- *Surapventricular tachycardia.*
- *Atrial tachycardia.* If the rate of supraventricular depolarization is about 150/min (one beat for every two large squares) the ventricles usually follow beat-for-beat. The P waves can sometimes be found in the preceding T wave.

If the atrial depolarization arises in or close to the AV node (*nodal* or *junctional tachycardia*) the P wave may be buried in the QRS complex.

If the rate of supraventricular depolarization is over 200/min, AV block occurs and only some (2:1 or 3:1) episodes of atrial depolarization are followed by ventricular depolarization—the ventricles cannot keep up with the atria (Fig. 7.13).

At an atrial rate of 300/min (one to every small square) there is a saw-tooth baseline and the rhythm is called *atrial flutter* (Fig. 7.14). (The ventricular rate is then 150/min in 2:1 block and 100/min in 3:1 block).

Fig. 7.13 Supraventricular tachycardia with varying atrioventricular block.

Fig. 7.14 Atrial flutter with saw-tooth atrial waves.

- *Atrial fibrillation* (Fig. 7.15). Uncoordinated contraction of separate atrial muscle fibres. Unless controlled by digoxin it is usually fast (>120/min), totally irregular without P waves, and has an irregular baseline.

Broad-complex tachycardia. Wide and abnormal QRS complex, i.e. depolarization, starts above the AV node with abnormal conduction below it (*supraventricular tachycardia with aberrant ventricular conduction*) or depolarization starts below the AV node (*ventricular tachycardia*).
- *Ventricular tachycardia* (Fig. 7.16). P waves are absent or dissociated from QRS complexes; the QRS complexes vary in shape and are often very broad. It can be difficult to distinguish from supraventricular tachycardia with aberrant conduction. The diagnosis is favoured by the presence of a known cardiac abnormality (ischaemic heart disease or cardiomyopathy). Supraventricular tachycardia is

Fig. 7.15 Atrial fibrillation.

Fig. 7.16 Ventricular tachycardia with slightly irregular ventricular QRS complexes and variable T waves due to dissociated superimposed P waves.

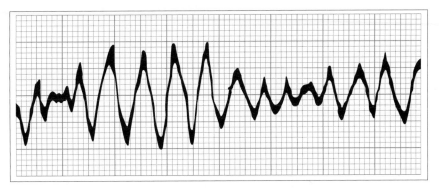

Fig. 7.17 Ventricular fibrillation. This is often seen in cardiac arrest and may be irreversible. It may sometimes alternate with ventricular tachycardia (and sinus rhythm).

Fig. 7.18 Atrial extrasystole.

usually terminated by a rapid intravenous injection of adenosine 3 mg, whereas ventricular tachycardia is not.

• *Ventricular fibrillation.* Very rapid irregular ventricular activation causes a saw-tooth appearance (Fig. 7.17). It is associated with no mechanical output resulting in cardiac arrest (p. 77).

Occasional *extrasystoles* (ectopic or extra beats which do not fit in the otherwise regular rhythm) occur normally. The QRS complex may be normal (atrial or supraventricular) (Fig. 7.18) or wide (ventricular or supraventricular with aberrant conduction; Fig. 7.19).

ECG patterns in common clinical conditions

Myocardial infarction

A characteristic pattern of ECG changes evolves:

• First few minutes—peaked T waves.
• First few hours—ST segment elevation, inversion of T waves.
• After the first few hours Q waves develop.
• After a few days the ST segment returns to normal (persistent elevation raises the possibility of left ventricular aneurysm).
• The T waves may eventually become upright but Q waves persist indefinitely.
• Rhythm abnormalities are common.

• Bundle branch block may occur at any stage, making further interpretation of the site, timing or extent of an infarct impossible.

Pulmonary embolism (Fig. 7.20)
• Tachycardia and transient arrhythmias (particularly atrial fibrillation).
• Right axis deviation.
• Right ventricular strain pattern — dominant R wave and inverted T waves in V1–4.

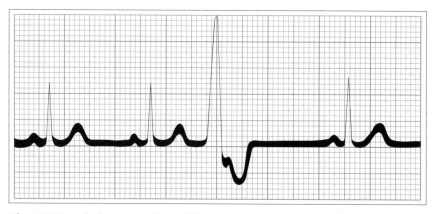

Fig. 7.19 Ventricular ectopic beat. A bizarre ventricular QRS complex. These are more ominous if multifocal, i.e. QRS of varying shape.

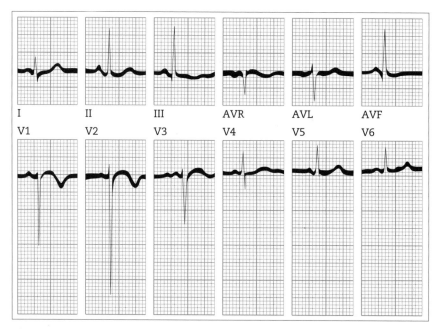

Fig. 7.20 Acute pulmonary embolism with S1, Q3, T3 pattern, a mean frontal QRS axis towards the right (+90°) and right ventricular (RV) strain pattern in leads V1–3.

- Right bundle branch block.
- Occasionally S1, Q3, T3 pattern (S wave in lead I, Q and inverted T in III).

Ventricular hypertrophy

Large R waves occur over the appropriate ventricle in the chest leads (V1–2 for right and V 5–6 for left). There tend to be large negative S waves in reciprocal leads (e.g. large S in V1 in left ventricular hypertrophy). If the sum of the S in V1 plus the R in V5 is greater than 35 mm, left ventricular hypertrophy is present on voltage criteria.

Digoxin

Sagging (reverse tick) ST segments, T wave inversion.

Metabolic abnormalities

Hyperkalaemia (Fig. 7.21). Flattened P wave, broad QRS complex, peaked T wave.

Hypokalaemia (Fig. 7.21). Prolonged PR, depressed ST, flattened T wave and prominent U wave.

Hypocalcaemia (Fig. 7.22). Prolonged QT interval.

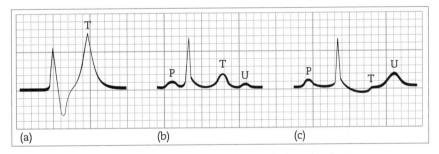

Fig. 7.21 (a) Hyperkalaemia; (b) normal and (c) hypokalaemia. The T-wave amplitude varies directly with the serum potassium and the U wave inversely (it is often normally present in V3–4). In hyperkalaemia the P waves become smaller and the QRS complex widens into the ST segment. In hypokalaemia the PR interval lengthens and the ST segment becomes depressed.

Fig. 7.22 Hypocalcaemia. Normal complexes apart from a prolonged QT_c (QT interval corrected for heart rate). Rate 95/min, QT 0.40, QT_c 0.50.

Fascicular block

There are three fascicles to the bundle of His: right, left anterior and left posterior. Block of one (unifascicular block) produces the following patterns:

1   Right: right bundle branch block (RBBB).
2   Left anterior: left anterior hemiblock: left axis deviation.
3   Left posterior: left posterior hemiblock: right axis deviation.

Hemiblock refers to a block in either the anterior or the posterior division of the left bundle. The QRS duration is usually at the upper limit of normal. Unlike LBBB, septal depolarization remains present (small q in the anterior leads; and r in the inferior leads—II, III, AVF).

Bifascicular block refers to the combination of RBBB and one of the unifascicular blocks. The QRS is lengthened, but the evidence of septal depolarization should still be present.

1 + 2 = RBBB + left anterior hemiblock, i.e. RBBB pattern + left axis deviation (Fig. 7.23)

1 + 3 = RBBB + left posterior hemiblock, i.e. RBBB pattern + right axis deviation.

Sinoatrial disease (sick sinus syndrome)

This is a chronic disorder often associated with ischaemic heart disease in which sinus bradycardia and/or episodic sinus arrest may alternate with episodes of rapid supraventricular arrhythmia. Symptoms include dizziness, syncope, palpitations and dyspnoea. Permanent pacing may be necessary. Diagnosis is most easily made using 24-h ambulatory ECG monitoring.

Exercise testing

The most widely used method is the treadmill test using the Bruce protocol. The speed and incline gradually increase at 3-min intervals to a maximal at stage seven

Fig. 7.23 Bifascicular block. Right bundle branch block with left axis deviation.

when the patient is walking at 9.7 km/h at a gradient of 22%. The ECG, heart rate, blood pressure, symptoms and maximal workload are recorded during the test. The ECG signal is often averaged by computer to reduce noise due to movement. ST segment depression of greater than I mm (0.1 mV) is usually regarded as a positive test, but many other parameters can signify cardiac disease. These include inability to achieve maximum heart rate or workload, inappropriate response in blood pressure (normal response is a small rise) and symptoms of angina.

Chest X-ray

The standard view is a PA (X-rays passing posterior to anterior with the patient's chest against the film), in inspiration. The X-rays are diverging from the source and magnify structures furthest from the film (e.g. vertebrae). An anteroposterior (AP) view (taken if the patient is too ill to stand) magnifies the heart. Lateral views are used largely for localization of lesions visible on the PA film.

The maximum diameter of the heart on a PA film is normally less than half the maximum diameter of the thoracic cage (cardiothoracic ratio less than 0.5). Enlargement of the heart occurs with cardiac dilatation (heart failure, valvular disease, prolonged hypertension) or the presence of a pericardial effusion.

Left atrial enlargement (mitral stenosis) causes:
- prominence of the left atrial appendage (upper left heart border)
- double contour adjacent to the right heart border
- elevation of the left main bronchus.

Enlargement of other chambers is difficult to distinguish radiologically.

Main vessels. Look for aortic dilatation (hypertension, aortic valve disease, aneurysm) which causes a prominent aortic shadow to the right of the mediastinum. Enlargement of the pulmonary artery (right-to-left shunts, pulmonary hypertension) produces a prominent bulge on the left border of the mediastinum. Look for valvular calcification (rheumatic valve disease). Pericardial calcification usually indicates old tuberculosis.

Check the density and texture of the lung markings, including the apices (the only markings visible in normal lungs are blood vessels). Pulmonary venous hypertension causes prominence and dilatation of the upper-lobe pulmonary vessels. Pulmonary oedema causes mottling of the lung fields, areas of consolidation and fluid collections which become visible as pleural effusions or fluid in interlobar fissures or interlobular septa (Kerley B lines).

Echocardiography

Two-dimensional images are obtained by scanning the ultrasound beam rapidly across the heart to record a cross-section in which the anatomy and motion of the heart can be recorded. The motion of individual cardiac structures (such as valves) can be recorded in detail by M-mode cardiography in which the changes in echo signals in one particular direction of the beam are recorded over time.

Relatively stationary structures generate straight lines, whereas moving structures such as valves generate undulating lines (Fig. 7.24).

Continuous-wave Doppler is used to quantify blood velocity and quantify pressure gradients across valves.

The combination of two-dimensional, M-mode and Doppler echocardiography provides a non-invasive means of investigating ventricular function, myocardial disease, valvular lesions, congenital malformations and pericardial effusion.

Transoesophageal echocardiography uses a probe introduced into the oesophagus involving a procedure similar to upper gastrointestinal endoscopy. It is useful for visualizing cardiac structures, including left atrial appendage, prosthetic valves, intracardiac tumours and vegetations of infective endocarditis, and intrathoracic structures, including the thoracic aorta and paracardiac tumours.

Ventricular function is usually assessed from changes in cavity size or wall motion. The ejection fraction is derived from stroke volume (end-diastolic minus end-systolic volume) divided by end-diastolic volume. Normal ejection fraction is >60%.

The shortening fraction is a measure of the percentage reduction in left ven-

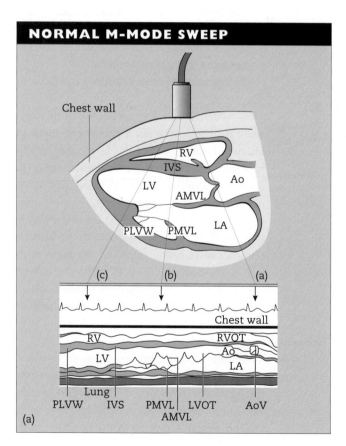

Fig. 7.24 (a) Normal M-mode sweep. IVS, Interventricular septum; RV, right ventricle; LV, left ventricle; AMVL, anterior mitral valve leaflet; Ao, aorta; PLVW, posterior left ventricle wall; PMVL, posterior mitral valve leaflet; LA, left atrium; RVOT, right ventricular outflow tract; LVOT, left ventricular outflow tract; AoV, aortic valve.

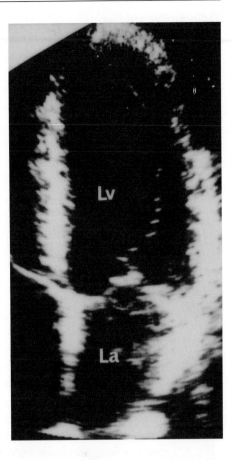

Fig. 7.24 (Continued) (b) Two-dimensional echocardiography through left vertricle (Lv) and left atrium (La).

NORMAL CARDIAC PRESSURES		
	Systolic/diastolic (mmHg)	Mean (mmHg)
RAP	7/3	<5
RVP	15–25/3–7	
PAP	25/10	<18
PCWP		6–12
LVP	120/7–12	
RAP, Right atrial pressure; RVP, right ventricular pressure; PAP, pulmonary arterial pressure; PCWP, pulmonary capillary wedge pressure; LVP, left ventricular pressure.		

Table 7.5 Normal cardiac pressures.

tricular cavity size during systole. It is used to follow changes in ventricular function in patients with valvular heart disease or cardiomyopathy.

Disturbances of wall motion (usually due to coronary artery disease) are assessed subjectively in different regions of the ventricle.

Radionuclide studies

Technetium (^{99}Tc)-labelled red cells are used to assess left ventricular function by gated radionuclide ventriculography (multiple uptake gated acquisition—MUGA). The ECG is used to gate the scan into different periods of the cardiac cycle.

Myocardial disease tends to cause dilatation of the heart, and the ejection fraction may fall on exercise—a poor prognostic sign.

Regional abnormalities of the ventricular muscle are recorded as areas of akinesia and hypokinesia. This is usually evidence of myocardial ischaemia or infarction.

Regional paradoxical movement suggests an aneurysm.

Thallium (^{201}Tl) behaves like potassium and is distributed through heart muscle in proportion to coronary blood flow. There is decreased uptake in areas of ischaemia, infarction or fibrosis. On exercise there may be areas of decreased perfusion which reverse after rest, indicating areas of reversible ischaemia.

Swan–Gantz catheterization

Right atrial pressure measured using a CVP line gives a poor indication of circulating intravascular volume in the presence of cardiac disease. A pulmonary artery flotation catheter (e.g. Swan–Gantz catheter) can be used to assess left atrial pressure.

A light flexible catheter with a balloon on the end is introduced through a central vein into the right side of the heart. The balloon is inflated with air, and 'floats' into the pulmonary artery and eventually wedges in a small pulmonary artery, where it registers a pressure similar to left atrial pressure (pulmonary capillary wedge pressure, PCWP).

Haematology

The commoner problems in clinical examinations, as in clinical practice, are to assess the significance of the data provided on a standard blood count (e.g. Coulter count), examine a patient with anaemia, purpura or ecchymosis, or to comment on the coagulation screen of a patient with a bleeding disorder.

Anaemia

It is essential to distinguish between pallor and anaemia. Pallor may be due to a deep-lying venous system and opaque skin. In the UK the commonest cause of anaemia is iron deficiency, due to chronic blood loss, especially in women during the child-bearing period. The second commonest cause is probably magaloblastic anaemia and most of these are due to intrinsic factor deficiency causing B_{12} deficiency. The malabsorption syndrome, including the post-gastrectomy syndrome, can give rise to deficiency in iron, vitamin B_{12} or folic acid. Myxoedema and chronic uraemia may present with a chronic anaemia. Anaemia may be a feature of many chronic conditions in which other clinical features are usually more obvious. These include the leukaemias, reticuloses and rheumatoid arthritis. In tropical countries chronic infections, especially chronic malaria and hookworm infestation, are common and the haemoglobinopathies should be considered.

'This patient is anaemic. What questions would you like to ask and what would you examine for?'

Ask patient

- Blood loss: menstrual loss, pregnancy, haemorrhoids, indigestion and melaena, salicylate or non-steroidal anti-inflammatory drug ingestion.
- History of drugs: aplastic anaemia, and megaloblastic anaemia from folate deficiency (anticonvulsants). Gastric irritants causing bleeding.
- History of gastric surgery, ulcerative colitis or malabsorption.

- Paraesthesiae and sore tongue of pernicious anaemia.
- Diet: the elderly pensioner may suffer from iron and/or ascorbic acid deficiency.
- Vegans may develop B_{12} deficiency and alcoholics folate deficiency.

Observe and assess degree of anaemia

- Face and conjunctiva: note the white hair and pale lemon-yellow skin of pernicious anaemia.
- Tongue: for glossitis of vitamin B_{12} or folate deficiency and angular stomatitis of iron deficiency.
- Nails and nail beds: brittle nails and koilonychia of iron deficiency and the splinter haemorrhages (sometimes with clubbing) of infective endocarditis.
- Note purpura (aplastic anaemia, leukaemia), mouth ulceration in neutropenia and the leg ulceration of the haemoglobinopathies.
- Note rheumatoid arthritis and consider uraemia and myxoedema.
- Note racial origin; thalassaemia and sickle-cell anaemia.

Examine also

- Neck for lymph nodes, which may be enlarged in chronic lymphatic leukaemia and reticuloendothelial diseases or be secondaries from carcinoma.
- Abdomen for splenomegaly, hepatomegaly and neoplasms (especially of the stomach, colon and uterus).

NB In the clinic, rectal examination is essential, and sigmoidoscopy should be performed for haemorrhoids, carcinoma and colitis in patients with a history of rectal bleeding.

There may be congestive cardiac failure from severe anaemia.

If you suspect pernicious anaemia, examine for peripheral neuropathy and subacute combined degeneration of the cord.

Retinal haemorrhage may occur in leukaemia and severe B_{12} deficiency.

Blood count (Table 8.1)

'Comment on this haemoglobin'
Check the haemoglobin for anaemia or polycythaemia.
NB A normal white cell and platelet count virtually excludes leukaemia and marrow aplasia.

Hypochromic anaemia

Check the indices for hypochromia (mean corpuscular haemoglobin (MCH)) and microcytosis (mean cell volume (MCV)). If present, they suggest iron deficiency.

Perform serum iron, transferrin, ferritin, faecal occult blood and proceed, if indicated, to sigmoidoscopy, barium enema, barium meal and follow through. A gynaecological examination may be indicated from the clinical history at the outset. Check other possible causes which normally produce normochromic but sometimes hypochromic anaemia (see below).

NORMAL VALUES

Hb (men)	13–17 g/dl
Hb (women)	11-16 g/dl
RBC (men)	4.5–6.4 m/mm³
RBC (women)	3.9–5.6 m/mm³
Haematocrit (PCV; men)	0.38–0.50
Haematocrit (PCV; women)	0.33–0.45
MCV	80–96 fl (PCV/RBC)
MCH	27–32 µg (Hb/RBC)
MCHC	32–36 g/dl (Hb/PCV)
Reticulocytes	$10–100 \times 10^9/l$
WBC	$4–11 (\times 10^9/l)$
Platelets	$150–400 \times 10^9/l$
Prothrombin time (INR)	Not more than 2 s longer than control
control time	11–13 s
Partial thromboplastin time	Not more than 7 s longer than control
control time	30–45 s
Bleeding time	Up to 11 min
Hess (tourniquet) test	Not more than 5 spots in a square inch
(80 mmHg for 5 min)	
Clotting time	Up to 10 min
Fibrinogen	2–4 g/l

Hb, Haemoglobin; RBC, red blood cell; PCV, packed cell volume; MCV, mean cell volume; MCH, mean corpuscular haemoglobin; MCHC, MCH concentration; WBC, white blood cells; INR, international normalized ratio.

Table 8.1 Normal haematological values.

Exclude thalassaemia and sickle-cell anaemia if indicated (haemoglobin electrophoresis and sickling tests).

Macrocytic anaemia

Check the indices for macrocytosis (MCV). In pernicious anaemia there is usually an associated low white blood cell (WBC) and low platelet count. Perform a serum B_{12} and red cell folate (or serum folate). A bone marrow examination shows megaloblastic change in vitamin B_{12} and folate deficiencies. Parietal cell and intrinsic factor antibodies may be present. An abnormal Schilling test (<6% in 24 h) is corrected by intrinsic factor in pernicious anaemia. Other causes of vitamin B_{12} and folate deficiencies, e.g. alcoholism, malabsorption, blind loops and ileal disease (Crohn's), are all rare. In ileal disease, the Schilling test is not corrected by intrinsic factor.

Investigate causes other than vitamin B_{12} and folate deficiencies with liver function tests and γ-glutaryl transferase for alcohol, thyroid function test for hypothyroidism and reticulocyte count (and bilirubin) for haemolysis. Check that the patient is neither pregnant nor using anticonvulsants. Aplastic and haemolytic anaemias are sometimes macrocytic but not megaloblastic.

Normocytic anaemia

If the indices are normal, consider anaemias secondary to chronic disease (such as rheumatoid arthritis, carcinoma, renal failure and chronic infection) and hypothyroidism (which may also give a macrocytic picture).

If the reticulocyte count is raised, this denotes marrow hyperactivity and usually (i) haemolytic anaemia, (ii) response to vitamin B_{12}, folate or occasionally iron therapy, or (iii) continued bleeding.

If the WBC and/or platelet counts are low and there is anaemia, this suggests marrow aplasia, usually secondary to drugs (and, rarely, toxic chemicals) or marrow infiltration (leukaemia, myelofibrosis, multiple myeloma, carcinoma).

Primitive white cells (blast) in the peripheral film indicate an acute leukaemia or occasionally a leukaemoid response to acute infection. The total WBC count is usually raised. The film usually shows whether the leukaemia is myeloid or lymphatic.

Eosinophilia suggests drug sensitivity, intestinal worms, allergy (e.g. asthma), including allergic aspergillosis and, rarely, polyarteritis nodosa, pulmonary eosinophilia syndrome and reticulosis such as Hodgkin's disease.

Polycythaemia rubra vera

The red blood cell (RBC), WBC and platelet counts are usually raised. There is an increase in red cell mass and haematocrit. Most have an increased neutrophil and platelet count with raised leukocyte alkaline phosphatase. Repeated venesection normalizes the haematocrit. Hydroxyurea is sometimes used. Both thrombosis and haemorrhage can occur. In secondary polycythaemia (secondary to hypoxia) only the RBC count is raised. Polycythaemia is also associated with renal carcinoma and cerebellar haemangioblastoma where there are raised erythropoietin levels.

NOTES

Hypochromic anaemia, unresponsive to oral iron therapy, occurs in:
- incorrect diagnosis or mixed deficiency;
- patients who do not take their tablets;
- continued bleeding (reticulocytosis persists);
- rheumatoid arthritis, systemic lupus erythematosus (SLE), infections (and other chronic illness);
- malabsorption;
- thalassaemia; and
- myelodysplastic syndrome—refractory anaemia (if ringed sideroblasts present = sideroblastic anaemia).

Megaloblasts are found in the marrow and only rarely in the peripheral blood. They are characterized by a large and inactive nucleus (maturation arrest) in a relatively hypermature, and even haemoglobinized, cytoplasm. They are not present in normal marrow and their presence denotes vitamin B_{12} or folate deficiency, which may be secondary to antifolate or phenytoin therapy.

Patients with pernicious anaemia (p. 420) which has been treated with vitamin B_{12} usually have normal peripheral blood, normal marrow (within 24 h) and normal serum folates and B_{12}. They may still be investigated with the Schilling tests and parietal cell and intrinsic factor antibodies are still present.

Vitamin B_{12} and folate deficiencies produce (if sufficiently severe) depression of all the marrow elements, including neutrophils and platelets. The polymorph nuclei appear hypersegmented. There is usually some haemolysis with a raised unconjugated serum bilirubin.

In folic acid deficiency consider pregnancy, dietary intake, malabsorption, drugs (phenytoin), alcoholism and haemolytic anaemia.

In haemolytic anaemia (p. 421) the serum bilirubin (unconjugated) is raised. There is no bile pigment in the urine (acholuric) but urobilinogen is present in the urine in excess. Reticulocytosis is present and its degree is an indirect measure of the rate of haemolysis. Haptoglobins in the blood are increased. The rate of disappearance of chromium-tagged red cells gives a more accurate measure of the rate of haemolysis. Splenomegaly and pigment stones may occur.

Haemolytic anaemias are rare in the UK. They are usually classified as:
1 Intracorpuscular defects (Coombs-negative). (Abnormal RBCs.) Thalassaemia, sickle-cell anaemia, hereditary spherocytosis, glucose-6-phosphatase deficiency, haemoglobinopathies.
2 Extracorpuscular defects. (Normal RBCs.)
    (a) Autoimmune haemolytic anaemias (Coombs-positive) are either primary, or secondary to drugs (methyldopa), leukaemia or reticuloses.
    (b) Rhesus-incompatibility (and mismatched transfusion) is an immune but not autoimmune disorder since the antibody is extrinsic (fetal).
    (c) Non-immune, e.g. burns, malaria, drugs.
    (d) Secondary to renal or liver disease.
    (e) Hypersplenism.
    (f) Red-cell fragmentation.

Primary aplastic anaemia. A pancytopenia with reduction in all the formed elements is rare.

Secondary bone marrow failure. Toxic factors acting on the marrow may affect one or all of the formed elements of the blood, red cells, white cells or platelets. Important recognized causes include drugs (gold, penicillamine, chloramphenicol, carbimazole), radiation and leukaemias.

NB   *Very high erythrocyte sedimentation rate* (ESR; i.e. over 100 mm/h suggests (i) multiple myeloma; (ii) SLE; (iii) temporal arteritis; (iv) polymyalgia rheumatica; or (v), rarely, carcinoma or chronic infection, including tuberculosis.

Skin haemorrhage

Purpura refers to small (pinhead) cutaneous bleeding. *Ecchymosis* refers to larger lesions (bruises). Bruising is very common; purpura is rare.

A useful working classification of the causes of skin (and other) haemorrhage is shown in Table 8.2. The commonest causes of skin haemorrhage are senile purpura, therapy with steroids or anticoagulants and, less commonly, thrombocytopenia due to leukaemia and marrow aplasia.

'Examine this patient's skin' (showing purpura or ecchymosis)

Quickly note

- Patient's age (senile purpura).
- If the patient is anaemic (marrow infiltration, aplasia and leukaemia).
- If the patient has rheumatoid arthritis (purpura usually due to drugs, steroids, gold).
- Ecchymoses of the lower limbs in the elderly may be due to scurvy. This is seen in persons living alone and on 'ulcer' diet. Potatoes are the usual source of vitamin C in those who cannot afford citrus fruits.
- Henoch–Schönlein or anaphylactoid purpura (rare) (p. 281). (This 'purpura' is actually a vasculitis and often most obvious around the buttocks and shins. It

CAUSES OF HAEMORRHAGE

Coagulation defects
Haemophilia
Christmas disease
Treatment with anticoagulants
Fibrinogen deficiency (defibrination: DIC)

Vascular purpuras (increased capillary fragility)
von Willebrand's disease
Hereditary haemorrhagic telangiectasia
Henoch–Schönlein purpura

Thrombocytopenic purpuras
Hypersplenism
Idiopathic thrombocytopenic purpura
Marrow suppression or replacement
DIC and microangiopathic haemolytic anaemia

Table 8.2 Causes of haemorrhage. DIC, disseminated intravascular coagulation.

usually follows an upper respiratory tract infection. It is commonest between the ages of 3 and 15 years and is rare in adults (in whom the prognosis is worse). The palpable rash is polymorphic and may be extensive, simulating a skin disease. It is associated with acute nephritic syndrome, arthralgia and abdominal pain.)

If invited to question the patient, ask about drugs (anticoagulant therapy, carbimazole, chloramphenicol, anticoagulants, steroids) and about a family history of bleeding (haemophilia and Christmas disease).

Examination

• Mouth and pharynx for the ulceration of neutropenia (marrow depression from leukaemia or drugs). For anaemia and lymphadenopathy (marrow aplasia and leukaemia).
• For splenomegaly (leukaemia and idiopathic thrombocytopenic purpura).
NB Platelet deficiency tends to result in multiple small bleeds (purpura, microscopic haematuria) and clotting-factor deficiency in isolated larger bleed (haemarthrosis, haematemesis, stroke, haematomata in muscles).

Coagulation defects

'Comment on this coagulation screen'
If the patient is present, no comment should be made before a good history has been taken and a thorough examination has been performed. You will wish to determine the type (skin, deep tissue, mucosa, joints), degree, precipitation and course of the haemorrhage. Ask about previous dental extractions, surgery, childbirth and trauma. A family and drug history is very important. Physical examination may suggest the underlying cause. Vascular abnormalities and platelet disorders tend to result in minor skin bleeding (purpura and petechia), especially in the lower limbs. Platelet disorders are associated with epistaxis, menorrhagia and gastrointestinal bleeding. Coagulation defects tend to result in prolonged post-traumatic bleeding (including that due to surgery) and bleeding into joints and muscle. A patient who has a convincing history of considerable haemorrhage and who is at special risk in surgery or biopsy procedures may nevertheless have a normal coagulation screen (Table 8.1). These simple tests cannot always exclude a bleeding abnormality and factors (Fig. 8.1) may have to be reduced to 10% of their normal level before they can be detected by them. Thus a patient with a bleeding history but a normal coagulation screen will require more detailed investigation, including assay of the individual factors.

Apart from those due to anticoagulant administration, 95% of serious coagulation defects are due to von Willebrand's disease and the haemophilias.

NOTES
The important factors to remember by number are shown in Table 8.3.

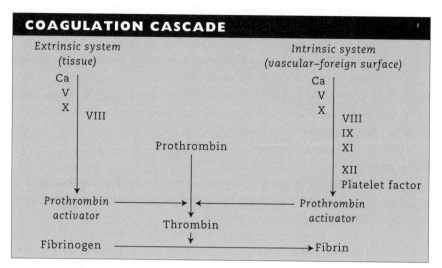

Fig. 8.1 Coagulation cascade.

COAGULATION FACTORS

Factor	Deficiency states
V	Very rare
VII	Warfarin therapy and liver disease
VIII (antihaemophilic globulin)	Haemophilia A and von Willebrand's disease
IX (Christmas factor)	Haemophilia B, warfarin therapy and liver disease

Table 8.3 Important coagulation factors.

Prothrombin time

Measures the *extrinsic system*. It is the time taken for the patient's citrated plasma to clot when a tissue factor (brain extract) and calcium are added. In a coagulation screen it is important because it measures deficiencies of V, VII, X, prothrombin and fibrinogen. It is normal in the haemophilias. It is relatively insensitive to reduction in prothrombin.

Partial thromboplastin time

Measures the *intrinsic system*. It is the time taken for the patient's citrated plasma to clot when kaolin (activates XI and XII), platelet substitute and calcium are added. In a coagulation screen it is important because it measures deficiencies of factors V, VIII to XII prothrombin and fibrinogen. It is prolonged in haemophilia.

A normal control is necessary because of the variable potency of the tissue factor.

Thromboplastin generation test

In difficult cases the thromboplastin generation test is used. In this test three components of the clotting mechanism 1–3 are mixed together. Of these three, either 1 or 2 is obtained from the patient. The other two components are either from a normal individual or are laboratory reagents.

1 *Absorbed plasma:* V and VIII are normally present (VII and IX were removed by absorption).

2 *Serum:* VII and IX (and X) are normally present (V and VIII were removed because used up in the clot).

3 *Platelets* (or platelet substitute) and *calcium*.

In classical haemophilia (factor VIII deficiency or haemophilia A) for instance, the mix containing the patient's absorbed plasma (1) with normal serum (2) would have an abnormal prolonged test.

Vitamin K and anticoagulants

Low levels of vitamin K and administration of coumarins (e.g. warfarin) or indanediones (e.g. phenindione) affect the synthesis of prothrombin and factor X plus:

- VII in the extrinsic system; and
- IX in the intrinsic system.

Similar deficiencies occur in cirrhosis due to hepatocellular failure (often unresponsive to vitamin K). In addition to cirrhosis with portal hypertension, bleeding may be exacerbated by the thrombocytopenia of hypersplenism.

Defibrination syndrome

Synonyms: consumption coagulopathy, disseminated intravascular coagulation (DIC). This occurs in obstetric practice, thoracic surgery and pulmonary embolism, and in shock, especially when associated with infection or bleeding, and following mismatched blood transfusion.

The syndrome may present more chronically as a disorder with intravascular coagulation rather than excessive bleeding. The thrombophlebitis migrans of malignancy may be an example.

Platelets and factor V and VIII are consumed in the pathological coagulation as well as fibrinogen. Fibrinolysis takes place simultaneously with coagulation and produces fibrin degeneration products which can be measured in the serum and urine.

Treatment is primarily that of the underlying disease, usually septicaemia. Replace the platelets and the deficient factors by fresh (12 h) whole blood or fresh frozen plasma and fibrinogen concentrates. Heparin may be given in normal (or lower) doses, progress being monitored by changes in the fibrinogen level.

Haemophilia

Haemophilia A is due to factor VIII deficiency and haemophilia B (Christmas disease) to factor IX deficiency. They are sex-linked recessive disorders of men, carried by women. All carriers who wish to have children should receive genetic counselling. The diseases can be detected *in utero*.

Therapy. As soon as possible after bleeding has started, purified factor VIII or IX is given as required. Cryoprecipitate, which contains VIII but not IX, is now seldom used. Purified factor VIII is also used to raise factor VIII levels in von Willebrand's disease. Fresh frozen plasma contains both factors but is best reserved for when the single factors are not available. Aspirin-containing preparations should be avoided because they impair platelet function and may cause gastric erosion. Desmopressin can be used to increase factor VIII levels in mild to moderate haemophilia.

von Willebrand's disease

This is an autosomal dominant disease of both sexes with variable clinical severity showing various types of abnormal bleeding, particularly from mucous membranes. There is a prolonged bleeding time, low factor VIII clotting activity and poor platelet adhesion. (von Willebrand factor is a cofactor for this adhesion.)

Thrombocytopenia

May result from decreased production (marrow aplasia, leukaemia or infiltration) or increased destruction (idiopathic thrombocytopenic purpura, hypersplenism and consumption coagulopathy).

Idiopathic thrombocytopenic purpura (ITP) is rare and not to be confused with thrombotic thrombocytopenic purpura, which is very rare indeed. ITP chiefly occurs in children following a respiratory or gastrointestinal viral infection. Patients present with purpura and a low platelet count. If the platelet count is very low, major bleeding may occur from the nose, gut, or into the brain. The bleeding time is prolonged but coagulation times are normal. Spontaneous recovery is the rule. Platelet counts down to 80 000 mm^3 do not need treatment. Steroids or intravenous immunoglobulin may be of benefit in the more severe cases, occasionally with lasting remission. Danazol 400–800 mg daily with a maintenance dose of 50 mg daily may be effective. Splenectomy should be avoided if possible especially in children, in view of the risk of pneumococcal septicaemia in asplenic patients, but may be curative when medical management is unsuccessful.

Thrombotic thrombocytopenic purpura is a very rare disease of young adults who present with fever, abdominal pain, purpura and focal neurological signs. Initial haematuria may progress to renal failure. The mechanism is unknown but it may be a disorder of vascular endothelium which is unable to produce a prostacycline platelet inhibitor (hence the widespread intravascular thrombosis). The mortality is high. Treatment consists of plasma exchange and renal dialysis, if indicated, with or without heparin and steroids.

Henoch–Schönlein purpura

See p. 281.

Osler's disease (Osler–Weber–Rendu)

- Hereditary haemorrhagic telangiectasia: autosomal dominant.
- May present as intermittent bleeding, usually gastrointestinal.
- There are small capillary angiectases throughout the gastrointestinal tract, including the buccal mucosa and tongue.

Lymphadenopathy

Localized

Usually results from:

- local infection (any age);
- carcinoma (usually over 45 years old);
- Hodgkin's disease (usually patients under 35 years; p. 427) and
- non-Hodgkin's lymphoma.

NB   Tuberculosis must be considered in all cervical lymphadenopathy. This is also a common site for stage I Hodgkin's disease, and also for neoplastic secondary deposits from the lung, testis, breast and nasopharyngeal carcinomas (ear, nose and throat examination must be performed before biopsy).

Examine this patient's neck for signs of goitre, and check lymph glands. Consider origin of swelling (including testicles).

Generalized

Usually results from:

- infectious mononucleosis and rubella;
- reticuloendothelial disorders;
- chronic lymphatic leukaemia; and
- other less common causes include toxoplasmosis, tuberculosis, sarcoidosis and brucellosis.

NB   If glandular enlargement persists, blood count is essential, particularly to confirm or exclude leukaemia, and a chest X-ray may show hilar lymphadenopathy. A biopsy usually supplies the diagnosis.

Diabetes

'This patient has diabetes mellitus: would you ask him/her some questions?' (also p. 221)

A similar approach is advised in the clinic. You should ask the patient's age and occupation and note if he/she is under- or overweight. Ask when the diabetes was first diagnosed. Ask about the common presenting symptoms of thirst, polyuria, fatigue and pruritus vulvae. In the young there is often loss of weight, even when the appetite is well-preserved. This combination also occurs in thyrotoxicosis (common), some malabsorption states, some tumours early in their course (e.g. carcinoma of the bronchus), some hypercatabolic states (e.g. leukaemia), and, to all appearances, in anorexia nervosa. You should take:
- family history for diabetes;
- obstetric history (big babies, stillbirths); and
- drug history (corticosteroids and adrencorticotrophic hormone, thiazide, diuretics).

NB   Always remember the four endocrine conditions which can present to a diabetic clinic: acromegaly, Cushing's syndrome, haemochromatosis and phaeochromocytoma.

Go quickly over the systems which can be involved in diabetes, asking questions about relevant symptoms.

Cardiovascular

Angina and myocardial infarct; intermittent claudication, cold feet, gangrene.

Nervous (p. 224)

Legs, feet. Numbness, pain or paraesthesiae, painless ulcers.

Eyes (p. 223). Failing vision (transitory with poor control), retinopathy, cataract.

Brain. Ischaemic attacks or strokes; hypoglycaemia.

Autonomic. Impotence, postural hypotension; diarrhoea (especially at night) and gastric distension.

Mononeuritis multiplex (pp. 152 and 224).

Respiratory
Cough, usually due to chronic bronchitis, but tuberculosis is commoner in diabetics than in the general population.

Renal (p. 224)
Polyuria (glycosuria, renal failure); frequency and/or dysuria of infection.

Skin (p. 225)
Sepsis, e.g. boils; xanthelasma (p. 233); necrobiosis lipoidica (rare; p. 225); vaginitis (usually monilial); balanitis; granuloma annulare.

Management

Define the outline of treatment and assess the adequacy of control (p. 225).

DIET
A controlled-caloric, low-fat, low-refined-sugar, high-fibre diet.

DRUGS
Insulin (Table 9.1)

Ask about the type of insulin and the frequency of injection. All insulin-dependent diabetics in the UK use U-100 insulin (100 units/ml), but this may not be so with visitors from other countries.

Human insulin is prepared either by a single amino-acid substitution in a pig insulin molecule (emp: enzymatic modification of porcine) or by genetic engineering (prb: pro insulin recombinant bacterial, or pyr: precursor yeast recombinant).

Most patients are best controlled with twice-daily injections of mixed insulins containing short- and medium-acting preparation (e.g. Actrapid/Monotard, or a premixed preparation, e.g. Mixtard), or tds preprandial short-acting (soluble) plus evening long-acting insulin (e.g. Ultratard).

Oral therapy
Try to determine the name, tablet size and frequency of administration. You should know whether they are sulphonylureas or the biguanide, metformin. Acarbose inhibits intestinal alpha glucosidase, delaying digestion of starch and sucrose.

INSULINS

Name	Onset (h)	Peak (h)	Duration (h)
Neutral soluble Actrapid Velosulin Humulin S	$\frac{1}{2}$–1	2–6	6–8
Isophane Protaphane Insulatard Humulin I	2	4–12	12–24
IZS (zinc suspension) Monotard Humulin Lente	2	2–8	16–24
Ultratard	4–8	12–20	24–28
Biphasic Mixtard (30% sol/70% isophane) Initard (50% sol/50% isophane) Humulin M1 (10% sol/90% isophane), M2 (20% sol/80% isophane, M3 (30% sol/70% isophane), M4 (40% sol/60% isophane), M5 (50% sol/50% isophane)	$\frac{1}{2}$–1 $\frac{1}{2}$–1	2–8 1–8	12–18

Table 9.1 Commonly used insulins.

ASSESSMENT OF DIABETIC CONTROL

Ask for the patient's routine blood or urine-testing charts. Persistent absence of glucose without hypoglycaemic symptoms suggests a high renal threshold and the charts may be useless for diabetic control. Conversely, persistent glycosuria can mean a low threshold and be similarly unhelpful. It is usually best for the patient to perform his or her own home blood glucose monitoring accurately and to keep a record. A glucose–oxidase-impregnated stick is read on a meter or by eye. Ideally the blood sugar should be normal (4–6 mmol/l) at all times and the patient symptomless. Realistically, aim to keep the blood glucose under 10 mmol/l at all times whilst avoiding hypoglycaemic symptoms.

Urine glucose measurements are helpful when blood glucose estimations are not available, usually because the patient refuses to prick a finger. Since the normal threshold is about 10 mmol/l, *any* glycosuria suggests poor control.

Glycosylated haemoglobin (HbA_{1c}) gives an index of average control over approximately the previous 2–3 months and fructosamine over 2–3 weeks.

INSULIN RESISTANCE

This is usually a phenomenon of non-insulin dependent (type 2) diabetes (p. 221).

SYMPTOMS OF POOR CONTROL

Hyperglycaemia

Polyuria (with nocturia) and thirst. Hospital admissions with ketoacidosis. Intermittent blurring of vision. Weight loss.

Hypoglycaemia

'Hypos' or 'reactions'. Determine at what time of day (in relation to food, exercise and insulin) they occur. Early-morning headaches may be the only indication of nocturnal hypoglycaemia. Weight gain.

Examination

'Would you examine this patient?'
You will probably be directed by the history. Otherwise, examination should include:

Obesity

In the clinic perform routine height and weight measurements. Calculate body mass index (p. 259).

Injection sites

Thighs, anterior abdominal wall and arms for fat atrophy or hypertrophy.

Eyes (p. 223)

Dilate pupils unless there is a history of glaucoma or raised intraocular pressure. Cataract and retinopathy (microaneurysms, exudates, retinal vessel proliferation, arteriosclerosis).

Legs and feet

Peripheral neuropathy (chiefly sensory). Test the tendon reflexes and for pin, light touch and vibration sense.

Peripheral vascular disease. Check the arterial pulses and temperature of the feet. Even if the pulses are present, the toes may be blue and cold due to small-vessel disease.

  Remember:
* necrobiosis (very rare);
* quadriceps wasting and tenderness (amyotrophy) improved by good control; and
* infection.

Chest

The history may indicate infection.

Abdomen

Feel for the liver, which may often be palpable in the long-standing insulin-dependent diabetic due to fatty infiltration. (NB Haemochromatosis is very rare.)

Test the urine for sugar, protein and ketones.

Autonomic function tests

Parasympathetic

1   Heart rate response to deep breathing.
2   Heart rate response to standing.
3   Heart rate response to the Valsalva manoeuvre.

Sympathetic

1   Blood pressure response to standing.
2   Blood pressure response to muscle exercise such as sustained hand grip.

Ask if you may see: (i) the result of a recent blood sugar series if control has deteriorated; (ii) a recent chest X-ray; and (iii) the result of a midstream urine specimen (MSU) if there is a history of dysuria. The measurement of blood levels of HbA_{1c} (glycosylated haemoglobin) may give a good indication of long-term diabetic control because it reflects the mean blood glucose level over the previous 1–2 months.

Establish the patient on a twice-daily mixed insulin or basal/bolus regime using a long-acting formulation such as Ultratard, usually at night, with Actrapid before each of the major meals, most conveniently with a cartridge in a pen device. Assess control with home blood glucose monitoring, checking before and after each of the three daily meals plus possibly bedtime and 3 a.m. samples. The patient should be seen regularly.

Screening in diabetes

'*What would you check at annual review?*'
•   Eyes. Visual acuity (Snellen chart) and examine retinae through dilated pupils (tropicamide and, possibly, pseudoephedrine eyedrops).
•   Blood pressure, lying and standing.
•   Feet for sensory neuropathy, including ankle jerks, and for arterial disease, including the four major arterial foot pulses and evidence of reduced capillary circulation. Note the temperature of the feet and check them for ulcers.
•   Injection sites for fat atrophy and hypertrophy (now uncommon).
•   Take blood for creatinine (and/or urea) and HbA_{1c}. Check the random blood glucose (with the timing of the last meal), and obtain the patient's own estimate of blood glucose at the same time, using the patient's own technique.
•   Urine for albumin and microalbumin (p. 224).

- Diet review and patient's understanding of his or her own diabetes.

NB   Management of diabetes: see p. 225.

Random screening of the whole population is probably not cost-effective although it does serve to increase its health-conciousness. People particularly at risk include those who have had gestational diabetes (where 60% become diabetic within 16 years), and siblings of type 2 diabetics, particularly after the age of 50.

Diabetes and pregnancy

The risks to the fetus are considerable, with a high perinatal mortality which is related to the degree of diabetic control. If fasting and postprandial blood glucose levels are within normal limits, fetal loss is probably no greater than in the normal population. The more rigid regimes insist on levels below 5.5 mmol/l for most of the day, with a postprandial level below 7–8 mmol/l. Urine testing is not useful because of the fall in renal glucose threshold. Insulin requirements tend to fall in the first trimester, stabilize in the second trimester, and rise again in the last trimester, only to fall abruptly on delivery. The patient may be admitted for accurate diabetic control and delivery at term (see *Diabetes and surgery*, below).

Diabetes and illness

Even with vomiting, hepatic glycogenolysis can provide enough glucose during most illnesses. Normal doses of insulin are continued and blood glucose estimated 2–4-hourly. Soluble insulin is taken 5 units 2-hourly if the blood glucose is in the range 12–20 mmol/l and not climbing. Ketonuria must be monitored every time urine is passed. Diabetics who have been properly educated in diabetes will know a number of suitable 10 g carbohydrate exchanges, such as a 5 ml spoonful of glucose or sucrose, 50 ml Lucozade or 200 ml whole milk.

Diabetes and surgery

The main danger is that the patient becomes hypoglycaemic whilst anaesthetized. However, with increases in cortisol, glucagon, growth hormone and catecholamines, plus a decrease in insulin, surgery tends to produce hyperglycaemia even in the non-diabetic subject. With elective surgery, the patient should be first on the operating list. No food or insulin is given on the morning of the operation. Routine bladder catheterization is not indicated.

NON-INSULIN-DEPENDENT DIABETES MELLITUS – NIDDM
(type 2, maturity-onset)

- *Before surgery.* Stop drugs 24h before (48h for chlorpropamide and glibenclamide).

• *During surgery.* Treat as insulin-dependent if blood glucose >10 mmol/l, or major surgery. Otherwise, no therapy.
• *After surgery.* Unless now on insulin, or postoperative blood glucose >15 mmol/l or patient is ill, reinstate oral therapy.

INSULIN-DEPENDENT DIABETES MELLITUS — IDDM (type 1)

• *Before surgery.* Continue 'bd mixed' or basal/bolus regimes. Convert others to tds preprandial if well-controlled; if not, delay surgery and stabilize.
• *During surgery.* Arrange for blood glucose every 2 h. Give 500 ml 4-hourly of 10% glucose with 10 mmol KCl in each. Add as many units soluble insulin to the (500 ml) bag as the patient's current blood glucose (to the nearest 5 units). Adjust KCl dose to suit patient.
• *After surgery.* Slow above regime to 6-hourly and return to normal regime when patient starts eating again.

Diabetes and driving

The licensing authority and insurance company must be informed when diabetes is diagnosed. Diabetic patients will be given a 'private driver's licence' for up to 3 years depending upon the quality of control, the regularity of medical surveillance and the state of complications. Patients with NIDDM and without complications are given 3-year licences. Patients with IDDM are given a licence when glycaemic control is good, the patient's understanding of the condition is good, and the patient is not subject to frequent or sudden attacks of hypoglycaemia. This implies that the patient must carry glucose tablets (or equivalent) and know and avoid situations in which there is increased risk of hypoglycaemia. The complications of reduction of visual acuity, sensory neuropathy and peripheral vascular disease must be assessed. Patients with IDDM will not normally obtain a vocational driving licence (for heavy goods vehicles and public service vehicles), but NIDDM patients normally will.

Skin

In examinations it is usual to show cases of common disorders such as acne, eczema, athlete's foot and drug eruption and those that have complications such as psoriasis and bullous eruptions (p. 406). Remember that several skin disorders are manifestations of systemic disease, e.g. purpura and lupus erythematosus.

History

'What do you think of this rash?'
Diagnosis depends on the history, examination of the skin, examination for underlying systemic disorder with special investigations for this, and special investigations of the skin, such as skin biopsy and scrapings for fungi.

If you are allowed to question the patient:
• Ask when the rash started and whether it has altered in character or progressed.
• Ask where the rash began. This is especially important in contact dermatitis and with pityriasis rosea (herald patch).
• Ask what drugs have been taken, especially over-the-counter drugs. The rash may have been treated topically and as a result may have altered in character and be either better or worse as a result. Discover if possible what drugs, e.g. steroids, antibiotics or antihistamines have been applied to the skin. Some substances in foods can cause urticaria. Many prescription drugs cause rashes.
• Does the rash itch? Insect bites and scabies (worse in bed) are relatively common. Dermatitis (p. 408) usually gives irritation and itching. Itching is also given by the lesions of urticaria and fibreglass (common) and by lichen planus and flexural psoriasis (rare).
• Enquire about occupation and hobbies, particularly with contact dermatitis (p. 408) and about changes in lifestyle such as visits abroad or to relatives and friends. Is anyone else in the household affected and what pets does the patient have? Is there a family history, for example, of eczema, psoriasis?
• Ask about the general state of health. Many conditions, some relatively rare, have skin manifestations. Remember the exanthems, e.g. rubella, but these are not

seen in the clinic or in examination. Ask the patient for his or her theories about the cause of the rash.

Examination

You will usually need to look at the entire skin so the patient will have to be completely undressed. Remember the back, buttocks and genitalia (ask the examiner before examining these), and special areas such as scalp, eyes, mouth, fingernails and toenails.

- Categorize the type of lesion as macule (flat), papule (slightly raised), nodule, vesicle, bulla, pustule, scaling and crusting, pigmentation, lichenification (thickening of the skin with increased skin makings due to continued scratching), purpura.
- Determine the distribution of the lesions. Generalized lesions suggest systemic disease or a drug rash. Some diseases, e.g. psoriasis (p. 406) and acne (p. 409) show a predilection for certain sites on the body. Localized lesions occur in contact dermatitis and some fungal infections. Fixed drug eruptions recur at the same site every time the drug is taken. The flexures are involved in intertrigo, seborrhoeic dermatitis, psoriasis and some fungal infections.
- Describe the configuration. Some lesions may be annular, e.g. ringworm, pityriasis rosea. Bullae occur in groups in herpes simplex and dermatitis herpetiformis.
- The more common special investigations include:

    (a) inspection under Wood's light, which will show green fluorescence in most cases of tinea capitis;

    (b) in scabies, extract mite by scraping the burrow and examine with low-power microscopy;

    (c) patch testing to chemicals suspected of causing contact dermatitis; and

    (d) skin biopsy for histology, particularly where malignancy is to be excluded, but also for immunofluorescence and electron microscopy.

Essential Background Information

Neurology

Headache and giddiness constitute the most commonly presenting neurological symptoms. Faints, dizzy turns and blackouts are common and may originate from the cardiovascular system, e.g. aortic stenosis, dysrhythmias such as complete heart block and sick sinus syndrome (p. 87) and cerebral emboli. Cerebrovascular accidents are the commonest cause for hospital admission.

Physiology
Neurotransmitters

Amino acids. L-*glutamate* is the most important excitatory neurotransmitter in fast relay pathways of the motor and sensory systems. These include corticospinal, spinothalamic, lemniscal, somatosensory and specialized sensory (visual, auditory) pathways. It is also important in memory and learning. It acts through various receptors (e.g. the N-methyl-D-aspartate receptor) to open ion channels. Inactivation is through reuptake.

γ-Aminobutyric acid (GABA) is found in inhibitory interneurons throughout the central nervous system. $GABA_A$ receptors act through chloride channels to stabilize membrane potentials. Activation of $GABA_A$ receptors is potentiated by benzodiazepines and barbiturates. $GABA_B$ receptors are G protein-linked. Inactivation of GABA is through reuptake.

Pharmacology

- *Benzodiazepines* are thought to exert their effect by potentiating the effects of endogenous GABA.
- *Barbiturates* have similar effects, but at high doses they mimic the effects of GABA. Thus their action does not rely on endogenous GABA, and they can cause more profound central nervous system (CNS) depression. Recently developed antiepileptic agents influence amino-acid neurotransmission.
- *Gabapentin* is structurally similar to GABA, although its action may be independent of the GABA system.
- *Lamotrigine* probably acts through inhibition of excitatory amino-acid release.
- *Vigabatrin* (γ-vinyl GABA) inactivates the enzyme GABA-transaminase (GABA-T).

Monoamines

The catecholamines *dopamine, noradrenaline* and *adrenaline* are synthesized from L-tyrosine:

Dopamine in brainstem neurons, particularly within the substantia nigra, is important for motor control. In the hypothalamus its principal neuroendocrine function is the inhibition of prolactin synthesis. Dopaminergic neurons in the mesolimbic system are thought to control emotions. Dopamine interacts with a number of receptors, including the D_1- and D_2-receptors, which are abundant in the corpus striatum.

Noradrenaline- and *adrenaline*-containing neurons originate in the pons and medulla oblongata, and connect with the limbic system, hypothalamus and spinal cord. In the peripheral nervous system noradrenaline is the principal neurotransmitter in postganglionic sympathetic fibres. Adrenaline is also released into the circulation as a hormone from the adrenal medulla. Noradrenaline and adrenaline

SYNTHESIS OF CATECHOLAMINES

$$\begin{array}{ccccc}
 & Tyrosine & Dopamine & & \\
 & hydroxylase & \beta\text{-}hydroxylase & & \\
\text{L-tyrosine} \longrightarrow & \text{Dopa} \longrightarrow & \text{Dopamine} \longrightarrow & \text{Noradrenaline} \longrightarrow & \text{Adrenaline} \\
 & Dopa & & Phenylethanolamine\text{-} & \\
 & decarboxylase & & N\text{-}methyltransferase &
\end{array}$$

Fig. 11.1 Synthesis of catecholamines.

interact with α_1-, α_2- and β-adrenergic receptors in the brain and spinal cord. α_1- and β-receptors mediate the sympathetic effects of noradrenaline.

Inactivation of catecholamines is through reuptake, and enzymatic breakdown by monoamine oxidases and catechol-O-methyltransferase. Dopamine is catabolized to homovanillic acid. In the brain adrenaline and noradrenaline are catabolized to 3-methoxy-4-hydroxy-phenylethyleneglycol, whereas in the peripheral nervous system the principal metabolite is vanillylmandelic acid.

Serotonin (5-hydroxytryptamine; 5-HT) is synthesized from L-tryptophan in neurons arising in the brainstem raphe nuclei which project throughout the brain and spinal cord. It is also present in the myenteric plexus, and circulates as a hormone. The four main receptor subtypes ($5\text{-}HT_1$, $5\text{-}HT_2$, $5\text{-}HT_3$, $5\text{-}HT_4$) are differentially distributed throughout the brain and spinal cord. $5\text{-}HT_1$ receptors can be subdivided into $5\text{-}HT_{1A-1E}$. $5\text{-}HT_{1D}$-receptors are abundant in cerebral vessels where they mediate vasoconstriction. Inactivation of serotonin is through reuptake or metabolization by monoamine oxidase to 5-hydroxyindoleacetic acid.

Histamine is synthesized from L-histidine in hypothalamic neurons which innervate various parts of the brain and spinal cord. It is also stored in and released by mast cells and basophils. Histamine interacts with H_1-, H_2- and H_3-receptors. Cerebral H_1-receptors are important in controlling arousal. Reuptake of histamine does not occur. Inactivation is through metabolism by histamine-N-methyltransferase and monoamine oxidase to methylimidazoleacetic acid.

Pharmacology

Drugs which antagonize the effects of adrenaline and noradrenaline generally have sedative effects, whereas dopamine antagonists cause drug-induced parkinsonism.

Major tranquillizers (e.g. *phenothiazines*) are thought to exert their effects by antagonizing the effects of dopamine in the cerebral cortex and limbic system.

Monoamine oxidase inhibitors increase all cerebral catecholamines by reducing their metabolism. *Tricyclic antidepressants* potentiate the action of brain amines by preventing reuptake at nerve terminals. However, their delayed action suggests that other mechanisms are involved in their antidepressant activity.

Antiparkinsonian drugs potentiate the effects of dopamine. *Levodopa* is the treatment of choice. It is given with a dopa-decarboxylase inhibitor (e.g. carbidopa or benserazide) to prevent the peripheral effects of dopamine. *Selegiline* is a *monoamine oxidase B inhibitor* which can be used in severe parkinsonism. *Bromocriptine* is a *dopamine receptor agonist*. Dopamine deficiency results in a relative excess of acetylcholine, and *antimuscarinic agents* (e.g. *benzhexol*) are sometimes effective in mild parkinsonism. Dopamine agonists reduce prolactin secretion.

Drugs which affect the actions of 5-HT are used in the treatment of migraine and depression. *Sumatriptan*, a 5-HT$_{1D}$ agonist, provides symptomatic relief from migraine by constricting cerebral blood vessels. *Pizotifen* antagonizes 5-HT$_1$- and 5-HT$_2$-receptors and is used in migraine prophylaxis. The antidepressant *mianserin* is a 5-HT-receptor antagonist. Agents which block reuptake of 5-HT are effective in the treatment of depression. They include *fluoxetine* (Prozac), *paroxetine* (Seroxat) and *sertraline* (Lustral). The hallucinogen LSD is a partial agonist at 5-HT$_2$-receptors.

Antihistamines are commonly used in the treatment of allergy. Drowsiness is a common problem.

Acetylcholine

Acetylcholine interacts with nicotinic receptors at the neuromuscular junction and autonomic ganglia, and with muscarinic receptors in the CNS and in post-ganglionic parasympathetic pathways. Inactivation is through hydrolysis by acetylcholinesterase. Cholinergic transmission is thus potentiated by anticholinesterases.

Pharmacology

Anticholinergic agents are used to inhibit peripheral effects of acetylcholine. *Atropine* acts at postganglionic (muscarinic) receptors and is used in the treatment of bradycardia and as a premedication to dry secretions. *Hyoscine* is structurally related to atropine, but differs by causing CNS depression and amnesia. Drugs which block the actions of acetylcholine at the neuromuscular junction are used as muscle relaxants in anaesthesia. They act by either competition (*non-depolarizing agents*, e.g. *pancuronium, tubocurarine*) or by depolarization (e.g. *suxamethonium*). Competitive muscle relaxants can be reversed by *anticholinesterases* (e.g. *edrophonium, neostigmine*). Anticholinesterases are also used in the treatment of myasthenia gravis.

In the eye *cholinergic agents* (e.g. the alkaloid *pilocarpine* or *anticholinesterases*) cause pupillary constriction, whereas *antimuscarinic agents* can be used to dilate the pupil (e.g. *homatropine, tropicamide*).

Neuropeptides

Neuropeptides occur throughout the central and peripheral nervous systems. Many act as hormones and have vasoactive actions (e.g. vasopressin, somatostatin) or gastrointestinal effects (e.g. vasoactive intestinal polypeptide, cholecystokinin). They are particularly important in regulating hypothalamic function (e.g.

THE INTERNAL CAPSULE, THALAMUS AND THIRD VENTRICLE IN CORONAL SECTION

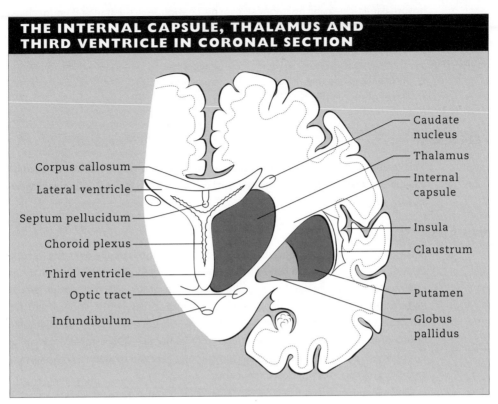

Fig. 11.2 Coronal section through the third ventricle.

LATERAL SURFACE OF THE LEFT CEREBRAL HEMISPHERE

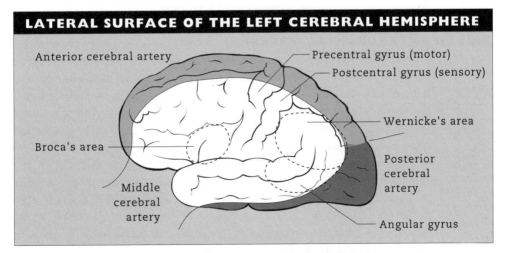

Fig. 11.3 Surface anatomy of the left cerebral hemisphere.

hypothalamic-releasing hormones), pain perception (e.g. substance P, endorphins) and autonomic pathways (e.g. neuropeptide Y).

Anatomy
- Internal capsule (Fig. 11.2)
- Arterial supply (Fig. 11.3).

Headache

This is one of the commonest of all presenting symptoms. The aim is to exclude treatable underlying intra- or extracranial disease and to make a definitive diagnosis (e.g. migraine).

TENSION HEADACHE

A severe continuous pressure is characteristically felt bilaterally over the vertex, occiput or eyes. It may be band-like or non-specific and of variable intensity. It is commonest in middle-aged women but may occur at any age or in either sex in association with stress or depression (ask about family, work, money and for symptoms of depression). The headache may be described with considerable drama and standard analgesics are invariably ineffective. Occasionally it may be symptomatic of worry about a brain tumour and relieved by definite reassurance and thorough normal physical examination.

POST-CONCUSSION HEADACHE

This has many features of tension headache but is usually associated with dizziness (not vertigo) and loss of concentration. There is often a history of inadequate recovery following the head injury, and of impending litigation.

RAISED INTRACRANIAL PRESSURE

This is most often due to intracranial tumour, haematoma or abscess. The pain is worse on waking in the morning after lying down and is associated with vomiting. It improves 1–2 h after rising and is exacerbated by coughing, sneezing or straining. Visual deterioration may not occur despite papilloedema. The pain usually responds to standard analgesics. NB (for teetotallers) Alcoholic hangovers also cause early-morning headaches.

Patients whose histories do not fit into one of these categories usually have either an obvious diagnosis (meningitis, subarachnoid haemorrhage, sinusitis, otitis media) or a less obvious local cause (teeth, cervical spine, skull, orbits). Benign hypertension, defects in visual acuity, glaucoma and ocular muscle imbalance seldom present as headache.

Preliminary investigation

Patients with headache of more than 6 weeks' duration and without abnormal clinical signs probably do not require investigation. Most hospital physicians, when seeing the patient referred from a family practitioner, would request:

• full blood count, including erythrocyte sedimentation rate (ESR; to exclude temporal arteritis in the over-50s);

• chest X-ray for bronchial carcinoma;

• computed tomographic (CT) scan should be performed to exclude a space-occupying lesion where clinically indicated, especially in the presence of:

(a) frontal headache on waking with nausea, i.e. symptoms suggestive of raised intracranial pressure

(b) occipital headache of sudden onset (subarachnoid haemorrage)

(c) abnormal, and in particular progressive, neurological signs including confusional dementia.

Unilateral facial pain

MIGRAINE

Migraine is episodic and affects approximately 10% of the population. It usually begins around puberty and continues intermittently to middle age. It is commoner in females than males (3:1) and there is often a family history. There may have been episodes of unexplained nausea and/or abdominal pain in childhood. It may be associated with periods and the contraceptive pill, with various foods (especially chocolate, cheese and red wine) and emotions (anger, tension, excitement). A characteristic attack starts with a sense of ill health and is followed by a visual aura (shimmering lights, fortification spectra, scotomas) usually in the field opposite to the side of the succeeding headache. The throbbing unilateral headache is associated with anorexia, nausea, vomiting, photophobia and withdrawal. There may be transient hemiparesis or sensory symptoms. It is very rarely associated with organic disease and CT scan with contrast is only indicated if of late onset (over 45 years) or to exclude arteriovenous malformation if abnormal physical signs persist or progress.

Management

Precipitating causes should be identified and removed—a patient's diary of symptoms and diet may help—and simple analgesia taken early (aspirin, paracetamol). Metoclopramide or domperidone may be given with them to reduce nausea. If attacks are frequent and interfere with work and social life, treat prophylactically with pizotifen 1.5 mg nocte, propranolol 80–160 mg daily, or if severe, sumatriptan (p. 122) may be injected by the patient at the onset of the prodrome.

CLUSTER HEADACHES (migrainous neuralgia)

These are a form of migraine. Attacks occur in clusters every 12–18 months and consist of very severe pain around an eye occurring often at night for 1–3 weeks. The eye becomes red and watery and the nostril of the same side blocked up. It often responds to ergotamine.

NEURALGIAS

Neuralgias are intermittent, but brief, severe, lancinating pains occurring along the distribution of a nerve.

Trigeminal neuralgia (tic douloureux)

This occurs almost exclusively in the elderly. In a patient under 50 years old it may be symptomatic of multiple sclerosis. The agonizing pain is usually triggered from a place on the lips or the side of the nose. It tends to get worse with age but may be specifically relieved by carbamazepine (Tegretol). Phenytoin may also be useful. A small aberrant vessel overlying the nerve (or ganglion) can be the cause, and dissection or cryotherapy of this completely relieves the symptoms. A patient may need thermocoagulation or section of the sensory root of the 5th nerve. Tumour can be a rare cause which can be excluded by CT scan. Suicide is a definite risk.

Glossopharyngeal neuralgia

Precipitated by swallowing, which produces pain in the pharynx.

Auriculotemporal neuralgia

Precipitated by swallowing, and may be treated by correcting malocclusion.

Postherpetic neuralgia

Occurs in patients with a history of herpes zoster infection (shingles) and the scars of the healed disease are usually obvious. The pain may be almost impossible to relieve.

GIANT CELL ARTERITIS

In giant cell arteritis the pain is usually severe and intractable. The pain is felt in the temples or over the entire scalp, and jaw claudication and/or visual changes may be present. Temporal or scalp arteries may be swollen and tender. The patient usually feels ill, and the ESR is greatly raised. Some 25% of patients have features of polymyalgia rheumatica. Temporal artery biopsy is performed if it can be done rapidly and the patient given high-dose steroids (prednisolone 40 mg daily) to prevent sudden blindness (uncommon). After 2 years 30–50% of patients are able to discontinue steroids.

ATYPICAL FACIAL PAIN

This refers to episodic aching in the jaw and cheek, lasting several hours and usually occurring in young to middle-aged women who are frequently depressed. It is often bilateral. It may respond to antidepressants or antihistamines.

UNILATERAL PAIN

Local pathologies involving the eyes, sinuses, teeth or ears may give unilateral pain, as may tumours involving the 5th nerve (cerebellopontine angle tumours). Pain from herpes zoster may occur before the rash appears.

NB   Patients with headache and facial pain may not give histories which fit conveniently into any well-recognized category. They should be seen at intervals to determine:

- symptoms of increasing anxiety or depression;
- symptoms of changing pain patterns; and
- developing abnormal clinical signs.

In the absence of these, treatment is with reassurance and simple analgesics.

Stroke

Stroke affects about 1 in 600 patients per year, and approximately 5% of the population over 65 will suffer from stroke. Approximately 85% are ischaemic (thrombosis or embolism), and 10% are due to intracerebral haemorrhage, and 5% subarachnoid haemorrhage.

Risk factors include smoking, hypertension, hyperlipidaemia, atrial fibrillation, ischaemic heart disease, valvular heart disease and diabetes.

In stroke units 5–13% of cases have a non-vascular lesion (tumour, subdural haematoma, post-ictal paresis, migraine, intracranial infection, metabolic disturbance, hysteria).

Investigations to confirm the diagnosis

The distinction between cerebral haemorrhage and infarction cannot be made on the basis of clinical or cerebrospinal fluid (CSF) findings, but requires CT scanning. A low-density area appears within a few hours of a cerebral infarct, whereas a high-density area appears immediately after a bleed. Brainstem, cerebellar and small cortical infarcts are often not visible. Magnetic resonance imaging (MRI) is more sensitive for detecting ischaemic stroke, but is more expensive, takes longer to perform, and requires more cooperation from the patient.

CT scanning should be performed if:

- diagnosis of stroke is in doubt (slow onset, unexplained unconsciousness or deterioration after stroke);
- cerebellar stroke (with declining consciousness to exclude secondary obstructive hydrocephalus);
- treatment with anticoagulants or antiplatelet agents is considered prior to carotid endarterectomy (exclusion of intracranial haemorrhage);
- subarachnoid haemorrhage is suspected; or
- the patient is young with no risk factors.

Investigations to establish the aetiology

Less common causes of stroke should be considered, particularly in young patients and those without risk factors.

The following investigations are usually performed:

- full blood count (FBC), ESR, coagulation screen, urea and electrolytes, glucose, cholesterol, syphilis serology;

- electrocardiogram (ECG) and cardiac enzymes;
- chest X-ray;
- echocardiography to detect cardiac source of embolus (25–30% of ischaemic strokes are caused by cardioembolism); and
- duplex imaging of the extracranial carotid and vertebral arteries provides information on arterial occlusion or source of emboli.

Other investigations which may be indicated include serum protein electrophoresis/viscosity, autoantibody screen (for anticardiolipin antibody, antinuclear antibody, antineutrophil cytoplasm antibody), protein C, S and antithrombin III levels, sickle test, blood cultures, urine for homocystinuria.

Cerebral angiography may be helpful in detecting cerebral vasculitis.

Management

General care to maintain comfort and an adequate airway. Ensure swallowing is safe, and keep the patient hydrated and nourished. Swallowing should be assessed (watch the patient trying to drink) and if there is difficulty, fluids should be given by nasogastric tube or intravenously.

Prevention and treatment of complications

- *Cardiovascular*: cardiac arrhythmias and hypertension are common. Most physicians do not treat high blood pressure in the early stages for fear of lowering cerebral blood flow and exacerbating ischaemia. Urgent treatment is required if hypertensive encephalopathy or hypertensive cardiac or renal failure is suspected.
- *Chest infections* account for 20–40% of deaths. Aspiration is common and treatment with antibiotics and physiotherapy should be started if the diagnosis is suspected.
- *Deep venous thrombosis* occurs in 50% of patients, and may be difficult to diagnose in a paralysed leg.
- *Hypertension* occurs, even in the absence of previously diagnosed hypertension.
- *Pressure sores* are common in bed-ridden patients. Avoidance requires careful positioning and regular turning.
- *Urinary infections* are associated with catheterization.
- *Seizures* occur in 5% of patients, and may require treatment with anticonvulsants (p. 134).
- *Hyperglycaemia* in non-diabetic patients suffering an acute stroke results from increased cortisol, catecholamine and glucagon levels. Insulin may be required temporarily.
- *Hyponatraemia* may result from excessive use of intravenous dextrose. In 10% of patients it is due to inappropriate antidiuretic hormone secretion, which usually resolves spontaneously.

Recovery and rehabilitation require an integrated approach between physicians, nurses, physiotherapist, speech therapist, occupational therapist and social worker.

LATERAL MEDULLARY SYNDROME (see Fig. 1.2, p. 6)

This is the commonest brainstem vascular syndrome and presents acutely with vertigo, vomiting and ipsilateral facial pain. Dysphagia and dysarthria may occur. The following features may be present.

Ipsilateral

- Palatal paralysis.
- Horner's syndrome.
- Spinothalamic sensory loss in the face.
- Cerebellar signs in the limbs.

Contralateral

- Spinothalamic loss in the body.

EXTRACEREBRAL HAEMORRHAGE
Extradural

This results from traumatic damage to the middle meningeal artery as it passes upwards on the inside of the temporal bone. Classically, momentary loss of consciousness is followed by apparent recovery and death 1–7 days later. Not every fracture of the temporal bone results in middle meningeal haemorrhage but suspicion alone warrants CT scan of the head and admission of the patient to observe conscious level. Should signs of local haemorrhage ensue, burr holes are performed, the clot is removed and the vessel tied.

Subdural

This occurs most frequently in the elderly, alcoholics and children. It often follows trauma. A small venous haemorrhage occurs and the clot slowly enlarges in size, absorbing fluid osmotically from the CSF.

Clinical presentation

The symptoms may develop over a period of weeks to months. Headache, confusion and progressive loss of conscious level occur with fluctuation of consciousness. The other signs are of a one-sided intracranial mass with contralateral weakness and hemiplegia, possibly with signs of raised intracranial pressure (falling pulse rate, rising blood pressure, papilloedema).

Management

CT scan may show the haematoma and removal may give full recovery, irrespective of the patient's age. Subdural haematomata may be bilateral.

SUBARACHNOID HAEMORRHAGE

Subarachnoid haemorrhage presents with abrupt onset of severe generalized headache. There may be loss of consciousness, vomiting or seizures. Meningeal irritation causes neck stiffness and photophobia. Focal neurological signs suggest local compression (e.g. 3rd-nerve palsy due to posterior communicating artery aneurysm) or associated intracerebral haematoma. Rising blood pressure, falling pulse and papilloedema indicate raised intracranial pressure.

Many patients give a history of previous similar but milder episodes, possibly due to smaller leaks.

Diagnosis

Unenhanced CT scan shows intracranial blood in over 90% of cases and reveals any associated haematoma. It may indicate the site of a leaking aneurysm, and any associated hydrocephalus. If CT scan is unavailable, or intracranial blood is not seen but clinical suspicion is high, lumbar puncture is performed to examine CSF for raised pressure, uniform blood staining and xanthochromia. Lumbar puncture can precipitate coning, and should not be performed if signs suggest raised intracranial pressure or cerebral or cerebellar haemorrhage.

Complications

Some 25% of patients die on the first day, and a further 25% die in the first month.

Hydrocephalus occurs in 20% of patients, and may require ventricular drainage. It results from obstruction to CSF flow by blood. Delayed *ischaemia* due to cere-

---

TRIALS

British aneurysm nimodipine trial compared placebo with nimodipine 60 mg 4-hourly, started within 96 h of subarachnoid haemorrhage and continued for 21 days, in 554 patients. Nimodipine improved outcome and reduced the incidence of cerebral infarction. *Br Med J* 1989; **298**: 636–642.

In the **MAST-E** (Multicentre Acute Stroke Trial–Europe), streptokinase increased mortality compared with placebo when given in the first 6 h after an ischaemic stroke. *N Engl J Med* 1996; **335**: 145–150.

The **International Stroke Trial (IST)** studied the effect of aspirin, subcutaneous heparin, both, or neither in 19 435 patients with acute ischaemic stroke. Heparin did not offer a clinical advantage, but aspirin 300 mg daily reduced death or non-fatal recurrent stroke. *Lancet* 1997; **349**: 1569–1581.

The **Chinese Acute Stroke Trial (CAST)** studied 21 016 patients in a randomised placebo-controlled trial. Aspirin 160 mg/day started within 48 h of suspected acute ischaemic stroke reduced mortality and non-fatal stroke. *Lancet*; **349**: 1641–1649.

bral vasospasm presents with deteriorating conscious level or focal neurological signs. It can be prevented by prophylactic treatment with oral (or nasogastric) nimodipine 60 mg 4-hourly. Sudden deterioration suggests *rebleeding*, which can be confirmed by repeat CT scan. *Haematoma*, if compressing, requires evacuation.

TRIALS

The **Canadian Cooperative Study Group** compared placebo with aspirin 1300 mg daily, sulphinpyrazone 800 mg daily, or aspirin and sulphinpyrazone in combination in 585 patients with TIA or minor stroke. Aspirin significantly reduced the risk of stroke in men but not women, possibly because fewer women were enrolled. Sulphinpyrazone provided no benefit either alone or in combination with aspirin. *N Engl J Med* 1978; **299**: 53–59.

The **UK-TIA aspirin trial** compared placebo with two doses of aspirin (300 and 1200 mg daily) in 2435 patients with TIA or minor stroke. Aspirin reduced the risk of the combined end-points of stroke, myocardial infarction and death. There was no significant difference between the two doses of aspirin but gastrointestinal symptoms were commoner with the higher dose. *J Neurol Neurosurg Psychiatry* 1991; **54**: 1044–1054.

The **Dutch TIA trial** compared carbaspirin calcium at a dose of 30 mg daily with 283 mg daily in 3131 patients with TIA or minor stroke. Both doses were equally effective in reducing the risk of stroke, but the 30 mg dose caused fewer gastrointestinal problems. *N Engl J Med* 1991; **325**: 1261–1266.

The **Swedish Aspirin Low-dose Trial** compared placebo with aspirin 75 mg daily in 1360 patients with TIA or minor stroke. Low-dose aspirin reduced the risk of stroke or death compared with placebo. *Lancet* 1991; **338**: 1345–1349.

The **Antiplatelet Trialists' Collaboration** performed a meta-analysis of 145 randomized trials involving nearly 100 000 patients with coronary cerebral or peripheral vascular disease. They found a 23% reduction in non-fatal stroke, non-fatal myocardial infarction and vascular death in patients with a history of stroke or TIA. There was no evidence that any antiplatelet drug, alone or in combination, was more effective than medium-dose aspirin (75–325 mg daily). Higher doses of aspirin were as effective but caused more unwanted effects. *Br Med J* 1994; **308**: 81–106.

TRANSIENT ISCHAEMIC ATTACKS

Transient ischaemic attacks (TIAs) are focal brain or retinal deficits caused by vascular disease which resolve within 24 h. Most clear within 1 h. The risk of stroke following TIA is approximately 5% within 1 month, 12% during the first year and 25% over 5 years.

The commonest cause is atherosclerosis of large arteries supplying the brain. Cardioembolic strokes may also be preceded by TIAs. Rarely, cerebral vasculitis, hypercoagulable states and arterial dissection present as TIAs. Non-vascular causes which may mimic TIA include seizures, migraine, tumour, subdural haematoma and hypoglycaemia.

• Carotid artery TIAs affect the cortex and produce ischaemia to the ipsilateral eye or brain, resulting in blurring of vision, or contralateral weakness or sensory disturbance.

• Vertebrobasilar TIAs affect the brainstem and cause dizziness, ataxia, vertigo, dysarthria, diplopia, and unilateral or bilateral weakness and numbness in the limbs.

Reduction of risk factors

• Treat hypertension.

• Stop smoking.

• Treat underlying heart disease (arrhythmias, valvular heart disease, coronary artery disease and heart failure).

Improving diabetic control, treating hyperlipidaemia and reducing excessive alcohol intake are all advisable, although the effect of each on reducing stroke risk

TRIALS

The **North American Symptomatic Carotid Endarterectomy Trial (NASCET)** studied 659 patients with TIA or minor stroke and 70–99% with carotid artery stenosis. Endarterectomy reduced the risk of non-fatal and fatal stroke. NASCET is continuing for patients with 30–69% stenosis. N Engl J Med 1991; **325**: 445–453.

The **European Carotid Surgery Trial (ECST)** studied 2518 patients with mild (0–29%), moderate (30–69%), or severe (70–99%) stenosis. Surgery reduced the risk of stroke or death in patients with severe stenosis, but medical treatment was better than surgery in patients with mild stenosis. Lancet 1991; **337**: 1235–1243.

The **European Carotid Surgery Trialists Collaborative Group** investigated the risk of stroke in the distribution of asymptomatic carotid artery stenosis in 2295 patients. The risk of stroke over 3 years was 2.1%, and neither screening nor endarterectomy for asymptomatic lesions was felt to be justified. Lancet 1995; **345**: 209–212.

is unclear. Mild to moderate alcohol consumption reduces the risk of coronary artery disease, and may have a mild protective effect on stroke risk.

Medical treatment

Antiplatelet agents are effective in preventing stroke in patients with TIAs. Aspirin in a daily dose of 75–325 mg daily is as effective as or better than any other agent or combination of agents. In the absence of risk factors for cardioembolism (atrial fibrillation, valvular disease) there are no conclusive data to support the use of oral anticoagulants.

Surgical treatment

The indications for carotid endarterectomy in patients with TIA depend on many factors, including the severity of the stenosis and the surgical morbidity and mortality at the centre involved. In centres with a low surgical morbidity and mortality (<6%) surgery is of proven value in patients with a stenosis of greater than 70% and a history of TIA.

Glasgow Coma Scale

Conscious level may be charted using the Glasgow Coma Scale (Table 11.1).

GLASGOW COMA SCALE

Category	Score
Eye opening	
None	1
To pain	2
To speech	3
Spontaneous	4
Best verbal response	
None	1
Incomprehensible	2
Inappropriate	3
Confused	4
Oriented	5
Best motor response	
None	1
Extending	2
Flexing	3
Localizing	4
Obeying	5

Patients are scored for each of the three categories. The sum of the three scores gives a measure of their overall conscious level, the range being from 3 (completely unresponsive) to 14 (fully conscious).

Table 11.1 Glasgow Coma Scale.

Brain death (two independent medical opinions are required)

The three main criteria essential to this medicolegal diagnosis are:

1   a known untreatable cause such as cardiac arrest, intracerebral haemorrhage or severe trauma. Patients with hypothermia or drug overdose are not acceptable;

2   absent cortical function: deep coma, as shown by absent response to any stimulus (other than spinal reflexes); and

3   absent brainstem function. This is demonstrated by:

(a) fixed dilated pupils;

(b) absent corneal, gag and cough reflexes;

(c) absent eye movements and no movement on rolling the head (i.e. the normal 'doll's eye movements', in which the eyes lag behind head movement, are absent);

(d) absent caloric responses. Ice-cold water into an external auditory meatus causes eye movements towards the stimulated ear in normal people;

(e) lack of spontaneous respiration.

Epilepsy

A paroxysmal electrical discharge in the cerebral neurons resulting in a wide variety of clinical patterns. Most commonly there is a continuing tendency to experience episodes of altered movement, sensory phenomena and odd behaviour, usually with altered consciousness.

Many patients who present following a 'fit' have only had an episode of unconsciousness. It is important to consider and exclude other conditions which are commonly confused with epilepsy.

Classification

Partial seizures

Partial seizures have a single focus (origin) of activity. This may be scar tissue following trauma or a stroke, or a tumour. Either:

• *simple* — no impairment of consciousness. Symptoms may be illusional, olfactory, psychic, cognitive, aphasic, sensory or motor (Jacksonian)

• *complex* — in which consciousness is impaired.

NB   Partial seizures may proceed to generalized seizures.

Generalized seizures

Generalized seizures in which there is widespread activity affecting both cerebral hemispheres. They include:

• childhood absence seizures (petit mal)

• myoclonic epilepsy — sudden convulsive movements of the limbs and trunk, usually in children

• tonic–clonic (grand mal) seizures (see below).

Also tonic (spasm) and clonic (jerking) seizures; atonic or akinetic seizures. Many seizure patterns remain unclassified.

Aetiology

Usually no cause is identified and the epilepsy is termed idiopathic. This probably includes patients who have suffered intrauterine, perinatal or neonatal insults. There may be a strong family history, suggesting genetic susceptibility, particularly with petit mal seizures.

Seizures may be secondary to cerebral disorders, metabolic disorders and drug intake.

Cerebral disorders

- Cerebral tumour or arteriovenous malformation.
- Sequel to severe head injury or birth injury.
- Cerebrovascular disease.
- Infection — encephalitis, bacterial meningitis, cerebral abscess, toxoplasmosis (the commonest intracranial lesion in acquired immunodeficiency syndrome (AIDS)), cysticercosis, syphilis. Falciparum malaria should be considered in travellers (examine blood film).
- Inflammatory lesions — systemic lupus erythematosus (SLE), vasculitis, multiple sclerosis.
- Degenerative—Alzheimer's disease, Huntington's chorea.

Metabolic disorders

- Hypoglycaemia.
- Hypocalcaemia or hypomagnesaemia.
- Renal or hepatic failure.
- Hyponatraemia.

Drugs (particularly following overdose)

- Alcohol: severe intoxication, rapid withdrawal by habitual heavy drinker, or following head injury while intoxicated.
- Amphetamines, tricyclic antidepressants, phenothiazines.

Provocation of seizures

Many aetiological factors (e.g. drug overdose, hypoglycaemia) can provoke seizures in patients not usually prone to epilepsy. In known epileptics, seizures can be provoked by sleep deprivation, stress, alcohol and occasionally stimuli such as television or disco lighting. In women seizures may increase in frequency around the time of menstruation.

Differential diagnosis

It is important to consider other causes of loss of consciousness, including:

- vasovagal fainting attacks;

- cerebrovascular disease — TIAs, carotid artery stenosis, vertebrobasilar ischaemia;
- low cardiac output—Stokes–Adams attacks in heart block, sinoatrial disease, aortic stenosis;
- postmicturition and cough syncope;
- postural hypotension may be due to hypotensive or sedative drugs, particularly in the elderly.

An account of the fit from a witness is invaluable.

In the differential diagnosis from faints, epileptics are stiff and not floppy in the fall, usually have staring open eyes rather than half-closed, have no memory of the fall and take over 30 s to recover.

Drop attacks occur only past middle age, usually in women in whom there is no loss of consciousness but there is a sense of surprise about the lack of external cause.

A hysterical episode is exacerbated by witnesses, is associated with coarse dramatic movement rather than neat jerking, and clenched flickering eyelids with the eye rolled up (if the lids can be prised apart). Also recovery is rapid with full mental alertness ('What happened, where am I?') and no neurological signs.

Clinical features

Grand mal (generalized tonic–clonic seizures)

In over 50% of cases a fit is preceded by an aura. This is followed by loss of consciousness and the tonic phase, which usually lasts up to 30 s. Cyanosis may occur as the respiratory muscles are also tonically contracted. The clonic phase follows in all limbs. Micturition and tongue-biting (and fingers if unwisely inserted into the mouth to pull the tongue forwards) which is followed by sleep, lasting for 1–3 h. During sleep the corneal and limb reflexes may be absent and the plantar responses upgoing.

The patient should be protected from injury during the acute phase. Rectal or intravenous diazepam (5 mg/min for 2–4 min) will control most fits. Status epilepticus may require continued diazepam or a chlormethiazole or phenytoin infusion with close attention to breathing. General anaesthesia with muscle relaxants and artificial ventilation are sometimes needed to suppress abnormal cerebral electrical activity.

Petit mal

This presents in childhood and is characterized by brief (10–15 s) moments of absence without warning and with immediate recovery. The electroencephalogram (EEG) shows typical spike-and-wave complexes at 3 s. It virtually never continues beyond adolescence, but about 5% of children will develop adult grand mal seizures.

Temporal lobe epilepsy

This is characterized by temporary disturbances of the content of consciousness. Hallucinations may occur (e.g. *déjà-vu* phenomena), as may visual disturbance such as macropsia and micropsia. Unreasoning fear and depersonalization may be present. Olfactory or gustatory auras may be the only symptom and are related to abnormal foci in the uncinate lobe. Automatism may follow the aura. Patients perform a complex movement pattern, repeated with each attack (psychomotor epilepsy).

Jacksonian (focal) epilepsy

Epileptic activity originates in one part of the precentral motor cortex. Fits begin in one part of the body (e.g. the thumb) and may proceed to involve that side of the body and then the whole body. Subsequent paresis of the affected limb may last up to 3 days (Todd's paralysis). Sensory epilepsy is a parallel condition originating in the sensory cortex.

Investigation

The object is to detect treatable underlying brain disease and to exclude factors which may be provoking attacks.

A full history and clinical examination are taken to exclude other causes of loss of consciousness (see above).

Check blood for evidence of *alcohol* (mean corpuscular volume, γ-glutamyl transferase), *hypoglycaemia* or *hypocalcaemia*.

All patients should have a chest X-ray.

An *EEG* may be helpful by demonstrating the type of epilepsy, site of an epileptic focus (slow-wave activity may suggest the presence of a tumour) and guide drug therapy. A diagnosis of epilepsy cannot be made from an EEG alone — epilepsy is a clinical diagnosis, not an electrical one. Of the general population, 10–15% have an abnormal EEG.

If there is a possibility of a transient cardiac arrhythmia as a cause of fits, 24-h ambulatory ECG monitoring should be performed.

In the absence of an obvious precipitating cause (e.g. drug overdose, hypoglycaemia in a diabetic), most doctors would proceed to *brain CT scanning* to exclude focal brain disease. CT scanning is of particular value in late-onset epilepsy, partial seizures and in patients with generalized epilepsy where the EEG discloses a focal abnormality, particularly if this is accompanied by slow waves.

Management

A single fit rarely requires treatment. Any underlying cause should be identified and patients should be advised about driving (p. 462).

Antiepileptic treatment should be reserved for those who have two or more seizures within a year. It is essential that the diagnosis is confirmed before starting treatment.

About 200 000 people in the UK are taking antiepileptic drugs. The aim is to prevent seizures without causing adverse effects. The initial choice depends on the type of epilepsy, and the risk of unwanted effects, and the likelihood of compliance. Seizure control with minimal adverse effects can be achieved using a single agent in about 80% of patients. The remaining 20% require a second agent, and a number of new add-on drugs have recently become available.

Established antiepileptic therapies

Carbamazepine is often regarded as the drug of first choice for simple and complex partial seizures, and for tonic–clonic seizures. Side effects include gastrointestinal disturbances, dizziness, hepatitis and skin rashes (5–10%). It induces its own metabolism, so increased doses may be needed to achieve therapeutic levels — optimum response occurs at plasma concentration of 4–12 mg/l (20–50 μmol/l). It is ineffective in absence seizures, which may be exacerbated.

Sodium valproate can be effective in controlling simple and complex partial seizures and all forms of generalized seizures, including tonic–clonic seizures, myoclonic seizures, atonic and tonic seizures and absence attacks. Because of its widespread use, some recommend it as the drug of choice for new-onset epilepsy. Unwanted effects include weight gain (one of the commonest reasons for non-compliance), hair loss and tremor. Hepatotoxicity, thrombocytopenia and pancreatitis (check amylase if abdominal pain) are rare adverse effects. Plasma concentrations are unhelpful in monitoring efficacy.

Phenytoin is effective in both partial and tonic–clonic seizures, but its usefulness is limited by a narrow therapeutic index and adverse effects. Cosmetic changes (gum hypertrophy, hirsutism, coarsening of facial features) are particularly undesirable in adolescents. Optimum plasma concentrations are 10–20 mg/l (40–80 μmol/l).

Phenobarbitone is effective in partial and generalized seizures, but causes sedation in adults and behavioural changes and hyperkinesia in children. It is usually reserved for patients who are intolerant of other therapies.

Ethosuximide is the drug of choice for simple absence seizures. It may also be used in myoclonic seizures. It can cause sedation, but skin rashes, liver changes and haematological disorders are rare. Optimum plasma concentration is 40–100 mg/l (300–700 μmol/l).

Benzodiazepines are useful for the treatment of status epilepticus, but sedation and tolerance limit their usefulness in chronic treatment. *Clobazam* is a 1,5 benzodiazepine (differing in structure from other compounds such as diazepam and clonazepam, which are 1,4 benzodiazepines). It may cause less sedation and psychomotor impairment, but tolerance is still a problem. *Clonazepam* is occasionally used in tonic–clonic or partial seizures.

New antiepileptic drugs

New antiepileptic drugs can form useful adjunctive therapy in uncontrolled epilepsy.

Gabapentin is structurally similar to the inhibitory neurotransmitter GABA, although it does not appear to interact with the GABA system. It is effective as an adjunctive treatment of partial seizures, with or without secondary generalization. Side-effects are uncommon, although somnolence, dizziness and ataxia can occur.

Lamotrigine probably acts through inhibition of excitatory amino acid release. It is used as adjunctive treatment in partial or tonic–clonic seizures. It is generally well-tolerated, although headache, dizziness, ataxia and gastrointestinal disturbance occur.

Vigabatrin (γ-vinyl GABA) inactivates the enzyme (GABA-T). It is used in partial or tonic–clonic seizures which are not controlled by other antiepileptics. Sedation, depression, weight gain and gastrointestinal symptoms limit its usefulness in some patients.

EPILEPSY AND PREGNANCY

Maternal epilepsy is associated with an increased risk of fetal malformation, which increases further if the mother is taking antiepileptics. Common anomalies include finger nail hypoplasia, facial deformities such as low-set eyebrows, broad nasal bridge, irregular teeth and low-set ears. More serious abnormalities, including cleft lip and palate, congenital heart disease and spina bifida, are less common. The incidence of neural tube defects is particularly common with sodium valproate (1.5%) and carbamazepine (1%). The newer antiepileptics (gabapentin, lamotrigine and vigabatrin) are not licensed for use in pregnancy, although there is no evidence to date that they are teratogenic in humans.

Epileptic women who wish to become pregnant should receive advice about the risk of congenital abnormality, and also about the need to continue treatment. The lowest dose of a single agent should be used wherever possible. Folic acid should be given before and for 12 weeks after conception. Screening for neural tube defects (α-fetoprotein levels and ultrasound) should be performed if sodium valproate or carbamazepine is used.

Most antiepileptics are excreted in breast milk, but concentrations are usually low and not harmful to the infant.

NB   Carbamazepine, phenytoin and phenobarbitone all induce hepatic microsomal enzymes and increase metabolism of oestrogens and progestagens, making oral contraception unreliable. Sodium valproate and the newer add-on agents (gabapentin, lamotrigine and vigabatrin) do not affect the efficacy of oral contraceptives.

Prognosis in epilepsy

Six years after diagnosis, 40% of patients will have been fit-free for 5 years. Relatively poor prognoses are associated with combinations of grand mal with other seizures, traumatic epilepsy, clustering of episodes, physical signs and mental

> **TRIAL**
>
> The **Medical Research Council Antiepileptic Drug Withdrawal Study Group** randomized 1013 patients to continuation or slow withdrawal of treatment. A total of 78% of those still on treatment and 59% of those in whom it had been withdrawn were seizure-free after 2 years. *Lancet* 1991; **337**: 1175–1180.

retardation. Attempts to withdraw treatment in patients who are symptom-free should be considered on an individual basis.

EPILEPSY AND DRIVING

See p. 462.

Advice to the patient with epilepsy

There are no rules, but it seems sensible to avoid heights, ladders, unsupervised swimming and cycling for 2 years from the last episode. Fires should be guarded and children should not be left in the bath unattended. Patients with epilepsy are unable to perform certain occupations (e.g. the armed forces, jobs involving driving), but epilepsy should not be a bar to most occupations.

Narcolepsy

This rare condition usually starts in late puberty. The onset is sudden, with episodes of irresistible and inappropriate sleep usually without fatigue, though often in sleep-provoking circumstances such as medical lectures. It is associated with cataplexy—attacks of sudden, brief muscle atonia without loss of consciousness often precipitated by laughter (also in medical lectures?). There may be abnormal mental states while passing between awake and asleep: sleep paralysis like cataplexy, and pre-sleep hallucinations like vivid dreams. These are disorders of rapid eye movement (REM) sleep and are strongly associated with human leukocyte antigen (HLA) DR2. Narcolepsy may respond to amphetamines, and cataplexy to clomipramine.

Multiple sclerosis

A demyelinating disease characterized by episodes of neurological deficit appearing irregularly throughout the CNS both in anatomical site and time. Prevalence is 50–80/100 000 with a slight preponderance in females. First episodes usually occur in young adulthood, with a peak at around 30 years.

Aetiology

Current evidence suggests an acquired autoimmunity against myelin proteins. This is determined in part by genetic susceptibility as evidenced by:
- racial variation;
- clustering in families, and excess concordance in monozygotic versus dizygotic twins; and
- HLA associations—in particular between multiple sclerosis in white patients and HLA DR15, DQ6, Dw2.

Geographical variations, with a high prevalence in temperate climates, emphasize the importance of environmental factors. Individuals who migrate before the age of 15 acquire the risk of the country to which they have migrated.

Experimental autoimmune encephalomyelitis (EAE) has provided a model for studying multiple sclerosis. EAE is a T-cell-mediated disease which is produced by immunizing animals with myelin basic proteins.

Pathology

Patches of demyelination occur in discrete areas (plaques) in the white matter of the brain and spinal cord, especially in:

- optic nerves—the commonest initial site;
- brainstem;
- cerebellar peduncles; and
- dorsal and pyramidal (lateral) tracts.

Oedema around acute lesions contributes to the neurological deficit. Function typically improves as oedema resolves. Later, scarring gives rise to the characteristic white plaque.

Clinical presentation

Plaques can occur at any site, so presentation is extremely variable. Symptoms include visual disturbance, clumsiness, weakness, numbness, tremor, cognitive impairment, bowel or bladder disturbance and sexual dysfunction.

Typical features

- *Visual disturbance* — almost all patients have visual loss or diplopia at some stage. Between 30 and 70% of patients with isolated optic neuritis subsequently develop multiple sclerosis. Recovery from optic neuritis is characterized by optic atrophy or temporal pallor of the disc.
- *Upper motor neuron deficit* with weakness, as a paraparesis, hemiparesis, or monoparesis.
- *Sensory deficit* with paraesthesia and proprioceptive loss in a limb or half of the body.
- *Cerebellar signs* with intention tremor, nystagmus, vertigo and dysarthria.
- *Bladder dysfunction* is common, and is occasionally the presenting complaint. Initially there is urgency and frequency, followed by incontinence. Constipation is the usual *bowel disturbance*, but urgency of defecation can occur. *Erectile impotence* and *ejaculatory failure* are common.
- *Cognitive impairment* — IQ and language skills often remain until late in the disease. However, memory, learning and the ability to deal with abstract concepts often deteriorate in chronic forms.

Chronic progressive forms are characterized by evidence of optic atrophy, cerebellar lesions and spastic paraparesis, frequently with posterior column loss. There is dementia with altered mood—both depression and euphoria occur.

Symptoms are commonly made worse by exertion and heat (patients may be able to get into a hot bath but not out of it).

Diagnosis

Clinically the diagnosis is made on the basis of at least two characteristic episodes of neurological dysfunction.

Visually evoked potentials (VEP) test the integrity of the visual pathways. Demyelination causes an abnormality (usually delay) in occipital EEG tracings in response to a stimulus such as a chessboard pattern presented to the eyes. Abnormalities are present in 95% of patients with multiple sclerosis but it is not specific. Sensory and auditory evoked potentials may also show delay.

Lumbar puncture reveals a raised CSF protein (up to 1 g/l) in 50% of patients. The most useful test in CSF is immunoelectrophoresis, which shows an increased proportion of immunoglobulin G (IgG) in 60% and oligoclonal bands in 90%.

MRI is the imaging procedure of choice for the diagnosis of multiple sclerosis. Plaques of demyelination appear as bright lesions, which are especially numerous in the periventricular area. Clinically silent lesions are frequently revealed. Refinements such as fluid attenuation inversion recovery (FLAIR) MRI can be used to suppress the signal from CSF and detect lesion in the spinal cord.

Prognosis

The average duration of life from onset of symptoms is 20–30 years. Overall, 80% experience steadily progressive disability, 15% follow a relatively benign course and 5% die in 5 years. There may be a long latent period (15–30 years) after an episode of optic neuritis before further neurological symptoms occur. Patients whose disease onset is sensory rather than motor tend to have a better prognosis. Poor prognostic factors are older age of onset, early cerebellar involvement and loss of mental acuity.

Management

Physiotherapy, rehabilitation, pharmacological treatment, surgery and psychological support all have a role. Support for the family should be provided.

Visual loss. High-dose intravenous steroids accelerate visual recovery in isolated optic neuritis (see Trials below), and delays the onset of further neurological signs.

Weakness. Physiotherapy and rehabilitation are important. Several studies have shown a benefit from aminopyridines, which promote nerve conduction by blocking potassium channels in excitatory nerve membranes.

Spasticity. This responds to stretching exercises, alone or in combination with antispasmodic agents such as benzodiazepines or baclofen. Baclofen is a GABA analogue that binds to GABA receptors in the dorsal horn of the spinal cord. Dantrolene sodium acts directly on skeletal muscle to reduce spasm. Intractable spasticity may require tendonotomy or neurectomy.

Bladder dysfunction. Antimuscarinic agents (e.g. oxybutinin, flavoxate) increase bladder capacity by diminishing unstable detrusor contractions. α-Adrenoceptor blockers (e.g. prazosin, terazosin) relax smooth muscle and may also be of benefit.

TRIALS

The **IFNβ multiple sclerosis study group** compared interferon-β (IFN-β) and placebo in a double-blind multicentre study of 372 ambulatory patients with relapsing–remitting multiple sclerosis. IFN-β was effective in reducing relapses over a 3-year period, but did not significantly affect disability. Neurology 1993; **48**: 655–661.

The **optic neuritis study group** compared intravenous steroids (methylprednisolone 250 mg qds for 3 days followed by oral prednisone for 11 days), oral steroids and placebo in 457 patients with optic neuritis. Intravenous steroids accelerated visual recovery from optic neuritis, and delayed subsequent development of multiple sclerosis over a 2-year period. By 4 years the rate of developing multiple sclerosis was similar in all three treatment groups. N Engl J Med 1993; **329**: 1764–1769.

Antidiuretic hormone (vasopressin), and its synthetic analogue desmopressin, have been used to control disabling nocturia. Self-catheterization enables some patients to remain free from a permanent indwelling catheter.

Sexual dysfunction. Counselling should be provided. Intracavernosal injection of papaverine may be of value in erectile impotence.

Psychological support. This is essential. Patients often remain surprisingly euphoric, but not infrequently there is marked depression.

Motor neurone disease

This disease involves progressive degeneration of:
- anterior horn cells in the spinal cord;
- cells of the lower cranial motor nuclei; and
- neurons of the motor cortex with secondary degeneration of the pyramidal tracts.

Clinical presentation

Motor neurone disease usually presents between the ages of 50 and 70 years, slightly more frequently in men than women (1.5 : 1), with the clinical features of one of the above groups but usually progresses to produce features of the other two as well. It is rare in all its forms: UK prevalence is 5/100 000 of the population (incidence 1.5/100 000). It is characterized by:
- muscular weakness and fasciculation; and
- absence of sensory signs.

There are three classical forms of clinical presentation.

1 Lower motor neuron weakness, with wasting and fasciculation of the small muscles of the hand. This is followed by wasting of the upper and lower limb muscles. This lower motor neuron wasting and fasciculation is termed *progressive muscular atrophy*.

2 Lower motor neuron weakness, fasciculation and wasting of the tongue and pharynx producing dysarthria, dysphagia, choking and nasal regurgitation (*progressive bulbar palsy*).

3 Upper motor neuron spastic weakness starting in the legs, and later spreading to the arms (*amyotrophic lateral sclerosis*).

Any combination of the above three groups can occur. In most cases upper and lower motor neuron lesions are combined at the time of presentation.

Fasciculation of some limb musculature is a hallmark of this disease. Lower limb lesions are usually of upper motor neuron type, and the upper limb lesions of lower motor neuron type. The limbs may demonstrate marked muscular wasting but still have exaggerated reflexes. The abdominal reflexes are usually preserved until late in the disease. Pseudobulbar palsy (p. 15) may occur but is very uncommon. The bladder is not affected.

Parkinson's disease and extrapyramidal disorders

PARKINSON'S DISEASE

James Parkinson, 1755–1824, London
Prevalence: 1–1.5/1000 in the UK (1/200 in those over 70 years).

Clinical presentation

This is a disturbance of voluntary motor function characterized by the triad of *rigidity*, *tremor* and *bradykinesia* (slow movements) plus postural abnormalities. Vague muscle ache and clumsiness with physical and mental fatigue may be seen, in retrospect, to have been early evidence.

The classical picture of parkinsonism is of immobile flexion at all joints (neck, trunk, shoulders, elbows, wrists and metacarpophalangeal joints) except the interphalangeal. Even in the early case, on walking, the arms do not swing fully and later in the disease the gait is stuttering and shuffling and the patient may show festination. He or she is slow and unstable on the turn and may freeze. The face is expressionless and unblinking, and speech slurred and monotonous. In the longstanding case, other symptoms are commonly present: difficulty in initiating movement (starting to walk, rising from a chair or turning in bed), poor balance with a tendency to fall because of slow correcting movements, small hand-writing, seborrhoea especially of the face, rarely increased salivation (which, with dysphagia, may give rise to drooling), and a soft unintelligible voice (dysarthria). Constipation and urinary frequency occur, sometimes with incontinence.

Oculogyric crises (forced upwards deviation of the eyes) occur characteristically in drug-induced and postencephalitic parkinsonism. These patients may also have symptoms of the side effects of treatment (see below).

The tremor (4–6/s) is usually most obvious in the hands ('pill-rolling'), improved by voluntary movement and made worse by anxiety. Titubation refers to tremor involving the head. Repeated movements, such as tapping with the fingers, though regular in rate and amplitude (unlike those with cerebellar disorders), are reduced in both amplitude and speed. The rigidity may be lead-pipe or, with the tremor superimposed, cogwheel. The patient may demonstrate a glabellar tap sign —the patient continues to blink when the mid-forehead between the eyebrows is repeatedly tapped. False positives are fairly common. Parkinsonism is usually asymmetrical. Patients are frequently, and understandably, depressed. Dementia with confusion and hallucination may supervene later.

Aetiology of parkinsonism

Idiopathic Parkinson's disease (paralysis agitans)

This is of slow onset and inexorably progressive. It presents in the 50–60-year age group and in males more often than females. It results from deficiency of dopamine in the substantia nigra and relative excess of acetylcholine stimulation in the corpus striatum as a consequence. Dopamine granules are reduced in the cells of the substantia nigra. It is asymmetrical, particularly at first, and may be familial.

Atherosclerosis

This is often associated with other manifestations of vascular disease (stroke, dementia, ischaemic heart disease, intermittent claudication and hypertension). There tends to be less tremor and more festination than in idiopathic parkinsonism.

Drugs

Neuroleptics, e.g. chlorpromazine and, less commonly, reserpine, may produce parkinsonism. The high doses used in psychiatry make it relatively common in schizophrenics. Dystonic movements—facial grimacing, involuntary movements of the tongue and oculogyric crises—are more common than in idiopathic parkinsonism, and are usually symmetrical. Tremor is less common.

NB   Acute extrapyramidal syndromes (grinding teeth, masseter spasm) may result from phenothiazines used as sedatives (e.g. perphenazine) and other dopa antagonists such as metoclopramide. They respond rapidly to intravenous procyclidine.

Poisoning

Rarely, Parkinson-like disorders may result from poisoning with heavy metals e.g. manganese and copper (NB Wilson's disease, p. 147) and after carbon monoxide poisoning.

Postencephalitic

Parkinsonism occurred following outbreaks of encephalitis lethargica (between 1917 and 1925—before even we were born) and still occurs sporadically.

Punch-drunk syndrome
This is due to brain damage in boxers.

Management
The object is to reduce each of the symptoms—rigidity, tremor and bradykinesia. This debilitating chronic illness requires specific drug therapy and expert supportive physiotherapy, occupational and speech therapy.

Levodopa is the drug of choice for idiopathic parkinsonism. It is effective in 75% of patients (excellent in 20%), particularly in those with bradykinesia, less so in those with tremor. It is not used in drug-induced parkinsonism. It is not given alone because the side effects of levodopa (anorexia, nausea and vomiting) are reduced by concomitant administration of a peripheral dopa-decarboxylase inhibitor. It is therefore usually given as Madopar (with benserazide) or Sinemet (with carbidopa).

The monoamine oxidase (B) inhibitor, *selegiline*, used in conjunction with levodopa may slow the disease process.

Late side effects of levodopa include the sudden unpredictable swings of the on/off syndrome, peak-dose dyskinesias (often welcomed), early-morning akinesia and end-of-dose failure. This is managed by increasing the dose frequency (but not the total daily dose) of the levodopa preparation using a slow-release preparation and adding selegiline and/or bromocriptine. Hallucinatory psychosis and dementia may develop. Anticholinergic therapy can be effective in the elderly who are at risk of confusion.

Transplantation of fetal neuronal tissue (high in dopa) into the caudate lobe of patients with Parkinson's disease has produced variable and, more recently, disappointing results.

Notes

• *Anticholinergic drugs.* Standard atropine-like drugs can be used first in mild disease and patients intolerant of dopa, e.g. benzhexol (Artane 2 mg bd increasing to 5 mg bd), benztropine (Cogentin) and orphenadrine (Disipal). They have more effect on tremor. Side effects include blurred vision, dry mouth, tachycardia, urinary retention, constipation and glaucoma. There may be confusion and loss of concentration, especially in the elderly.

• *Amantadine* may be added to the other two groups of drugs in a dose of 100 mg bd, but helps only a few and tolerance quickly develops.

• *Bromocriptine*, a dopamine agonist, can be of value in those patients who cannot tolerate levodopa or those in whom control is unsatisfactory. It tends to be ineffective in those who are not primarily improved by levodopa. Its chief indication therefore is for late failure of levodopa. It is started in small doses (1.25 mg) before bed and the dose is gradually increased. The commonest side effect is nausea: domperidone can be added to control the nausea if necessary.

• *Pergolide* is a D_2 receptor agonist which can be useful in reducing 'off' periods.

- *Apomorphine* stimulates D_1 and D_2 receptors. It can only be given parenterally.
- *Stereotactic thalamotomy* is used only for intractable symptoms of rigidity and tremor in the non-dominant limbs on the contralateral side.
- *Depression* is easy to overlook in parkinsonism due to reduced emotional expression. It should be treated with a tricyclic antidepressant but not with monoamine oxidase inhibitors since the combination with levodopa may induce acute hypertension.

The remaining extrapyramidal disorders are very uncommon.

Neurodegenerative diseases

A number of these have parkinsonism as a component.

1 Alzheimer's disease with gross early cognitive impairment.
2 The 'Parkinson-plus' syndromes:
   (a) Steele–Richardson–Olszewski syndrome with failure of voluntary gaze (see below);
   (b) Shy–Drager syndrome with autonomic failure and postural hypotension; and
   (c) multi-system atrophy with cerebellar and pyramidal involvement.

Steele–Richardson–Olszewski syndrome

This is a very rare condition which affects males more than females (2:1) in late middle age. It is a degenerative condition of the upper brain stem akin to Parkinson's disease and often confused with it in the early stages. It may start with no more than an expressionless facies and a rigidly-held spine, though the patient should stand straight rather than stooped. There may be lead-pipe rigidity and cog-wheeling. Characteristically, voluntary vertical eye movements become progressively more fixed, and then laterally and with convergence. Pseudobulbar palsy leads to dysphagia, dysarthria and emotional lability. Falls are common. As with parkinsonism, there may be some mild dementia.

HEPATOLENTICULAR DEGENERATION

(Wilson's disease).

Aetiology

It is an autosomal recessive disorder where the primary defect is a failure to excrete copper into the bile. Accumulation of hepatic copper inhibits the formation of caeruloplasmin, the copper-binding serum protein. When the storage capacity of the hepatocytes is exceeded, copper is released into the blood and is deposited in the:

- liver producing cirrhosis, hepatosplenomegaly and jaundice;
- basal ganglia producing choreoathetosis;
- cerebrum producing dementia and emotional lability;
- eyes producing Kayser–Fleischer rings (a green–gold 'fuzz') around the cornea, and cataract in the lens;

- renal tubules (rarely) producing the effects of heavy metal poisoning and renal tubular acidosis (aminoaciduria, phosphaturia, glycosuria and hypercalciuria);
- bones to produce osteoporosis and osteoarthritis; and
- red cells to produce haemolytic anaemia.

The cerebral type is commoner than the hepatic type.

Management

- Low dietary copper intake.
- D-penicillamine (1–2 g daily for 6 months to 2 years followed by maintenance treatment) — a chelating agent to increase 24-h urinary copper excretion.

The prognosis for improvement is very good. Siblings should be examined and screened for low serum copper and caeruloplasmin plus increased 24-h urinary copper output.

CHOREA

This term describes jerky, explosive involuntary movements, usually of the face and/or arms, which appear pseudopurposive unless very marked. They may interfere with voluntary movements of limbs and with speech, eating and respiration. They cease during sleep.

Chorea may follow a stroke or kernicterus. It may occur in pregnancy (chorea gravidarum) and with the oral contraceptive, and may be congenital.

Huntington's chorea

George Sumner Huntington, 1851–1916, America.

This is a Mendelian dominant disorder on the short arm of chromosome 4 and there is usually a family history. GABA and acetylcholine are reduced in the substantia nigra and globus pallidus. The symptoms usually start between 30 and 45 years of age. The chorea is distal initially and involves the legs (with ataxia), arms (with clumsiness) and face. The movements are rapid and jerky. Epilepsy occurs. Mental changes develop gradually, usually without insight, and progress to dementia and death in about 10–15 years. The chorea may respond to tetrabenazine.

The Huntington's disease gene (chromosome 4) contains an expanded CAG trinucleotide repeat (p. 174). Identification of the genetic mutation increases the precision of genetic testing.

Presymptomatic testing for Huntington's disease must be approached with great care because of the implications of a positive test for the patient and family.

Sydenham's chorea

Thomas Sydenham, 1624–1689, English.

A child of 5–15 years (female more often than male) is described as restless, clumsy or fidgety. There is proximal chorea of the arms (and less so, the legs) and grimacing. It is associated with rheumatic fever and usually recovers completely in

2–3 months. It must be differentiated from a nervous tic. It is very rare now in the UK.

Cerebral tumours

They are rare with a UK incidence of 1/20 000 and may be primary (20%) or secondary (80% from bronchus, breasts, kidney, colon, ovary, prostate or thyroid). Primary tumours originate from:

- supporting tissues such as gliomas (50%; or astrocytomas), oligodendrogliomas and ependymomas (both benign);
- meninges producing meningiomas (25%);
- blood vessels—angiomas and angioblastomas; and
- nervous tissue (very rare).

Symptoms and signs

Caused by raised intracranial pressure

- Headache, classically throbbing bilateral frontal and early-morning, associated with nausea, vomiting and later papilloedema and increased by stooping.
- Mental confusion, change in personality, apathy, drowsiness and dementia.
- 6th-nerve palsy results from pressure on the nerve as it crosses the petrous temporal bone (a 'false localizing sign').

Epilepsy

Occurs in 30% of tumours, particularly of the frontal or temporal lobe.

Progressive focal signs

These depend upon the site of the tumour.

- *Prefrontal.* Progressive dementia with loss of affect and social responsibility. Anosmia may be present and the grasp reflex is present in the contralateral hand.
- *Precentral.* Contralateral hemiplegia and Jacksonian epilepsy.
- *Parietal.* The chief parietal signs are falling away of the contralateral outstretched arm, astereognosis and tactile inattention. Apraxia and spatial disorientation may occur. Low-sited tumours may produce lower quadrantic homonymous hemianopia rather than complete homonymous hemianopia (or visual inattention). Dysphasia occurs with lesions in the dominant temporoparietal region.
- *Temporal lobe.* Symptoms of temporal lobe epilepsy with aphasia (if on the dominant side) and an upper quadrantic homonymous hemianopia.
- *Occipital lobe.* Lesions produce homonymous hemianopia, either complete or quandrantic, with macular sparing.

Investigation

Screen for primary neoplasms at the sites which most frequently metastasize to the brain (bronchus, breast and kidney). Perform fluorescent treponemal antibody absorption (FTAA) and *Treponema pallidum* haemagglutinin (TPHA) tests for syphilis and plasma protein electrophoresis for myeloma.

Raised alkaline phosphatase and calcium suggest associated secondary bone deposits. CT or nuclear magnetic resonance scanning is the investigation of choice. Lumbar puncture is dangerous because of the risk of coning.

ACOUSTIC NEUROMA

A neurofibroma of the acoustic (8th) nerve. It is relatively rare and is more common in neurofibromatosis.

Clinical presentation

Typically, symptoms begin at 35–45 years with progressive deafness and diminished reaction on caloric testing, sometimes with tinnitus and mild vertigo. Pressure on other nerves and the brainstem of the same side at the cerebellopontine angle produce:
- 7th nerve: facial palsy;
- 5th nerve: weakness of mastication, loss of corneal reflex and facial sensory loss;
- 6th nerve: lateral rectus palsy;
- cerebellar syndrome (ipsilateral).

Investigation

Skull radiology may reveal erosion of the internal auditory meatus and/or petrous temporal bone. CT scanning will confirm the diagnosis. CSF protein is usually considerably raised to above 1 g/l. It is a slowly enlarging tumour and by the time it presents may be large (3–6 cm in diameter). Because of this and its vascularity, it is easily seen on an enhanced CT scan.

NB   Check for associated neurofibromata, especially of adrenal medulla, thyroid, parathyroid, cranial nerves, spinal nerve roots and meninges.

BENIGN INTRACRANIAL HYPERTENSION

This mimics cerebral tumour with headaches and papilloedema. It may be due to impaired absorption of CSF by the arachnoid villi. It is commoner in obese young women and is associated with oral contraceptives and pregnancy, and may follow head injury and treatment of infection (e.g. otitis media). The blind spot can enlarge and sight may be threatened. Lumbar puncture shows normal CSF under high pressure. CSF pressure is uniform in the cerebrum, so a CT scan shows normal ventricles and sulci. The absence of pressure gradient reduces the risk of coning on lumbar puncture. It tends to recover spontaneously in a few months, but carbonic anhydrase inhibitors (e.g. acetazolamide), steroids or peritoneal shunting may be required.

Peripheral neuropathy

A disorder of peripheral nerves, either sensory, motor or mixed, usually symmetrical and affecting distal more than proximal parts of the limbs. By convention isolated cranial nerve palsies and isolated and multiple peripheral nerve lesions (median, ulnar, lateral popliteal palsies and mononeuritis multiplex) are excluded.

Aetiology

In general medical practice four disorders must be considered: diabetes mellitus, carcinomatous neuropathy, vitamin B deficiency (including B_{12}) and drugs or chemicals. Only the first is common.

Diabetic neuropathy

Apart from causing isolated cranial and peripheral nerve lesions (including mononeuritis multiplex), diabetes causes a distal, predominantly sensory, neuropathy affecting commonly the distal lower limbs in a stocking distribution. Symptoms of numbness, paraesthesiae and sometimes pain in the feet are associated with loss of vibration and position sense. Characteristically the ankle reflex is lost (see p. 224).

Carcinomatous neuropathy

Carcinoma may be associated with either a sensory neuropathy affecting the 'glove-and-stocking' regions or motor neuropathy in which there is muscle weakness and wasting, usually of the proximal limb muscles. The neuropathy may be mixed. If distal muscles are affected, the neuropathy may be indistinguishable from any motor neurone disease.

Vitamin B deficiency

Sensory neuropathy characterizes deficiency of vitamin B_1. Patients, often alcoholics, present with numbness ('walking on cotton wool') and paraesthesiae. Pain and soreness of the feet may be a feature. In vitamin B_{12} deficiency the peripheral neuropathy may be associated with subacute combined degeneration of the cord (p. 164) and megaloblastic anaemia (p. 420).

Drugs

Peripheral neuropathy may result from treatment for tuberculosis with isoniazid, which is pyridoxine-dependent and occurs in 'slow acetylators'. Other drugs include vincristine, vinblastine, phenytoin and nitrofurantoin.

Other rare causes

Uraemia, myxoedema, polyarteritis nodosa, heavy-metal and industrial poisoning (e.g. lead, triorthocresyl phosphate), infectious disorders (leprosy, diphtheria, Guillain–Barré syndrome), amyloidosis, sarcoidosis and porphyria.

NB   Investigation of patients with peripheral neuropathy is aimed at excluding underlying carcinoma and confirming the other common and treatable disorders. In about 50% of cases the aetiology remains unknown.

Brachial neuralgia (neuralgic amyotrophy)

This may follow a presumed virus infection and presents with pain in a shoulder (C5 dermatome) and root pain down the arm with rapidly progressive weakness and wasting (usually of C5–6 innervated muscles). Sensory loss is segmental in distribution. Adjacent nerve roots may be involved. The sensory symptoms usually resolve completely but the weakness and wasting may not.

Mononeuritis multiplex

A disorder affecting two or more peripheral nerves at one time, producing symptoms of numbness, paraesthesiae and sometimes pain in their sensory distribution with associated muscle weakness and wasting. The lower limbs are more commonly affected and the neuropathy is asymmetrical. This uncommon syndrome occurs in diabetes mellitus, carcinoma, amyloidosis, polyarteritis nodosa and, less commonly, in other collagen diseases. Leprosy is the commonest cause worldwide but the diagnosis is then usually obvious.

Hereditary ataxias

These are familial disorders, usually transmitted as Mendelian dominants. Pathological changes of degeneration are present in one or more of the optic nerves, cerebellum, olives and long ascending tracts of the spinal cord. Each family presents its own particular variants. All are rare.

FRIEDREICH'S ATAXIA
Pathology
Degeneration is maximal in the dorsal and lateral (pyramidal) columns of the cord and the spinocerebellar tracts. It is autosomal recessive.

Clinical presentation
Cerebellar ataxia is noted at 5–15 years affecting first the lower and then upper limbs. Pes cavus and spinal scoliosis may be present. Pyramidal tract involvement produces upper motor neuron lesions of the legs, and dorsal column involvement sensory changes and absent ankle jerks. Arrhythmias and heart failure are common due to cardiomyopathy. There may be optic atrophy. Mild dementia occurs late in the disease and patients die from cardiac disease in their 40s.

CEREBELLAR DEGENERATIONS
This group of hereditary ataxias affects primarily the cerebellum and the cerebel-

lar connections of the brainstem. All are rare. These disorders may present in late middle age and must be distinguished from:

- tumours of the posterior fossa;
- primary degeneration secondary to bronchial carcinomas; and
- myxoedema.

HEREDITARY SPASTIC PARAPLEGIA

The pyramidal tracts are affected and the patients develop progressive spasticity. The onset occurs from childhood to middle age. The disorder, when first seen, must be distinguished from cord compression (which may require emergency decompression) and multiple sclerosis in the elderly. Dantrolene sodium or baclofen reduces spasticity.

Meningitis

Aetiology

Besides the bacterial and viral causes listed in Table 11.1, the following points should be considered.

- Tuberculosis meningitis is easily missed and should be considered in the differential diagnosis of all cases of viral meningitis.
- Cerebral tumours, lymphomatous infiltration, abscesses and venous sinus thrombosis may produce a lymphocytosis and raised protein in the CSF.
- Neck stiffness and headache without more severe signs may follow a small sub-arachnoid haemorrhage.
- Diabetics may be precipitated into coma by meningitis.
- The confident diagnosis of meningism may mean failure to diagnose meningitis.
- If in doubt, lumbar puncture should be performed.
- Pneumococcal meningitis is often secondary to underlying pneumococcal infection in the lung, sinuses, or ear.

Clinical features

These are:

- infection;
- meningism ($\pm$ mild encephalitic features); and
- raised intracranial pressure.

MENINGOCOCCAL MENINGITIS

The meningitis is part of a septicaemia. The meningococcus is carried in the nasopharynx often asymptomatically (carriers) and tends to produce epidemics of infection chiefly in children and young adults. These occur in conditions of over-crowding and in closed communities. After a short incubation period of 1–3 days the disease begins abruptly with fever, headache, nausea, vomiting and neck stiff-ness. Mental confusion and coma may follow. There may be a characteristic rash

CAUSES OF MENINGITIS

Organism	Special clinical features	CSF	Microbiology	Antibiotic of choice
Common causes				
Meningococcus	Purpuric rash Septicaemic shock	Polymorphs: 0.5–2.0 × 10⁹/l Protein: 1–3 g/l Glucose: very low	Gram-negative intracellular diplococci Positive blood culture Positive CSF immunoelectrophoresis	Penicillin
Pneumococcus	Cranial nerve damage Otitis media Lobar pneumonia High mortality (10–20%)	Polymorphs: 0.5–2.0 × 10⁹/l Protein: 1–3g/l Glucose: very low	Gram-positive diplococci Positive blood culture Positive CSF immunoelectrophoresis	Penicillin
Haemophilus influenzae	Commonest in children under 5 years	Polymorphs: 0.5–2.0 × 10⁹/l Protein: 1–3 g/l Glucose: very low	Gram-negative bacilli	Cefotaxime (ampicillin)
Coxsackievirus and echovirus	Paralysis (very rare)	Lymphocytes: 0.05–0.5 × 10⁹/l Protein: 0.5–1 g/l Glucose: normal	Positive throat swab Positive stool culture Serum antibody: rising titre	None
Mumps virus		Lymphocytes: 0.05–0.5 × 10⁹/l Protein: 0.5–1 g/l Glucose: normal	Positive throat swab Positive stool culture Serum antibody: rising titre	None
Rare causes				
Mycobacterium tuberculosis	Subacute onset Altered personality Strokes Cranial nerve lesions Fits in children Pyrexia of unknown origin	Lymphocytes 0.1–0.6 × 10⁹/l Protein: 1–6 g/l Glucose: low, <1.4 mmol/l	Acid- and alcohol-fast bacilli Ziehl–Neelsen staining and fluorescence microscopy	See pp. 157 and 346
Leptosptra ictero-haemorrhaglae (Weil's disease)	Follows exposure to rat urine (sewers) Associated hepatitis and nephritis High peripheral white blood cell count: 10–20 × 10⁹/l	Lymphocytes: 0.2–0.3 × 10⁹/l Protein: raised by 0.5–1.5 g/l Glucose: normal	Serum antibody: rising titre	Penicillin
Lyme disease	Associated with cranial nerve lesions (unilateral or bilateral seventh nerve and asymmetrical arthalgia and erythema chronicum migrans	Immunofluorescent antibody tested		Penicillin
Poliovirus	Meningitis (common) Asymmetrical paralysis (rare) Polio incidence increasing with decrease in immunization	Lymphocytes: 0.05–0.5 × 10⁹/l Protein: 0.5–1 g/l Glucose: normal	Positive throat swab Positive stool culture Serum antibody: rising titre	None

NB   Other rare causes: acquired immunodeficiency syndrome (AIDS), herpes simplex virus, arbovirus, *Staphylococcus*, *Listeria*, *Pseudomonas*, *Cryptococcus* in immunosuppressed; *Escherichia coli*, streptococci and *Listeria* in neonates.

Table 11.2 Bacterial and viral causes of meningitis.

with widespread irregular petechiae of variable size. There is risk of cardiorespiratory collapse and consumption coagulopathy (p. 105).

Vaccines are only available against groups A and C. Most cases in the UK are group B. Travellers to at-risk areas should be immunized.

Lumbar puncture

The CSF is purulent and shows a raised protein to about 1–3 g/l (100–300 mg/100 ml), 500–2000 polymorphs/mm^3 and a low or almost absent sugar. Intracellular and extracellular Gram-negative diplococci are present. The organism can also be isolated in blood culture.

Treatment

Drug of choice
Benzylpencillin 2–4 g infusion 6-hourly.

Second-line treatment (when the patient is allergic to penicillins)
Cefotaxime (1–2 g, 8-hourly) or chloramphenicol (20 mg/kg body weight, 6-hourly).

Supportive therapy with fluids, inotropes and clotting factors may be needed.

In hospital they should be isolated for 24 h from the onset of treatment and close family contacts should be given rifampicin.

PNEUMOCOCCAL MENINGITIS

Infection may be secondary to pneumococcal pneumonia or it may spread from infected sinuses or ears or through fractures of the base of the skull. It is commoner in paediatric and geriatric practice, and after splenectomy. Symptoms develop rapidly, sometimes within hours, and fever, headache, nausea and vomiting may quickly proceed to coma.

Lumbar puncture

The CSF is purulent with a raised protein, high polymorph count and low sugar. Gram-positive diplococci are present. Blood culture is often positive (as it is in pneumococcal pneumonia).

Treatment

Drug of choice
Benzylpenicillin, as for meningococcal meningitis. The dose can be reduced after about 3–4 days provided the fever has fallen and there is clinical improvement. Treatment should continue for 10 days.

Second-line treatment
Cefotaxime or chloramphenicol, as for meningococcal meningitis.

Pneumococcal meningitis is extremely serious and especially so if the patient is in coma before therapy is started. The overall mortality is high (20–30%).

HAEMOPHILUS INFLUENZAE MENINGITIS

This usually occurs in children under 5 years old because after that age they develop specific antibodies. It may be insidious in onset with a longer incubation period than in the meningitides described above (5 days). It usually follows an influenzal-type illness and presents with fever, nausea and vomiting.

Lumbar puncture

The CSF is purulent with a high protein and polymorph count and low sugar. Gram-negative bacilli can be seen, and grown on culture.

Treatment

Drugs of choice

Cefotaxime 1–2g 8-hourly; chloramphenicol 3–5g daily (children 50–100mg/kg per day for 10 days, though a lower dose is required in the neonate) is an alternative.

   The overall mortality is 5–10%.

Intrathecal penicillin therapy

There is little evidence to support the use of intrathecal benzylpenicillin therapy through the lumbar puncture needle on finding a purulent CSF. Some physicians consider daily intrathecal and intraventricular therapy of value in pneumococcal meningitis if the patient is unconscious on admission, as the mortality is so high (50%). There is no good evidence that this improves the outlook.

ACUTE BACTERIAL MENINGITIS OF UNKNOWN CAUSE

This problem occurs when a purulent CSF is obtained from a patient with meningitis but no organisms are seen with Gram staining. This is most frequently due to pre-admission antibiotic therapy. There is no time to wait for the results of culture and antibiotics should be started immediately. In adults there are a number of recommended courses of action, any of which should treat effectively the common organisms found (i.e. pneumococcus, meningococcus, *Haemophilus influenzae*), i.e.:

- Cefotaxime is the drug of choice.
- Chloramphenicol with penicillin is an alternative.

   The use of chloramphenicol with penicillin, although theoretically inadvisable (bacteriostatic drug with a bactericidal one respectively), is used in some centres with considerable success.

TUBERCULOUS MENINGITIS   (see also Tuberculosis, pp. 346 and 460)

This may present as acute meningitis but more commonly as an insidious illness with fever, weight loss and progressive signs of confusion and cerebral irritation leading to mental deterioration and finally coma.

   The CSF looks opalescent and by investigation resembles viral meningitis but the glucose is very low.

Three of four drugs (rifampicin, isoniazid with pyridoxine, ethambutol and pyrazinamide) should be given initially and the dose of isoniazid doubled. If streptomycin is used, blood levels must be monitored to prevent ototoxicity. (There is no place for intrathecal streptomycin.)

VIRAL MENINGITIS

A large number of viruses have been implicated, including enteroviruses (coxsackie A and B, echoviruses, polioviruses), herpesviruses (herpes simplex virus-1, (HSV-1), HSV-2, Epstein–Barr virus, varicella-zoster virus), mumps, measles and adenoviruses. The CSF is clear with normal or raised protein content, and normal glucose. Mononuclear cells may be seen, but there are no organisms. The symptoms of headache and meningism are self-limiting.

HERPES SIMPLEX ENCEPHALITIS

Encephalitis implies infection of the brain parenchyma. The commonest cause is HSV. Most episodes are thought to result from reactivation of latent virus. It occurs in otherwise healthy individuals, but is commonest in the immunosuppressed. A brief prodrome of headache, fever and malaise is followed by severe CNS dysfunction, with focal signs, seizures and coma.

CT shows low-density lesions with ring enhancement and EEG may show focal abnormalities. Lesions are commonest in the temporal lobes. CSF findings are similar to those in viral meningitis. Identification of HSV in CSF by polymerase chain reaction, rising titres to HSV and/or brain biopsy may all aid diagnosis, but treatment with acyclovir 10 mg/kg tds should be started if the diagnosis is strongly suspected.

Intracranial abscess

The primary source of the infection is usually chronic middle-ear infection (50%), the paranasal sinuses or the lungs. There may be a history of head trauma or neurosurgery. The clinical presentation is usually that of a space-occupying lesion (headache, nausea, vomiting and papilloedema, with or without focal signs) plus the evidence of the primary infection. A CT scan defines the lesion. Lumbar puncture is potentially dangerous because of the risk of coning. Neurosurgical advice should be sought concerning the optimum time for aspiration and/or open drainage. Mixed infections occur in 50%. Blood cultures and aspiration of any other infected sites help to identify the organisms.

Initial treatment is with intravenous cefotaxime with metronidazole to cover *Staphylococcus*, *Streptococcus* and anaerobes until sensitivities are known. Even with modern management the mortality is 30%. Of those who survive, a third develop epilepsy and many physicians give anticonvulsants to survivors.

Guillain–Barré syndrome

A syndrome of acute weakness and reduced tendon reflexes, with or without sensory loss. Most commonly there is an inflammatory demyelinating polyradiculoneuropathy affecting predominantly motor nerves.

Aetiology

Some patients give a history of an infectious illness preceding the onset of weakness by 1–2 weeks. Associations with enteroviruses, *Haemophilus influenzae*, *Mycoplasma*, measles and *Campylobacter jejuni* have been reported. Antibodies to ganglioside GM1 are found in 20–30% of patients. A particular strain of *C. jejuni* (Penner serogroup 19), which has been implicated in pathogenesis, contains β-*N*-acetylglucosamine residues homologous to the terminal carbohydrate residue of ganglioside GM1.

There is a strong association between antibodies to ganglioside GQ1b and the Miller–Fisher syndrome.

Clinical features

Typically paraesthesia, followed by numbness, begins in the toes and is rapidly (hours) followed by flaccid paralysis of the lower limbs which ascends to involve the arms and sometimes the facial muscles, the muscles of the palate and pharynx (causing dysphagia) and the external ocular muscles. Less commonly, the disease affects the upper limbs or the cranial nerves alone, or proximal more than distal muscles, and sensory symptoms are not always present.

Paralysis is of lower motor neuron type with flaccidity and early loss of reflexes. Maximal disability occurs at 3–4 weeks.

The major complications are:
*   respiratory failure from weakness of respiratory muscles;
*   autonomic involvement causing lability of blood pressure and arrhythmias; and
*   venous thromboembolism.

The *Miller–Fisher syndrome* is characterized by ataxia, ophthalmoplegia and areflexia in the absence of significant limb weakness.

Investigation

Lumbar puncture characteristically reveals a very high CSF protein (3–10 g/l) with no, or very few, white cells.

Differential diagnosis

Poliomyelitis is excluded by a known history of immunization, the presence of sensory symptoms, the symmetrical pattern of paralysis and the CSF findings (in polio the protein is lower and the white cell count raised).

Transverse myelitis usually causes sphincter disturbance, and is characterized by the presence of a sensory level.

The rapid speed of onset can suggest *brainstem stroke*, and in some cases myalgia is a prominent feature, raising the possibility of *muscle* or *joint disease*.

Management

The most important aspect of treatment is the prevention of complications. Complete recovery occurs over several months in 80–90% of patients.

Careful nursing with physiotherapy to maintain morale and prevent pressure sores, chest infection and contractures is required in all cases.

Anticoagulants may prevent deep venous thrombosis and death from pulmonary embolism.

TRIALS

Guillain–Barré Syndrome Trial Study Group compared intravenous methylprednisolone 500 mg daily for 5 days with placebo in 242 patients. Treatment was started within 15 days of onset of neurological symptoms. No beneficial effect of steroids was observed. *Lancet* 1993; **341**: 586–590.

The **French Cooperative Group in Plasma Exchange in Guillain–Barré Syndrome** studied the effect of four plasma exchanges with fresh frozen plasma or albumin replacement in 220 patients in a randomized controlled trial. Plasma exchange improved both short-term and 1-year functional status. Fresh frozen plasma showed no additional benefit compared with albumin. *Ann Neurol* 1992; **32**: 94–97.

The **Dutch Guillain–Barré Study Group** compared intravenous immunoglobulin with plasma exchange using a replacement fluid that did not contain immunoglobulin in 150 patients who were unable to walk independently. Treatment was started within 14 days of onset of neurological symptoms. Treatment with intravenous immunoglobulin was at least as effective as, and in some respects superior to, plasma exchange. *N Engl J Med* 1992; **326**: 1123–1129.

The **Plasma Exchange/Sandoglobulin Guillain–Barré Syndrome Trial Group** compared plasma exchange, intravenous immunoglobulin and combined plasma exchange and intravenous immunoglobulin started within 14 days of onset of neurological symptoms in 383 patients who had difficulty walking. Plasma exchange and intravenous immunoglobulin had equivalent efficacy, and the combination did not confer a significant advantage. *Lancet* 1997; **349**: 225–230.

Careful fluid balance and nutrition may be necessary if dysphagia occurs.

Peak expiratory flow rate and vital capacity should be monitored frequently. If paralysis ascends to involve respiratory muscles early ventilation is necessary. Shoulder adduction (C6, 7, 8) is a good clinical test of intercostal muscle function. Early tracheostomy is required in almost all patients with respiratory failure as muscle activity takes weeks or months to recover.

Several trials have shown that steroids have no beneficial effect. Plasma exchange is of benefit, but intravenous immunoglobulin may be as effective as, or slightly better than, plasma exchange.

Poliomyelitis

Poliovirus is one of the enteroviruses (with echovirus and Coxsackievirus) and a picorna (*pico* = small; rna = RNA) virus. The incidence in the UK has fallen dramatically since immunization began in 1957, but polio remains endemic in the tropics.

Immunization

Sabin vaccine is live attenuated poliovirus types 1, 2 and 3 given as a drop orally.

Clinical features

In areas without an immunization scheme infection with poliovirus is common, but the serious features of acute meningitis and muscle paralysis are rare.

About 90–95% of infected patients have mild upper respiratory or gastro-intestinal symptoms which settle completely. The rest have a more severe early infection with fever, sore throat, diarrhoea or constipation and muscle pains. This *minor illness* usually settles but 1–2% of patients go on to develop a *major illness* 5–10 days later with features of acute viral meningitis. A small number of patients who have acute poliovirus meningitis develop flaccid lower motor neuron muscle paralysis with loss of reflexes as a result of damage to the anterior horn cells. This may be preceded by muscular pain. The legs are most commonly affected and paralysis may spread to involve the arms and the medulla oblongata and lower pons, causing a bulbar palsy.

Respiratory failure is due to paralysis of the respiratory muscles and may be further complicated by aspiration pneumonia following the dysphagia and inability to cough caused by bulbar palsy. There are no sensory neurological changes.

Diagnosis

CSF is the same as other forms of virus meningitis (see p. 157) with raised protein (50–100 g/dl), increased cells, initially polymorphs, followed by lymphocytes 50–400/mm³. The sugar is normal.

The virus can be grown from throat, stool and CSF and paired sera will show a rising titre.

Paralytic poliomyelitis must be distinguished from the Guillain–Barré syndrome (p. 158).

Management

Patients should be isolated and contacts immunized. Artificial ventilation is required for respiratory failure — the most common cause of death. Careful nursing is necessary in all paralysed patients to prevent sores, combined with monitoring of fluid and electrolyte balance. Physiotherapy and progressive rehabilitation are started, after the fever has settled.

Full muscle recovery is rare if limbs are paralysed. Patients with isolated bulbar palsy usually recover completely but those with paralysis of the respiratory muscles rarely do, and may require continued artificial ventilation.

Syphilis of the nervous system

Tertiary syphilis of the CNS never develops in a syphilitic patient who has received early and correct treatment. All forms are now rarely seen in the developed world except as chronic cases with residual symptoms and signs, but it remains common worldwide. Tertiary syphilis may be divided into four groups:

1   meningovascular disease, occurring 3–4 years after primary infection;
2   tabes dorsalis— 10–35 years after primary infection;
3   general paralysis of the insane— 10–35 years after primary infection; and
4   localized gummata.

The first three produce symptoms by a combination of primary neuronal degeneration and/or arterial lesions.

Meningovascular syphilis

This affects both the cerebrum and the spine (*meningo*: producing fibrosis of the meninges and nipping of nerves; *vascular*: producing endarteritis and ischaemic necrosis). Headache is a common presenting symptom.

Cerebrum. Syphilitic leptomeningitis produces fibrosis and thickening of the meninges with nipping and paralysis of cranial nerves. The second, third and fourth nerves are most frequently involved.

Vascular endarteritis. Produces ischaemic necrosis. Hemiplegia may result. Syphilitic endarteritis is one cause of isolated cranial nerve lesions.

Spinal meningovascular syphilis. Meningeal thickening involves posterior spinal roots to produce pain and anterior roots to cause muscle wasting.

Endarteritis. May produce ischaemic necrosis, and transverse myelitis and paraplegia.

Tabes dorsalis

The signs result from degeneration of the dorsal columns and nerve roots.

Clinical presentation

Lightning pains due to dorsal nerve root involvement characterize the disease. There are severe paroxysmal stabbing pains (crises) which occur in the limbs, chest or abdomen. Paraesthesiae may also occur. Ataxia follows degeneration of the dorsal columns of the spinal cord. The gain is wide-based and stamping because position sense is lost.

Examination

The facies is characteristic. Ptosis is present and the forehead wrinkled due to overactivity of the frontalis muscle. Argyll Robertson pupils are small, irregular pupils which do not react to light, but constrict with accommodation. There may be optic atrophy. Cutaneous sensation is diminished typically over the nose (tabetic mask), sternum, ulnar border of the arm and outer borders of the legs and feet. Vibration and position sense are lost early in the disease. Deep pain sensation (pressure on testicles or Achilles tendon) may also be lost. Charcot's neuropathic joints are grossly disorganized from painless arthritis (also rarely seen in diabetes mellitus and syringomyelia when there is loss of pain sensation). Absence of visceral sensation results in overfilling of the bladder. The reflexes are diminished or absent in the legs. The plantar responses are flexor in pure tabes dorsalis. Romberg's sign (increased unsteadiness on closing the eyes) is present and is evidence of loss of position sense.

GENERAL PARALYSIS OF THE INSANE

A late manifestation of systemic syphilis. Pathologically the meninges are thickened, particularly in the parietal and frontal regions. Primary cortical degeneration produces a small brain with dilated and enlarged ventricles. The dorsal columns degenerate.

Clinical presentation

The pathological changes are associated with marked mental impairment. This may produce loss of memory and concentration with associated anxiety and/or depression. Later, insight is lost and the patient may become euphoric with delusions of grandeur and loss of emotional response. Epilepsy occurs in 50% of cases.

Examination

Euphoria may be present. The face is vacant and memory lost. Argyll Robertson pupils are present. The tongue demonstrates a 'trombone' tremor. Dorsal column involvement produces limb ataxia from loss of position sensation. Upper motor neuron lesions occur in the legs with increased reflexes and upgoing plantar responses.

NB   In taboparesis there is a combination of the lower limb upper motor neuron signs of general paralysis of the insane and the signs of dorsal root degeneration from tabes dorsalis. This produces a combination of absent knee reflexes with upgoing plantar responses.

FTAA and TPHA tests

The TPHA and FTAA tests are the most specific tests available for diagnosis. They may remain positive for years after adequate treatment.

Management

Penicillin by injection is the drug of choice for active syphilitic infection. Improvement, stabilization or deterioration may occur in any one case despite adequate penicillin therapy.

The Herxheimer reaction is an acute hypersensitivity reaction and results from toxins produced by spirochaetes killed on the first contact with penicillin. Death has been reported and some authorities give steroids during the first days of penicillin therapy.

Disorders of spinal cord

SYRINGOMYELIA

A longitudinal cyst in the cervical cord and/or brainstem (syringobulbia) occurs just anterior to the central canal and spreads, usually asymmetrically, to each side. It may be due to outflow obstruction of the fourth ventricle from a congenital anomaly such as the Arnold–Chiari malformation (also associated with spina bifida). It starts in young adults and is usually very slowly progressive over 20–30 years. It is very rare.

Damage to the cord (see Fig. 1.1, p. 6) occurs:
- At the root level of the lesion:
  (a) in the decussating fibres of the lateral spinothalamic tracts (pain and temperature) since they cross anteriorly (NB Fibres of the posterior column enter posteriorly and are not involved—hence the dissociated sensory loss.); and
  (b) the cells in the anterior horn where the lower motor neuron starts.
- Distant from the lesion in the upper motor neuron in the pyramidal tracts.

The classical case of syringomyelia therefore presents with:
- painless injury to the hands (sensory C6, 7, 8); and
- weakness and wasting in the small muscles of the hands (T1).

Examination may reveal more extensive dissociated sensory loss in the cervical segments, and upper motor neuron signs in the legs. These are usually asymmetrical. All signs and symptoms are ipsilateral to the lesion. Charcot's joints may occur in the upper limbs. In treatment, surgical decompression and aspiration of cysts should be considered.

SYRINGOBULBIA

In brainstem syringomyelia the descending root of the trigeminal nerve (pain and temperature) may be involved from the first division downwards and a Horner's syndrome from involvement of the cervical sympathetic tract. The motor nuclei of the lower cranial nerves may be involved in syringobulbia (true bulbar palsy) and there may be a rotary nystagmus from involvement in vestibular and cerebellar connections.

SUBACUTE COMBINED DEGENERATION OF THE CORD

The neurological consequences of B_{12} deficiency include subacute combined degeneration of the cord, signs of peripheral neuropathy and, very rarely, dementia and optic atrophy.

Combined degeneration refers to the combined demyelination of both pyramidal (lateral columns) and posterior (dorsal) columns, the signs and symptoms being predominantly in the legs. It is now rare.

Clinical presentation

Sensory peripheral neuropathy with numbness and paraesthesia in the feet are the usual presenting symptoms. Less commonly the disease presents as a spastic paraparesis. The signs are of:

- posterior column loss (vibration and position senses, with positive Rombergism);
- upper motor neuron lesion (weakness, hypertonia and hyperreflexia, with absent abdominal reflexes and upgoing toes); and
- peripheral neuropathy (absence of all the jerks, reduced touch sense and deep tenderness of the calves).

Investigation

Rarely, there is no anaemia or macrocytosis. The following are indicated:

- serum B_{12} and folate levels;
- marrow histology for megaloblastic change; and
- parietal cell and intrinsic factor antibodies.

These and the Schilling test are the only tests of value if the patient has been given vitamin B_{12} injections.

Management

Vitamin B_{12} (hydroxocobalamin 1 mg repeated five times at two-day intervals and then 1 mg every three months for life).

Prognosis

Neurological symptoms and signs usually improve to some degree. However, they may remain unchanged or, rarely, continue to progress. Sensory abnormalities resolve more completely than motor, the peripheral neuropathy more than the myelopathy.

PERONEAL MUSCULAR ATROPHY (Charcot–Marie–Tooth)

This condition is often confused with the muscle dystrophies. It is rare and genetic counselling is advisable.

Pathology

It may be transmitted as an autosomal dominant, or in some families is recessive and sex-linked. It may be classified into two groups of hereditary motor and sensory neuropathy affecting the peripheral nerves—type I with thickened peripheral nerves due to repeated demyelination and remyelination (ulnar at elbow, and common peroneal at the neck of the fibula), and type II due to axonal degeneration, without thickening.

Clinical presentation

It presents about the age of 20 years with wasting and weakness of all the distal lower limb muscles and pes cavus. Later, the upper limbs may be affected. The wasting stops at mid-thigh, producing an inverted champagne-bottle appearance, and at the elbows. Fasciculation and sensory loss are sometimes present, and reflexes depressed. The disease usually arrests spontaneously and life expectancy is normal. Contractions may produce talipes equinovarus.

CORD COMPRESSION

Aetiology

Disorders of vertebrae (extradural). These constitute 45% of cases:
- cervical spondylosis;
- collapsed vertebral body (usually secondary to carcinoma, myeloma or, rarely, osteoporosis);
- prolapsed intervertebral disc; and
- rarely, tuberculosis, abscesses, Paget's disease, reticuloses, angiomata, cervical and lumbar stenosis.

Meningeal disorders (intradural). Also constitute 45% of cases:
- neurofibroma (dumb-bell tumours); and
- meningioma (usually thoracic and more common in women).

Disorders of spinal cord (intramedullary). 5–10% of cases:
- gliomas; and
- ependymomas.

Clinical presentation

Patients present with a spastic paraparesis: there is upper motor neuron weakness in the legs, loss of sphincter control (an ominous sign) and loss of abdominal reflexes if the lesion is in or above the thoracic cord. The level of the sensory loss indicates the level of the neurological lesion which may, however, be up to two roots higher. Remember that, compared with the vertebral column, the cord is about one segment short in the lower cervical region, two segments short in the upper thoracic region, and three to five segments short in the lower thoracic region. The sacral segments and end of the cord lie opposite the L1 vertebra. Remember also, that the cervical spine has seven vertebrae and the cervical spinal cord eight segments.

It is important to consider the possibility of cord compression in all cases of spastic paresis. Cord compression is a neurosurgical emergency, particularly if of recent onset and rapid progression. Decompression must be performed as early as possible if recovery is to occur.

NB The tumours which commonly metastasize to bone arise in bronchus, breast, prostate, thyroid and kidney.

Investigation

- X-ray of the spine and CT scan or nuclear magnetic resonance to show the cord.
- X-ray of the chest for carcinoma of the bronchus.
- Lumbar puncture for spinal block and raised protein.
- Myelography to delineate the level and character of obstructing tissues — this investigation may increase the severity of transverse myelitis and should therefore be performed only after receiving expert advice.

Differential diagnosis

Other causes of spastic paraparesis are:
- Disseminated sclerosis. Demyelination may cause isolated slow progressive paraparesis in the middle-aged.
- Subacute combined degeneration of the cord.
- Transverse myelitis.
- Anterior spinal artery thrombosis.
- Motor neurone disease.
- Parasagittal cranial meningioma.

CERVICAL SPONDYLOSIS

Over 70% of the adult population in the UK have X-ray changes of osteoarthritis of the joints of the cervical spine. The most frequent and obvious abnormality is the presence of osteophytes. These radiological changes are unrelated to the presence or severity of symptoms.

Clinical features

Most patients are symptom-free. Pain in the neck, associated with and pre-cipitated by movements of the neck, is the commonest symptom. Occasionally compression of the cervical nerve roots causes root pain, paraesthesiae, numbness and sometimes segmental weakness with muscle wasting (even with fasciculation). Rarely, narrowing of the cervical canal with compression of the spinal cord or occlusion of the spinal cord vessels (spinal stenosis) produces brisk reflexes in the arms and upper motor neuron damage affecting the legs.

NB Lumbar spinal canal stenosis may produce weakness of the legs and sometimes pain in the calves on walking (intermittent claudication). It must be distinguished from femoral artery stenosis, the commonest cause of intermittent claudication (or limping).

Disorders of muscles

MIXED CONNECTIVE TISSUE DISEASE

A rare overlap disorder presenting with progressive weakness in the proximal limb muscles, usually more marked in the lower limbs. The disease merges with dermatomyositis and scleroderma in which skin manifestations are an obvious feature, with the other collagen disorders such as polymyositis, in which muscle weakness may be a marked or dominant feature, and SLE. Antibodies to ribonucleoprotein (RNP) are present.

POLYMYOSITIS AND ALLIED DISORDERS

Clinical presentation

The disorder presents at any age, but is more common in patients over 30 with muscle pain and tenderness with progressive weakness (50% of cases). Proximal muscles are affected more than distal ones, and patients may first notice difficulty climbing or standing from a sitting position, and difficulty lifting objects above their heads. Neck muscles are frequently involved (60%) but the facial and ocular muscles rarely (cf. myasthenia gravis). Dysphagia is common (50%) and involvement of the respiratory muscles may be severe and endanger life. Arthralgia occurs in about 25% of cases. Raynaud's phenomenon is common in the young (30%) and may proceed to scleroderma. Skin rashes are common (60%) and range from diffuse erythema to the manifestations of dermatomyositis (p. 186).

Prognosis

This is variable but generally worse in older patients. The disease may remit spontaneously, particularly in the young (under 30), but may recur and/or progress to a more diffuse systemic collagen disorder (30–50 years). In patients over 50 the prognosis depends on the underlying carcinoma if present. The overall mortality of untreated cases is about 50%.

Treatment

Corticosteroids (prednisolone 40–60 mg daily) are given initially, and the dose reduced gradually depending upon the patient's clinical state and the serum creatine phosphokinase level. Azathioprine is sometimes given as well and allows a reduction in steroid dosage. This is high during active disease but falls rapidly if therapy is successful. Steroid therapy is usually needed for 1–3 years before being gradually withdrawn. Physiotherapy is usually very helpful.

Differential diagnosis

The differentiation is from other causes of proximal myopathy (p. 26). *Trichinella spiralis* infection of muscles may produce acute myositis.

NB   Polymyalgia rheumatica usually presents with pain and stiffness. Wasting is not a characteristic feature (p. 185). All these conditions are relatively rare.

Investigation

Muscle biopsy

This shows muscle fibre necrosis and inflammatory cell infiltration.

Serum aldolase and creatine phosphokinase

These enzymes are greatly elevated in the muscular dystrophies during the most active stage of muscle degeneration (in the second and third decades of life). In polymyositis, the level of the enzymes is markedly elevated, gives a measure of active muscle destruction and should decline rapidly on corticosteroids coincident with improvement in muscle strength. There may be high titres to nuclear antigens, and the antinuclear factor (ANF) may be positive.

Electromyography

In the muscular dystrophies, evidence of decrease in active muscle is shown by the presence of short-duration, low-amplitude polyphasic action potentials. Polymyositis produces a similar picture but also with evidence of spontaneous fibrillation, possibly evidence of muscular irritability. Spontaneous fibrillation is characteristic of degenerated muscle undergoing active degeneration, and is associated with evidence of a decrease in the number of motor units on voluntary movement. Electromyograph (EMG) findings often do not fit neatly into the above patterns as the distribution of muscle involvement is patchy and as the EMG recording depends upon the particular region of muscle sampled.

MYASTHENIA GRAVIS

A very rare disorder of muscle weakness resulting from failure of neuromuscular transmission. There is a reduction in the number of functioning postsynaptic acetylcholine receptors (AChR) and a high titre of specific anti-AChR antibodies has been shown in most cases. Thymoma is associated in 10% of cases and thymus abnormalities in 75%. Excessive muscular fatigability may also occur in polymyositis and SLE, and there is an increased incidence of myasthenia gravis in thyrotoxicosis. The Lambert–Eaton myasthenic syndrome associated with carcinoma is clinically different (see below).

Clinical presentation

Painless muscular weakness is produced by repetitive or sustained contraction. It is usually most marked in the face and eyes producing a symmetrical ptosis and diplopia. Weakness of speech and swallowing may occur. The proximal muscles are more often affected than the distal, and the upper limb muscles more than the lower. There is no wasting and tendon reflexes are preserved.

Prognosis

The disorder may never progress beyond ophthalmoplegia and periods of remission up to 3 years occur. Death may be rapid if the respiratory muscles are involved. Thymectomy usually improves the outlook unless a thymoma is present.

Diagnosis

Edrophonium (Tensilon) 10 mg iv with cardiac monitor (in case of bradycardia/asystole) reduces the weakness of affected muscles for 3–4 min. The anterior mediastinum should be searched with chest X-rays and CT scan for thymoma. AChR IgG antibodies are present in 90% of cases.

Treatment

Therapy is achieved with long-acting anticholinesterases orally, such as neostigmine or pyridostigmine (Mestinon), preferably by increasing the dose slowly until measured muscular strength is optimal. Overdose may give depolarization block with weakness. Thymectomy at any age appears to increase the percentage of patients in remission. An alternate-day regime of steroids (between 10 and 80 mg alternate days) is of proven value and immunotherapy with azathioprine may be useful and allow a reduction in steroid dosage. Plasmapheresis has been used in intractable cases but the effect is short-lasting (days–months). The differential diagnosis is from other causes of ptosis (p. 4), muscular dystrophies involving the face, familial hypokalaemic paralysis and the Lambert–Eaton syndrome. In this, a disorder of acetylcholine release, the myasthenia is associated with a carcinoma, usually oat cell, of the bronchus. It differs from classical myasthenia gravis in that the eyes are less frequently affected, that proximal limb muscle weakness is common and their strength initially *increased* by repeated movement. There is no response to edrophonium but oral 3,4 diaminopyridine may help.

MYOTONIA

Myotonia is the inability of muscles to relax normally after contraction. This produces a reluctant release of handshake, and percussion contraction for instance of the thenar muscles.

Dystrophia myotonica

An autosomal dominant (chromosome 9) disorder producing progressively more severe symptoms and signs with succeeding generations, i.e. anticipation. It is rare.

Genetics

There is expansion of a CTG repeat in the 3' untranslated region of the myotonin protein kinase gene (19q13). Trinucleotide repeat is a novel form of genetic mutation in which there is expansion of a sequence of DNA which contains a series of repeated nucleotide triplets. In diseases identified so far the repetitive sequence is present in the gene of normal individuals, but is expanded up to 1000-fold in the gene of affected patients.

Clinical presentation

Both males and females are affected with usual onset at 15–40 years. UK incidence is 5/100000. The classical case demonstrates:
- Abnormal facies — with frontal balding, ptosis, a smooth expressionless forehead, cataracts and a lateral smile or sneer.
- Wasting of the facial muscles, sternomastoids, shoulder girdle and quadriceps.
- The forearms and legs are involved and reflexes lost. There is no fasciculation.
- Myotonia which increases with cold, fatigue and excitement and may reduce with repeated activity.
- Testicular or ovarian atrophy with impotence and sterility.
- Mental deficiency.

NB   The heart may be involved (e.g. heart block) and diabetes mellitus may develop. Phenytoin may reduce myotonia.

Myotonia congenita

This is a hereditary disorder, transmitted as a Mendelian dominant, which affects both sexes equally, and first presents in childhood. There is no muscle wasting and no long-term effects. It is very rare. The myotonias should not be confused with two disorders of children amyotonia congenita and progressive spinomuscular atrophy.

Amyotonia congenita

A congenital disorder producing weakness and hypotonia which is first noticed in children at the head-lifting stage. The muscle disturbance becomes less severe as the children grow older, although contractures may produce scoliosis.

Progressive spinomuscular atrophy (Werdnig–Hoffmann)

A hereditary disorder involving progressive degeneration of the anterior spinal horn cells starting in the first year of life and producing weakness, muscle wasting and fasciculation, and death within 6 months.

MUSCULAR DYSTROPHIES

Each family produces its own pattern of disease but some forms are more common than others. They are all rare. Genetic counselling is advised. There is no effective treatment. Chromosome studies may define the carrier state.

Pseudohypertrophic (Duchenne)

A sex-linked recessive disorder affecting males with a prevalence of 3:100000 and incidence of 25:100000 male births. The age of onset is 5–10 years with symptoms of difficulty in climbing stairs, or even walking, and the use of Gowers' manoeuvre to rise from the floor. On examination the posture is lordotic and the gait waddling due to weakness of the muscles of the pelvic girdle and proximal lower limb. The calves are hypertrophied but weak and the creatine phosphokinase level is raised. The EMG and muscle biospy are characteristic. In later stages muscle contracture of the legs may produce talipes equinovarus and muscle weakness may spread to the upper limbs, though not to the face. The child dies in the early teens, usually from chest infection or cardiomyopathy. Becker's dystrophy is a mild form.

Genetics

The cytoskeletal protein dystrophin (Xp) is either abnormal or absent. In Becker's muscular dystrophy a milder form of muscular dystrophy is caused by mutations of the dystrophin gene, resulting in partially functional dystrophin protein which is reduced in amount or size.

Facio-scapulo-humeral (Landouzy–Déjérine)

Transmitted as an autosomal dominant and affects both sexes equally. The onset is at puberty with progressive wasting in the upper limb-girdle and face. The disorder may abort spontaneously or progress to the muscles of the trunk and lower limbs. Individuals usually live to a normal age.

Limb-girdle (Erb)

Transmitted as an autosomal recessive and affects both sexes equally. It presents at 20–40 years. It involves the muscles of the shoulders and pelvic girdles and is slowly progressive, with death usually in middle age.

Other forms may affect the muscles of the face and eyes (oculomuscular dystrophy) or the distal limb muscles (Gower's muscular dystrophy). They are very rare.

Dementia

Dementia means loss of mind. The earliest feature is loss of memory for recent events. There is a global disruption of personality with the gradual development of abnormal behaviour, loss of intellect, mood changes often without insight, blunting of emotions and failure to learn. Eventually there is a reduction in self-care, restless wandering and incontinence. In patients under 60 years of age it is usually termed presenile dementia, though this distinction is not important.

The commonest causes are Alzheimer's disease and multi-infarct dementia, but treatable disorders must always be excluded.

Causes of dementia

Degenerative

- Alzheimer's disease.

- Huntington's disease.
- Pick's disease.
- Steele–Richardson syndrome.
- Spinocerebellar degeneration (including Friedreich's ataxia).
- Parkinson's disease (sometimes).
- Multiple sclerosis.

Vascular
- Multi-infarct dementia.
- Cerebral vasculitis (rare).

Toxic
- Poisoning with carbon monoxide, lead.
- Alcoholism.

Drug-induced
- Usually overmedication with sedatives.

Traumatic
- Head injury.
- Subdural haematomas.
- Boxers ('punch drunk').

Malignancy
- Primary cerebral tumour (meningiomata may grow very slowly).
- Posterior fossa tumour with hydrocephalus.
- Metastases.

Metabolic
- Uraemia.
- Hepatic encephalopathy.
- Hypothyroidism (myxoedema madness).
- Wilson's disease.
- B_{12} deficiency.

Infection
- AIDS.
- Herpes simplex encephalitis.
- Cerebral syphilis.
- Progressive multifocal leukoencephalopathy.
- Subacute sclerosing panencephalitis.
- Creutzfeldt–Jakob disease.

Pseudodementia
- In depression.

Investigation

Investigation is aimed at establishing the diagnosis and excluding treatable causes. Patients should have:

- Psychometric evaluation to establish the diagnosis and assess severity;
- FBC and ESR;
- Urea and electrolytes, glucose, calcium;
- Liver function tests;
- Thyroid function studies;
- Serological tests for syphilis;
- Vitamin B_{12};
- Chest X-ray (for bronchial carcinoma); and
- CT scan of the head is advisable in all patients, and essential in younger patients, to exclude tumour, hydrocephalus, subdural haematoma.
- In selected patients serological tests and examination of CSF to exclude toxicity or infection.

ALZHEIMER'S DISEASE

Alois Alzheimer, 1864–1915, Poland.

Alzheimer's disease affects about 10% of people over the age of 65, and between 25 and 40% of those over 85. About 50% of cases of severe dementia are due to Alzheimer's disease (most of the remaining cases are due to multi-infarct dementia, alone or in combination with Alzheimer's disease).

Pathology

Two characteristic features are found in the brain of patients with Alzheimer's disease:

1 *Senile plaques* consist of extracellular deposits of β-amyloid, a peptide formed by cleavage of β-amyloid precursor protein (genetic locus 21q21–22). Abnormal deposits of β-amyloid are also found in blood vessels.

2 *Neurofibrillary tangles* are dense bundles of abnormal fibres in the cytoplasm of neurons which contain an altered form of the microtubule-associated protein, τ. Neither senile plaques nor neurofibrillary tangles are specific to Alzheimer's disease. They occur in other chronic cerebral conditions and can be found in elderly patients without dementia.

Aetiology

Risk factors are:

- increasing age;
- head trauma;
- Down's syndrome (trisomy 21; p. 389); and
- genetic susceptibility. A family history can be obtained in 30–50% of cases. Rare familial forms in which young-onset Alzheimer's disease is inherited in an autosomal dominant pattern show linkage to chromosome 21, and in some cases chromosome 14. Associations between sporadic and familial late-onset Alzheimer's

> **TRIALS**
>
> Tacrine (a cholinesterase inhibitor) in high doses (160 mg/day) had a beneficial effect on Alzheimer's disease, assessed by both clinical impression and neuropsychological test scores, in a 30-week randomized placebo controlled trial. *JAMA* 1994; **271**: 985–991.
>
> However, the usefulness of tacrine may be limited by side effects, including hepatotoxicity. *JAMA* 1994; **271**: 992–998.

disease and polymorphisms of the apolipoprotein E gene on chromosome 19 have been reported.

Clinical features

Loss of memory for recent events is the usual presenting feature. Insight may be preserved in the early stages and depression is common. Later, more marked memory disturbance is accompanied by impaired motor abilities, often with extrapyramidal features. Disturbed sleep pattern, loss of sphincter control and personality change all contribute to the progressive social disintegration.

Management

It is important to exclude treatable causes of dementia. Management is largely supportive, towards both patient and family. Treatment of depression may be effective in the early stages. Recent trials have suggested benefits from cholinergic drugs.

MULTI-INFARCT DEMENTIA

In dementia resulting from cerebrovascular disease the onset may be abrupt with a stepwise progression, and other focal neurological signs may be present. Predisposing factors (e.g. smoking, hypertension, hyperlipidaemia, diabetes) and other evidence of vascular disease are often present. Postmortem studies have shown that pathological changes associated with vascular lesions and Alzheimer's disease often coexist.

HUNTINGTON'S DISEASE (see also p. 148)

George Sumner Huntington, 1851–1916, America.

Progressive dementia and involuntary movements (chorea) develop in middle age. Inheritance is autosomal dominant, although the disease is late and variable in its presentation. Death usually occurs 10–15 years after the onset of symptoms.

Disease-related gene

The Huntington's disease gene (chromosome 4p16) contains an expanded CAG trinucleotide repeat. *Trinucleotide repeat* is a genetic mutation in which there is expansion of a sequence of DNA which contains a series of repeated nucleotide triplets. The repetitive sequence is present in the gene of normal individuals, but is expanded up to 1000-fold in the gene of affected patients. The length of the tri-nucleotide repetitive sequence tends to increase as the gene passes from parent to offspring, providing an explanation for anticipation, the phenomenon by which the disease gets progressively more severe through successive generations.

The Huntington's disease gene encodes a novel protein of currently unknown function.

Management

Tetrabenazine may help the chorea by depleting nerve endings of dopamine. Extrapyramidal dysfunction and depression are common side effects. Identification of the genetic mutation has increased the precision of genetic testing. However, presymptomatic testing for Huntington's disease must be approached with great care because of the implications of a positive test for the patient and family.

NORMAL-PRESSURE HYDROCEPHALUS

Enlargement of all of the ventricles is associated with dementia, usually with pyramidal signs in the limbs, an ataxic gait and urinary incontinence. CSF pressure is normal, but continuous monitoring may reveal intermittent periods of raised pressure. Some patients respond to ventriculoperitoneal shunting.

PICK'S DISEASE

Pick's disease is a rare form of dementia in which focal neuropsychological deficits occur within the context of dementia. There is focal cortical atrophy with silver staining inclusion bodies (Pick's bodies) in surviving neurons. An earlier age of onset (around 60), a slight predominance in men and frequent impairment of speech help to distinguish the disease clinically from Alzheimer's disease.

CREUTZFELDT–JAKOB DISEASE

Creutzfeldt-Jakob disease usually presents in late middle age with dementia which progresses to death within months. Spongiform changes are found in the brain at postmortem. The agent of this and other transmissible spongiform encephalopathies such as scrapie and *bovine spongiform encephalopathy* is believed to be a prion protein which is resistant to inactivation by heat or chemicals.

Schizophrenia

The diagnosis of schizophrenia is based on the presence of a collection of symptoms such as delusions, hallucinations, disordered speech or behaviour, flattened affect and lack of volition. It usually presents in adolescents or young adults, and is associated with marked difficulties with work and social function. It is associated with an increased risk of alcoholism and suicide. The aetiology is unknown, but genetic factors are important. Monozygotic twins of schizophrenics have an almost 50% chance of developing schizophrenia.

First-rank symptoms

Schneider (1887–1967) defined a number of *first-rank symptoms* which allow a diagnosis of schizophrenia in the absence of an underlying organic pathology:
*   thought insertion, withdrawal or broadcasting (thoughts put into or taken out of the patient's mind, or being known to others);
*   voices discussing the patient's thoughts or behaviour;
*   voices repeating or anticipating the patient's thoughts;
*   passivity experiences (external control of emotions, sensations or movement); and
*   delusional perception (a delusion triggered by a normal observation).

Non-first-rank symptoms

*   Formal thought disorder in which there is impaired connection of thoughts, which may lead to incoherent speech.
*   Chronic negative symptoms—apathy, blunting of emotions, paucity of speech, social withdrawal.
*   Catatonic behaviour—extreme motor activity with bizarre posturing.

Associated features

Features which are common but not specific for schizophrenia are:
*   persecutory delusions;
*   ideas of reference (belief that events have a specific significance);
*   suspiciousness;
*   lack of insight; and
*   stereotypies (repetitive movements) or mannerisms.

Management

Admission to a psychiatric unit is often required in the acute illness. Antipsychotic drugs (neuroleptics) are the most effective treatment.
*   Chlorpromazine causes marked sedation and has muscarinic side effects, but relatively few extrapyramidal effects.
*   Flupenthixol is less sedating and may be useful if apathy or withdrawal is present.
*   Haloperidol, fluphenazine and prochlorperazine have fewer sedative and muscarinic effects, but more extrapyramidal effects.
*   Risperidone is a benzisoxazole derivative and has relatively few extrapyramidal effects.
*   Clozapine may be effective when other drugs have failed, but causes agranulocytosis, making frequent monitoring of blood counts essential.

The most troublesome side effects are extrapyramidal: parkinsonian symptoms, dystonia, tardive dyskinesia and akathisia (restlessness). Antiparkinsonian drugs (e.g. benztropine, procyclidine) are often used to treat or prevent these effects.

Affective disorders

Affective disorders are disorders of mood. Mild forms are common and usually self-limiting. They can be classified into depressive and manic and episodes.

DEPRESSIVE EPISODES

Depressive episodes are characterized by abnormalities of:
- mood—sadness, feelings of worthlessness, anxiety;
- speech and thought—slow speech, poverty of thought, suicidal ideas, impaired concentration;
- normal functions — insomnia, early-morning waking, anorexia, weight loss, reduced libido, psychomotor retardation;
- behaviour—loss of social interactions, poor performance at work, self-neglect;
- perception—illusions and in severe cases hallucinations.

MANIC EPISODES

Manic episodes are characterized by:
- elation and grandiosity;
- flight of ideas, pressure of speech, irritability, distractibility;
- insomnia, increased appetite, increased libido;
- illusions and in severe cases hallucinations; and
- hyperactivity, overspending.

In bipolar disorders there are recurrent episodes of mania and depression. Unipolar disorders are characterized by recurrent depressive episodes.

Management

Sympathetic support.

Depressive episodes. Tricyclic antidepressants and selective 5-HT reuptake inhibitors are generally preferred to monoamine oxidase inhibitors. In severe disorders electroconvulsive therapy may be necessary.

Manic episodes. Neuroleptic drugs (e.g. chlorpromazine, haloperidol) are used in acute episodes.

Lithium salts are used in the prevention of bipolar disorders, and may be useful in acute attacks. They are often continued indefinitely with regular monitoring of renal and thyroid function.

Rheumatic Disease

Musculoskeletal strains are very common and the cause of most referrals in general practice (sports injuries and back pain). Osteoarthritis affects most people who live past middle age.

Non-organ-specific autoimmune disorders, such as systemic lupus erythematosus (SLE) and systemic vasculitis, remain uncommon, but should come to mind in the clinical situations of:
- pyrexia of unknown origin, malaise and weight loss;
- multisystem disease; and
- renal disorders.

The following named diseases describe commoner clinical pictures. Lesions chiefly affect skin, glomeruli, joints, serous membranes and blood vessels.

Systemic lupus erythematosus

SLE commonly presents in women aged 20–40 years (90%) and is exacerbated by sunlight and infection. Hydralazine, usually in prolonged high dosage, may give a similar picture, as may procainamide. In the UK the prevalence is 36/100 000 white women, 90/100 000 Asian women, and 200/100 000 Afro-Caribbean women. The American Rheumatism Association criteria tend to exclude milder cases.

TRIALS

Subcommittee for Systemic Lupus Erythematosus Criteria of the American Rheumatism Association Diagnostic and Therapeutic Criteria Committee 1982 revised criteria for the classification of SLE. *Arthritis Rheum* 1982, **25**: 1271–1277.

The subcommittee proposed a diagnosis of SLE if four of the following 11 criteria are present, serially or simultaneously, during any interval of observation:

1   malar rash
2   discoid rash
3   photosensitivity
4   oral ulcers
5   arthritis
6   serositis (pleuritis, pericarditis)
7   renal disorder
8   neurological disorder (seizures or psychosis)
9   haematological disorder (haemolytic anaemia, leukopenia, thrombocytopenia)
10   immunological disorder
11   antinuclear antibody.

Clinical presentation

The commonest early features are fever (75% of cases), arthralgia and general ill health, with weight loss. It can mimic rheumatoid arthritis, subacute bacterial endocarditis, and may produce the nephrotic syndrome. Only one-third develop the typical butterfly rash on the face. One or more of the following systems may be involved.

Joints (90% of cases)

A migratory, usually symmetrical polyarthralgia, not unlike rheumatoid arthritis but very rarely erosive or deforming, and affecting the fingers, wrists, elbows, shoulders, knees and ankles. Avascular necrosis may follow prolonged steroid therapy.

Skin (80%)

Non-specific erythema, photosensitivity, alopecia and malar (butterfly) rash (30%) are the commonest features. Oral and mucosal ulceration is not uncommon (30%).

Nail fold infarcts may occur (10%). Follicles are blocked, and telangiectases present. It may involve the ears, neck, chest and upper limbs. Raynaud's phenomenon is present in 10%.

Kidneys (100% in some studies)
Renal involvement is common and associated with a poor prognosis. Clinical presentation is with almost any manifestation of renal disease, including hypertension, haematuria, proteinuria, nephrotic syndrome, acute renal failure and end-stage renal disease (p. 285).

Nervous system (50% at presentation)
The commonest abnormalities are headache and peripheral neuropathy. Cranial nerve abnormalities, strokes, psychoses and depression also occur. Central nervous system abnormalities are associated with a poorer prognosis. Rarely, epilepsy is the presenting feature. Symptoms mostly result from ischaemia due to vasculitis, coagulopathy, embolism, dissection and premature atherosclerosis.

Lungs (50%)
Pleurisy with effusions is relatively common. Patchy consolidation and plate-like areas of collapse, and/or diffuse reticulonodular shadowing on chest X-ray may be seen. Haemorrhagic lupus pneumonitis is rare, but often fatal.

Cardiovascular system (40%)
Pericarditis is sometimes the first indication of SLE. Raynaud's phenomenon (10%; p. 405), cardiac failure of cardiomyopathy and non-bacterial endocarditis of mitral (Libman–Sacks) and aortic valves all may occur.

Blood
The sedimentation rate is raised in active disease, and often leads to first suspicion of disease. Thrombocytopenia with purpura may be the first indication of SLE. Normochromic, normocytic anaemia of chronic disease occurs in over 70%. About 10% also have haemolytic anaemia (with reticulocytosis and hyperbilirubinaemia) and leukopenia may occur. There may be splenomegaly.

Lymphatic system
Generalized lymphadenopathy (50%) with or without hepatosplenomegaly (15%) may occur.

Investigation

The antinuclear factor (ANF) is positive in 98% of cases. Antibodies against double-stranded DNA are found in up to 90% of those with active disease. Low serum complement, particularly the C3 and C4 fractions, occurs, especially in lupus nephritis.

Management

Non-steroidal anti-inflammatory drugs may be sufficient to relieve joint symptoms.
    Antimalarials (chloroquine, hydroxychloroquine) are used when skin and joint

disease predominate. They can cause lens opacities which are not serious clinically (and resolve on stopping it) and retinal degeneration, which is rare but irreversible.

Steroids may be required when non-steroidal anti-inflammatory drugs and anti-malarials are insufficient to control symptoms, often in combination with *cytotoxic immunosuppressants* (azathioprine, cyclophosphamide, methotrexate). Steroids in combination with monthly pulsed intravenous cyclophosphamide have been used to induce remission in renal lupus.

Plasmapheresis is used in some centres to treat severe disease, but its benefit has not been proven in clinical trials.

General measures include avoidance of sunlight, antibiotics for intercurrent infection (C-reactive protein (CRP) is normal except when there is active infection) and blood transfusion for anaemia.

Prognosis

The history is of episodic relapses and remissions lasting months to years. Five-year survival is over 95% unless there is renal involvement. Death usually results from active generalized disease, sepsis or cardiovascular disease.

ANTIPHOSPHOLIPID SYNDROME

Although first described in SLE, most patients with the antiphospholipid syndrome do not meet the criteria for SLE. It is characterized by venous or arterial thromboses, and the presence of antiphospholipid antibodies which typically bind to charged phospholipids, the classical example used in assays being cardiolipin. These antibodies bind to phospholipids used in coagulation tests, paradoxically causing an anticoagulant effect *in vitro* (hence the term lupus anticoagulant). Other important features of the syndrome are thrombocytopenia and recurrent spontaneous abortion, usually in the second or third trimester. Histologically there is a bland thrombus without inflammation of the vessel wall. Lifelong anticoagulation is usually required.

TRIAL

Khamashta *et al.* retrospectively studied 147 patients with the antiphospholipid syndrome and a history of thrombosis. Treatment with high-intensity warfarin (international normalized ratio (INR) >3) with or without low-dose aspirin was more effective in preventing thrombosis than treatment with low-intensity warfarin (INR < 3) with or without low-dose aspirin, or treatment with aspirin alone. *N Engl J Med* 1995; **322**: 993–997.

Systemic vasculitis

Inflammation of small and medium-sized blood vessels occurs in a number of generalized inflammatory diseases. It can present as the primary feature of a disease (e.g. microscopic polyarteritis and Wegener's granulomatosis) or as a secondary feature of conditions such as rheumatoid arthritis (p. 188) or SLE (p. 178). The cause is unknown, although flare-up of disease is often associated with infection. Many organs can be affected; common sites are skin, lungs, kidney, joints, eyes and nervous system.

Clinical features

- Malaise, fever, rashes, uveitis, arthritis.
- Dyspnoea, cough, haemoptysis (from pulmonary haemorrhage).
- Haematuria, renal failure (glomerulonephritis).
- Psychiatric disturbance.
- Epilepsy, strokes, peripheral neuropathy.

Vasculitis may be classified according to the size of vessel involved, or the presence of serological markers. Antineutrophil cytoplasm antibodies (ANCAs) recognize cytoplasmic components (usually proteases) of neutrophils. The pattern of staining seen by immunofluorescence and the target antigen vary. Diffuse cytoplasmic staining (classical or cANCA) is seen with antibodies against proteinase 3 and is associated with Wegener's granulomatosis. Perinuclear staining (pANCA) occurs with antibodies against myeloperoxidase which occur in microscopic polyarteritis nodosa.

A number of different disease patterns are recognized:

POLYARTERITIS NODOSA

Polyarteritis nodosa is characterized by necrotizing inflammation of small and medium-sized arteries, leading to formation of small aneurysms. It is commonest in young males. Clinical presentation is usually with organ infarction in the presence of a systemic illness.

- Malaise, fever, weight loss, arthralgia.
- Hypertension (sometimes malignant) occurs almost invariably at some stage, and in 50% at presentation.
- Renal disease—over half of cases have an abnormal urinary sediment, but renal impairment is less common and usually mild.
- Nervous system (over 50%). Mononeuritis multiplex or polyneuritis. Occasionally stroke.
- Skin (25%)—tender subcutaneous nodules. Punched-out lesions occur around the ankles.
- Arteritic lesions around the nail bed and splinter haemorrhages can mimic bacterial endocarditis (particularly if combined with fever).
- Joints (10%)—a non-deforming polyarthritis.

Investigations

There is usually anaemia and leukocytosis. Proteinuria, microscopic haematuria and a raised erythrocyte sedimentation rate (ESR) are common. Biopsy of involved tissue (muscle, nerve, skin, kidney) demonstrates changes of segmental fibrinoid necrosis of the walls of medium-sized arteries and arterioles with cellular infiltration. Arteriography shows narrowing of vessels, pruning of the peripheral vasculature and the presence of aneurysms. Aneurysms are commonest in the renal and hepatic vasculature. ANCAs are present in fewer than 20% of cases.

MICROSCOPIC POLYARTERITIS

In microscopic polyarteritis the necrotizing vasculitis affects predominantly small vessels (capillaries, venules, arterioles). The kidney is most commonly affected (over 90%) with development of a rapidly progressive glomerulonephritis. Fifty per cent have lung disease (haemoptysis, pleurisy, asthma). Frank pulmonary haemorrhage is rare (5%), but potentially fatal. Other features include arthralgia (50%), vasculitic or purpuric rashes (40%) and hypertension (20%).

pANCA staining is seen in 50% of patients, usually with specificity against myeloperoxidase. Microaneurysms do not occur.

WEGENER'S GRANULOMATOSIS

In Wegener's granulomatosis tissue necrosis occurs as a result of both granulomatous inflammation and systemic vasculitis. Typically localized granulomatous inflammation, usually in the upper or lower respiratory tract, is followed by a systemic vasculitis and glomerulonephritis.

Clinical features

Ear, nose and throat involvement is a prominent early feature (95%). Nasal stuffiness, facial pain and epistaxis are common. Saddle-nose deformity results from erosion of the nasal septum and destruction of nasal cartilage. Middle-ear disease causes pain and deafness.

Lungs (95%). Cough, dyspnoea, haemoptysis and chest pain are common. Pulmonary nodules may cavitate or progress to diffuse infiltration. About 10% develop diffuse pulmonary haemorrhage. Bronchial stenosis, ulceration and inflammation are seen at bronchoscopy.

Kidneys (90%). Proteinuria, haematuria and renal impairment result from a focal, segmental, necrotizing glomerulonephritis.

Joints and muscles (70%). Transient arthralgia and synovitis are common, but chronic arthritis is not a feature.

Eyes (30%). Scleritis, episcleritis, uveitis and conjunctivitis all occur.

Involvement of *skin* (25%), *nervous system* (15%) and *gastrointestinal tract* (10%) also occurs.

Investigations

Eighty per cent of patients with active Wegener's granulomatosis have cANCA, usually with specificity against proteinase-3. Biopsy of affected tissue shows a necrotizing vasculitis with granuloma formation.

CHURG STRAUSS SYNDROME

Churg Strauss syndrome is distinguished by the presence of asthma, allergic rhinitis and eosinophilia, together with a systemic vasculitis affecting extrapulmonary organs. Eosinophils predominate in the inflammatory infiltrate, which may be granulomatous. Central and peripheral nerve involvement is common. Renal involvement tends to be mild. ANCA are not usually present.

HYPERSENSITIVITY VASCULITIS

This term is often used to describe inflammation of small vessels (usually post capillary venules) in which skin lesions predominate, with or without systemic features. Although most cases are idiopathic, it is associated with autoimmune diseases (rheumatoid arthritis, SLE), malignancy (lympho- and myeloproliferative disorders), infections (hepatitis B, human immunodeficiency virus, (HIV)), and drugs (e.g. penicillin, sulphonamides, thiazides).

HENOCH–SCHÖNLEIN PURPURA

Palpable purpura, arthritis and abdominal pain (haemorrhagic enteritis in severe cases) occur in association with a glomerulonephritis indistinguishable from immunoglobulin A nephropathy (p. 280).

BEHÇET'S SYNDROME

Aphthous ulceration of the oral mucosa is associated with involvement of other organs.
- *Genitalia* (90%). Scrotal or labial ulceration.
- *Skin* (80%). Erythema nodosum, acneiform lesions and vasculitic lesions all occur. A papule or pustule may form after puncture of the skin with a needle (*pathergy reaction*).
- *Eye* (50%). Anterior and posterior uveitis.
- *Joints* (50%). Non-deforming mono- or polyarthritis.
- *Neurological* (10%). Usually central nervous system involvement.

Treatment

Treatment of systemic vasculitis usually involves a combination of high-dose corticosteroids and cyclophosphamide to induce remission, followed by a maintenance regime in which other immunosuppressive agents (e.g. azathioprine) may substitute for cyclophosphamide.

Large-vessel vasculitis

TAKAYASU'S ARTERITIS

Takayasu's arteritis is a granulomatous arteritis affecting the aorta and its major branches, and sometimes the pulmonary arteries. It is commonest in young women. Systemic features (fever, arthralgia, myalgia, anaemia) usually precede the ischaemia/pulselessness which usually affects the upper limbs. Bruits may be audible over the aorta, carotids and subclavian vessels. The diagnosis is usually confirmed by angiography which shows diffuse narrowing of the aorta and main arteries. The ESR and CRP are elevated, with anaemia and leukocytosis. Treatment is with high-dose corticosteroids (60–80 mg daily), with gradual reduction guided by inflammatory markers.

GIANT-CELL ARTERITIS (temporal arteritis, cranial arteritis)

Clinical presentation

A disease in patients usually over 60 who develop severe headache, with burning and tenderness over the scalp and tenderness over the temporal arteries, sometimes with visual blurring and jaw claudication. Systemic manifestations are common with fever, weight loss, arthralgia and a myalgia identical to polymyalgia rheumatica in 50%. The ophthalmic arteries may be involved and blindness may result. Personality changes may occur from involvement of the cerebral vessels. The coronary arteries or other vessels can be involved.

Investigation

The ESR is markedly raised (often above 90 mm/h). The alkaline phosphatase may also be raised. Diagnosis is confirmed on temporal artery biopsy which shows patchy involvement of the arterial wall with areas of necrosis, large mononuclear cell infiltration and giant cells. As arterial involvement may be patchy, a negative biopsy does not exclude the diagnosis.

Management

Steroids in high doses (prednisolone 40–60 mg daily) are given urgently to suppress symptoms (this usually occurs within 2 days) and to prevent blindness. Treatment is given for 2–3 years or more, gradually reducing the dosage while monitoring symptoms and the ESR.

POLYMYALGIA RHEUMATICA

Clinical presentation

Occurs in patients usually over 60 years old and is more common in women. It presents with muscle pain, stiffness and occasionally tenderness, usually in the shoulder girdle and neck, but sometimes in the pelvic region. Symptoms are worse on waking. There is little, if any, weakness or wasting. The associated findings are headache, lassitude, depression and weight loss. It may be associated with giant-cell arteritis. The ESR is usually very high (>70 mm/h and rarely <30 mm/h).

Management

Steroids (10–20 mg prednisolone daily) are required urgently to relieve symptoms and prevent blindness in patients with associated giant-cell arteritis. The response is characteristically rapid. The dose is often reduced to a very low level, whilst monitoring symptoms and the ESR, which should be kept within normal limits. Treatment should be continued for 1–2 years.

Dermatomyositis

Mainly affects women of 40–50 years. About 20% of all cases are associated with underlying malignancy (bronchus, breast, stomach, ovary) and in men presenting over the age of 50 years, over 60% have carcinoma, usually of the bronchus. An acute form occurs in children and is often fatal.

Clinical presentation

The onset may be acute or chronic. Skin and muscle changes occur in any order, or together, sometimes with 2–3 months separating their appearance. General ill health and fever are common.

Skin involvement (60%)
- Classically purple heliotrope (a lilac-blue flower) colour occurs around the eyes. The remainder of the face may be involved.
- Violet, oedematous lesions over the small joints of the hands with telangiectasia.
- Arteritic lesions around the nails.
- There may be generalized telangiectasia, especially of the face, chest and arms.

Muscle involvement
Tenderness and weakness of muscles occur, commonly of the shoulder and proximal muscles of the upper limb, and if this predominates the disease closely resembles polymyositis (p. 167). Dysphagia is common. Muscle wasting and fibrosis with fixed joint deformity may occur in chronic disease.

Other systems
- Lungs with plate-like areas of collapse and diffuse fibrosis.
- Heart with cardiomyopathy and cardiac failure.
- Sicca syndrome (p. 194).

Investigation
Investigation of myositis (p. 168).

Management

Steroids are given in high doses (e.g. prednisolone 60–80 mg/day) in the acute stages but are relatively ineffective in the chronic cases. Immunosuppression with azathioprine if there is an inadequate response within 2 months.

Prognosis

Depends upon the underlying neoplasm if present. The disease may progress rapidly but exacerbations and remissions are the rule and continue for 10–20 years until respiratory or cardiac failure occurs.

Polymyositis

(See p. 167).

Scleroderma (systemic sclerosis)

A disease mainly of middle-aged people. There is excessive deposition of collagen and other matrix proteins in organs, including the skin. There is progressive fibrosis with atrophy of the skin structures (*scleroderma* literally means *hard skin*). There is vasomotor instability (usually manifest as Raynaud's phenomenon), and blood vessels also show proliferative intimal lesions leading to ischaemia.

Clinical presentation

The following systems may be involved:

General

Lassitude, fever and weight loss.

Skin (75%)

Raynaud's phenomenon with sclerodactyly and telangiectasia. In the early stages there is non-pitting oedema of the skin of the hands and feet, later involving the face, neck and trunk. The skin becomes smooth, waxy and tight and finally thin, atrophic and pigmented in 50%. Skin ulcers develop in 40%. Vitiligo may occur. Changes are maximal over the hands, ankles and face, producing a typical mask-like face. Subcutaneous calcification may be present (10%). The *sicca syndrome* (p. 194) develops in 5%. (Morphoea is a localized indurated sclerodermatous lesion usually on the trunk, neck or extremities. It is benign and only rarely proceeds to systemic sclerosis.)

Lungs

Diffuse interstitial fibrosis progressing to respiratory failure occurs later. Overspill pneumonitis from oesophageal dysfunction.

Oesophagus and intestine

Reduced motility can occur in any part of the gastrointestinal tract. Dysphagia is common (65%). Steatorrhoea and malabsorption are rare. Barium studies may reveal deformity and diminished peristalsis in the oesophagus, and dilatation of the second part of the duodenum.

Locomotor system

Polymyositis. Polyarthralgia later proceeds to a rheumatoid picture.

Heart

Pericardial effusion, cardiomyopathy and heart failure are rare.

Kidney

Progressive renal failure is usually associated with hypertension. Angiotensin-converting enzyme (ACE) inhibitors are useful in reducing blood pressure and preventing renal damage.

CREST syndrome

This is a syndrome which includes calcinosis cutis, Raynaud's phenomenon, oesophageal immobility, sclerodactyly and telangiectasia.

Investigation

There is no specific test. The ESR is often raised and antinuclear antibodies are present in 60%. Anticentromere antibodies tend to be found in patients with diffuse cutaneous systemic sclerosis associated with extensive visceral involvement. Antitopoisomerase antibodies (Scl-70) occur in patients with a more limited cutaneous disease, in whom involvement of other organs is a much later event.

Management

No treatment has been proven to alter the course of the disease. Most therapies are symptomatic. Antacids and sleeping upright may assist in preventing oesophageal reflux. Physiotherapy may help stiff fingers and joints and maintain muscle activity. Vasodilators and electrically heated gloves may reduce the symptoms of Raynaud's phenomenon. Non-steroidal anti-inflammatory drugs may be used for arthralgia (with caution if there is renal involvement). D-penicillamine has been used in some patients. Steroids and other immunosuppressants are sometimes tried, but are usually ineffective.

Rheumatoid arthritis

Women are more frequently affected than men (3 : 1). It is usually insidious in onset but may be an acute or a chronic relapsing disease marked by ill health and chronic joint deformity. The dominant clinical feature is a chronic synovitis.

However, the name 'rheumatoid disease' may be more appropriate since tissues other than the joints are frequently affected. The overall picture is of a systemic connective tissue disease with the brunt of the disease falling upon the joints. The extra-articular manifestations are very important in determining both the morbidity and mortality of the disease. There is often a family history.

Clinical features

Musculoskeletal

The small joints of the hands and feet are the most commonly affected, usually symmetrically, but other large synovial joints (hips, knees, elbows) are often also involved. The onset may be gradual with progressive pain, early-morning stiffness and swelling of joints. The acute onset is associated with fever and general constitutional illness. Examination may show:

• Tenderness and diminished movement of involved joints with characteristic fusiform soft-tissue swelling of the metacarpophalangeal and interphalangeal joints of the hands. (The metatarsophalangeal joints of the feet may also be tender on pressure.) The wrists are commonly involved. The terminal interphalangeal joints of the fingers are spared (unlike in psoriatic arthropathy; p. 195). The chronic disease may produce fixed deformities and ulnar deviation at the metacarpophalangeal joints.

• Wasting of the small muscles of the hand is common and results from a combination of disuse atrophy, vasculitis and peripheral neuropathy. Wasting may occur in the muscle around any affected joint.

• Inflammation of the soft tissues surrounding inflamed joints causes swelling, tenosynovitis (Achilles tendinitis, olecranon bursitis) and even tendon rupture. Localized subcutaneous nodules are present in 25%.

Joints less commonly involved are the ankles, which have relatively little synovial tissue, the costovertebral joints producing diminished chest expansion, temporomandibular joints, the cricoarytenoid joints (causing hoarseness and, rarely, acute respiratory obstruction) and the cervical spine. Laxity of the atlantoaxial joint ligaments with some erosion of the odontoid peg may result in acute or chronic cord compression and death. Atlantoaxial subluxation is present in 25% of patients, though only 7% have neurological signs. It may be necessary to X-ray the cervical spine in severe cases of rheumatoid arthritis prior to intubation for general anaesthesia.

NB Acute septic arthritis may occur in rheumatoid joints. Acute solitary effusions should be aspirated and examined microscopically and bacteriologically.

Lung

Lung involvement is clinically uncommon but lung function tests will show changes in nearly half of all patients with rheumatoid arthritis. They tend to be commoner in men than in women. It may occur before the arthritis and usually in seropositive disease. It presents as:

• isolated unilateral pleural effusion (must be differentiated from primary tuberculosis);
• rheumatoid nodules, single or multiple, which may be present throughout the lung parenchyma—commonly subpleural;
• diffuse fibronodular infiltration or fibrosing alveolitis; and
• Caplan's syndrome: the presence of large (up to 5 cm) rheumatoid nodules in the lungs of coal miners with silicosis but also occurring in other pneumoconioses. They may calcify, cavitate or coalesce and may precede clinical arthritis. The patients are seropositive.

Cardiac
Pericarditis (with or without effusion) is clinically uncommon, though found at postmortem in about 30%.

Vascular
Arteritic lesions characteristically produce nail fold infarcts and minute 'splinter' necrosis in the digital pulps. (This form of vascular necrosis is characteristic of arteritic lesions seen in the collagen disease, although multiple emboli in infective endocarditis may produce a similar picture.) Necrotizing arteritis may affect large vessels and give rise to digital gangrene, infarcted bowel or stroke. Chronic leg ulcers result from skin necrosis secondary to vasculitis—the ulcers are frequently on the lateral aspect of the tibia (cf. varicose ulcers). Raynaud's phenomenon (p. 405) may occur.

Neurological
• Peripheral neuropathy: this is usually predominantly sensory. Arteritis of the vessels supplying the nerves may be responsible.
• Neuropathy may also follow therapy with gold and chloroquine.
• Mononeuritis multiplex, particularly of digital nerves, ulnar nerves and lateral popliteal nerves.
• Entrapment neuropathy, e.g. carpal tunnel syndrome and the ulnar nerve at the elbow.
• Spinal cord lesions secondary to cervical disease.

Reticuloendothelial
The spleen is enlarged in about 5% of cases but only 1% develop leukopenia. Generalized lymphadenopathy is present in 10%.

Infection
Of all kinds (except urinary tract infections) and in all sites (especially joints) is much commoner and should be looked for in all patients who deteriorate suddenly.

Blood

Normochromic normocytic anaemia is common and its severity relates to that of the disease. Iron deficiency may result from bleeding secondary to salicylate or other non-steroidal anti-inflammatory therapy but this is uncommon and peptic ulceration and colonic neoplasms should be excluded. The height of the ESR reflects the activity of the disease. The CRP is raised even in the absence of infection (see SLE; p. 178).

Renal

Amyloidosis, though common on biopsy, is seldom clinically important in rheumatoid disease. Proteinuria or nephrotic syndrome may complicate treatment with pencillamine and gold.

Ocular

- Keratoconjunctivitis sicca occurs in 15% of patients with rheumatoid arthritis: see *Sjögren's syndrome* (p. 194).
- Scleritis presents as pericorneal injection with pain and tenderness in 0.6% of cases of rheumatoid arthritis. It may lead to uveitis and glaucoma.
- Scleromalacia perforans is even less common and occurs in long-standing rheumatoid arthritis: a rheumatoid nodule in the sclera may perforate.
- Iatrogenic: lens opacities and retinal degeneration with chloroquine and cataracts from steroids.

Iatrogenic

From gold (proteinuria, nephrotic syndrome, skin rash, marrow suppression); aspirin and most non-steroidal anti-inflammatory drugs (gastric erosion); penicillamine (nephropathy), steroids (p. 214) and chloroquine (cataract, retinopathy, photosensitivity).

Investigation of inflammatory polyarthropathy

There is often a normochromic normocytic anaemia. The ESR is performed to assess the activity of the disease and to monitor therapy. Perform ANF and DNA antibodies to exclude collagen disease. The serum uric acid helps to exclude gout, particularly if the distribution is asymmetrical. A chest X-ray helps to exclude the hypertrophic arthropathy of bronchial carcinoma and the arthropathy of acute sarcoid, which usually affects the ankles and knees. Human leukocyte antigen (HLA) B27 supports the diagnosis of Reiter's disease and the arthropathy of ulcerative colitis or Crohn's disease.

Rheumatoid factor

This is a circulating immunoglobulin of the IgM class which is an antibody to the patient's own IgG. It fixes complement and aids phagocytosis of immune complexes by neutrophils. It agglutinates sensitized sheep red cells (sheep cell agglutination test; SCAT) and also latex particles which have been coated with denatured γ-globulin (latex agglutination tests, e.g. F_2LP test, in which the F_2 fraction of denatured γ-globulin is used to coat the latex particles). High titres correlate with more severe arthritis with a worse prognosis, and with a higher incidence of extra-articular disease (nodules, arteritis, leg ulcers, digital gangrene, neuropathy, Felty's syndrome and fibrosing alveolitis).

Rheumatoid factor is positive in:
- 50–70% of outpatients with rheumatoid arthritis (100% in patients with nodules and Sjögren's syndrome);
- 25–35% of patients with collagen disease;
- 15% of patients with juvenile rheumatoid arthritis (Still's disease); and
- 4% of the general population, rising with age. Its presence does not necessarily indicate that rheumatoid disease will develop later.

Rheumatoid factor is usually negative in ankylosing spondylitis, Reiter's syndrome, psoriatic arthropathy and colitic arthropathy.

Radiology

The joints may be normal in early rheumatoid disease. The characteristic sequence of abnormalities is:
1 soft-tissue swelling and periarticular osteoporosis;
2 narrowing of joint space and periarticular erosions;
3 subluxation and osteoarthritis occur in long-standing disease; and
4 fibrosis or bony ankylosis.

Management

The assessment of disease activity depends on both clinical and laboratory findings.
- *Mild disease* is characterized by slight joint swelling and pain, with brief morning stiffness. Haemoglobin and platelet count are normal and ESR normal or marginally elevated.
- *Active disease* has more severe symptomatology, and the laboratory findings are abnormal (haemoglobin low, platelets often high and ESR >40 mm/h). The rheumatoid factor is more likely to be positive.

The objects of therapy are first, symptom control of pain and stiffness, enabling the patient to maintain as near normal existence as possible; and second, suppression of synovitis and systemic inflammation in more severe disease. A social assessment of occupation, of family help and home conditions is essential when planning therapy.

Rest disease joints in splints, especially at night to reduce pain and prevent deformity.

Physiotherapy to maintain full joint movement and strengthen weak muscles. Early attention and advice regarding posture may prevent chronic deformity and degeneration of all involved joints.

Drugs used in rheumatoid arthritis can be broadly divided into those aimed at pain relief and disease suppression.

Pain relief

Analgesics. Simple, such as paracetamol, or a compound such as co-proxamol or co-codamol.

Non-steroidal anti-inflammatory drugs. Aspirin, although inexpensive and effective, is less well-tolerated than newer non-steroidal anti-inflammatory drugs. Ibuprofen has fewer gastrointestinal side effects than other similar drugs, but tends to be less effective. Piroxicam, ketoprofen, indomethacin, naproxen and diclofenac have an intermediate risk of side effects, whereas azapropazone carries the highest risk. If there is gastrointestinal tolerance H_2-blockade or the prostaglandin E_1 analogue misoprostol may be added.

Disease-suppressing drugs

Corticosteroids are effective at producing symptomatic relief and suppressing disease activity, although concerns over side effects (osteoporosis, weight gain, hypertension, diabetes, cataracts; p. 214) have limited their use. Local injection of steroids into joints (or other painful sites) may give relief.

Gold. Sodium aurothiomalate is given by intramuscular injection at a dose of 50 mg weekly until there is evidence of remission (usually after about 500 mg). If there is no response after a total of 1 g, treatment is usually stopped. In patients who respond, the dosage interval is gradually increased to monthly. Treatment may be continued for up to 5 years, although only one-half of patients remain on therapy after 2 years. Regular blood counts and urinalysis are required. Leukopenia and thrombocytopenia, or proteinuria (due to membranous glomerulonephritis; p. 281), are usually reversible if gold is discontinued. Rashes may necessitate discontinuation of treatment.

Penicillamine has a similar action to gold. Side effects of thrombocytopenia, proteinuria and rashes are common, but in some cases treatment can be continued at a reduced dose, or stopped and then reintroduced.

Chloroquine and *hydroxychloroquine* tend to be better tolerated than gold or penicillamine. Retinopathy is rare if recommended doses are not exceeded (4 mg/kg daily for chloroquine 6 mg/kg per day for hydroxychloroquine).

Sulphasalazine is split into 5-aminosalicylic acid and sulphapyridine by bacteria in the large intestine. Its use is limited by gastrointestinal intolerance, rashes and hematological abnormalities. Leukopenia and thrombocytopenia usually occur in the first 3–6 months, and are reversible on cessation of treatment.

Immunosuppressant drugs (*methotrexate, azathioprine, cyclophosphamide, cyclosporin A, chlorambucil*) have all been used in active rheumatoid arthritis, either alone or in combination with corticosteroids or other agents to allow use of lower doses.

Surgical management

Synovectomy (especially of the knee joint), realignment and repair of tendons,

TRIALS

The **Arthritis and Rheumatism Council Low-Dose Glucocorticoid Study Group** compared prednisolone 7.5 mg daily with placebo in 128 adults with active rheumatoid arthritis of less than 2 years' duration. Over a 2-year period steroids reduced the rate of radiologically detectable disease progression. *N Engl J Med* 1995; **333**: 142–146.

The **Methotrexate–Cyclosporine Combination Study Group** compared methotrexate alone or in combination with cyclosporin in 148 patients who had previously demonstrated partial responses to methotrexate. Over a 6-month period patients receiving combination therapy demonstrated clinically important improvement, without substantial increases in side effects. *N Engl J Med* 1995; **333**: 137–141.

joint prostheses (hip, knee, fingers) and arthrodesis may be required for severe pain or deformity.

Advice of an expert in *rehabilitation* may allow a severely disabled patient to continue a tolerable and even happy existence at home. Depression should not be missed.

Diseases resembling rheumatoid arthritis

STILL'S DISEASE

Adult-onset Still's disease, like the juvenile form (p. 198) is characterized by a high spiking fever (85%), an evanescent rash (80%) and arthritis (100%), but occurs after the age of 15 years. Other features include splenomegaly (35%), pleurisy (30%), pericarditis (20%), neutrophil leukocytosis (100%), lymphadenopathy (70%) and hepatic abnormalities (85%). Roughly half go into remission off medication. Non-steroidal anti-inflammatory drugs are the treatment of choice, e.g. naproxen. Steroids are often needed in the acute phase.

SJÖGREN'S SYNDROME

It is commoner in women than in men (9:1). The major clinical features (sicca syndrome) result from reduced secretions from the lachrymal and salivary glands which produce dry gritty eyes and corneal ulcers (keratoconjunctivitis sicca) and a dry mouth (xerostomia) with dysphagia. Recurrent respiratory infections occur from diminished bronchial secretions. About 50% are associated with rheumatoid arthritis, 30% are uncomplicated and 20% associated with other autoimmune disease (mostly non-organ-specific). Rheumatoid factor is usually present, ANF frequently present (70%), anti-Ro is often present (40–60%), and lupus erythe-matosus cells are seldom present (15%). In Schirmer's test, filter paper is hooked over the lower eyelid; in normal people at least 15 mm is wet in 5 min and in the sicca syndrome usually far less. Fluorescein demonstrates corneal ulceration. Labial salivary gland biopsy may show diagnostic histology. Treatment is sympto-matic with artificial tears (hypromellose) and the arthritis is treated as uncompli-cated rheumatoid arthritis.

FELTY'S SYNDROME

Some patients with severe rheumatoid arthritis have enlarged lymph nodes, splenomegaly and hypersplenism (anaemia, leukopenia and thrombocytopenia). Removal of the spleen often reverses blood abnormalities but the underlying rheumatoid process is not affected and operation is seldom indicated. Leg ulcers are common due to vasculitis. The ANF is usually positive.

PSORIATIC ARTHRITIS

An arthritis similar to but distinct from rheumatoid arthritis may complicate psoriasis (p. 406). The clinical picture resembles rheumatoid arthritis and may be clinically indistinguishable from it in 30% but:

- psoriasis is present;
- joint involvement is usually asymmetrical and deforming and involves the terminal interphalangeal joints which may be the only affected joints (50%);
- pitting occurs in the nails (80%);
- subcutaneous nodules do not occur;
- sacroiliitis is more common (30%); and
- tests for rheumatoid factor are negative.

Ankylosing spondylitis (sacroiliitis)

Clinical features

A disease mainly of young adult males (20–40; cf. rheumatoid arthritis) with a 6% familial incidence. Joint involvement affects the sacroiliac joints, causing low back pain with morning stiffness. The disease may involve the spine, producing pain and stiffness initially of the lumbosacral region and eventually of the thoracic and cervical spine. The hips are involved in 50% of patients. Examination reveals decreased spinal movements and loss of the normal lumbosacral curvature. 'Springing' the pelvis (i.e. pressing the iliac crests towards each other) causes sacroiliac pain.

Peripheral joints are involved in 25%, especially the knees and ankles. The ribs fuse to the vertebrae. Up to 15% may present with a peripheral arthropathy. The arthropathy differs from rheumatoid arthritis in that it is asymmetrical and affects large joints more than small joints.

Other features of ankylosing spondylitis are:

- general ill health;

- uveitis (in 25–30% of cases and up to 40% in long-standing cases);
- ulcerative colitis — more common in patients with ankylosing spondylitis and vice versa;
- aortic regurgitation due to aortitis; and
- respiratory failure may result from the fixed ribcage with kyphoscoliosis, and from fibrosing alveolitis.

Investigation

Tests for rheumatoid factor are usually negative. The ESR is raised in 80%. HLA B27 is present in 96% (compared with 7% in the general population, and 50% of asymptomatic relatives).

Radiology

The sacroiliac joints are irregular with sclerosis of the articular margins. Bony ankylosis occurs late. The intervertebral ligaments calcify and finally ossify to produce a 'bamboo' spine.

Differential diagnoses

- Osteoarthritis of the spine.
- Prolapsed intervertebral disc.
- Tuberculosis which may affect only one sacroiliac joint.

Rarely:

- Psoriatic arthritis.
- Reiter's disease.
- The sacroiliitis of ulcerative colitis.

    All these may be variants of ankylosing spondylitis.

Management

Bed rest is contraindicated because it increases stiffness and ankylosis.

Careful posture with spinal muscle exercises is essential to prevent chronic deformity. Sleeping on a firm bed without pillows should help prevent fixed spinal flexion.

Analgesics. Phenylbutazone (Butazolidine) 200–300 mg/day is particularly effective but must now be reserved for specialist use.

Indomethacin or other non-steroidal anti-inflammatory drugs may be given as an alternative.

Radiotherapy, although effective in reducing pain, is inadvisable except in those with intractable pain as there is an increased risk of leukaemia (0.3%).

Sulphasalazine (500 mg starting dose to maintenance dose of 2–3 g/day), as in rheumatoid arthritis, offers symptomatic improvement more of peripheral joints than sacroiliitis in 2–3 months, probably by altering the immune process.

Prognosis

Many mild cases may never present to a physician. With expert care 70–80% will maintain complete or almost complete activity. More severe cases develop moderate to severe bony ankylosis of the spine to produce fixation of mobility and rounded kyphosis of the cervical and thoracic spine. This may impair ventilation. In severe cases extreme rigidity of the spine may occur within 3–5 years. The disease may remit at any stage but recurrent episodes may occur.

Reiter's syndrome

A disease usually of young men presenting with urethritis, arthritis and conjunctivitis (only 30%). There is usually a history of sexual intercourse 2–4 weeks previously. It occurs in <1% of patients with non-specific urethritis. The disease may, less commonly in the UK, follow bacillary (*Shigella*) dysentery.

Clinical features

- Arthritis: typically acute or subacute and usually polyarticular and asymmetrical, affecting large joints of the lower limbs.
- Sacroiliitis occurs in 30%. Plantar fasciitis, calcaneal spurs and Achilles tendinitis may occur (20%).
- Conjunctivitis is common in the acute disease. Iritis is associated with chronic recurrent disease, particularly when associated with sacroiliitis.
- Skin lesions: mouth ulcers are common. Urethritis and prostatitis are associated with superficial skin ulceration around the penile meatus (circinate balanitis).
- Pustular hyperkeratotic lesions of the soles of the feet and less frequently the palms of the hands (keratoderama blennorrhagica) may occur (15%).
- Cardiovascular lesions may occur.
- Tests for rheumatoid factor are by definition negative.
- HLA B27 is present in 70%.

Differential diagnosis

- Gonococcal arthritis (the gonococcus is present in up to half the cases and is detected in urethral discharge or blood culture).
- Ankylosing spondylitis.
- Behçet's disease.
- Psoriatic and rheumatoid arthritis.

Management

- The treatment of the acute stage is symptomatic.
- Rest and aspirate the inflamed joints.
- Indomethacin is the drug of first choice.
- The majority of cases settle spontaneously within 4–10 weeks, but the disease may recur in 50%. (The urethritis may respond to tetracycline 2 g/day for 10 days.)

Acute generalized arthritis

STILL'S DISEASE — JUVENILE FORM

A childhood disease, usually of acute onset with fever and skin rashes. Joint pain is not an essential feature (absent in 25% at onset) and may be monarticular (30%) at the onset. Subcutaneous nodules are rare. Eye changes include chronic irido-cyclitis (10%), corneal band opacity and complicated cataract. Lymphadenopathy is present in 30%, splenomegaly in 20% and simple pericarditis in 10%. One-third of patients present with a history of insidious polyarthritis as in adult rheumatoid arthritis. Tests of rheumatoid factor are usually negative (85%).

Prognosis

The majority of cases settle spontaneously with minimal or no disability. Bone growth may be retarded. In one-third the disease continues into adult life.

Acute rheumatic fever

An acute febrile systemic disorder affecting mainly the heart and joints following a streptococcal infection (group A, β-haemolytic), occurring usually between the ages of 5 and 15 years. The disease is now very rare in developed countries.

Diagnosis

In the text below, double asterisks denote major criteria, single asterisks minor criteria. The diagnosis is made if there are one major and two minor, or two major with evidence of previous streptococcal infection.

Symptoms

The disease usually presents with flitting polyarthropathy** or carditis** (40%), the former being more common in adults and the latter in children. Both may be present at the same time but carditis is uncommon over the age of 20. The involved joints may be exquisitely tender*. There may be a history of streptococcal infection of the throat or skin 10–20 days previously. Rarely, children may present with chorea**.

Examination

General

The dominant features are fever* (90%) and flitting arthropathy of large joints (small joints may be affected in the elderly) which are exquisitely tender. Erythema nodosum and erythema marginatum* (5%) are more common in children. Symmetrical subcutaneous nodules** (10%) lying over bony prominences and extensor surfaces occur virtually only in children and their presence probably correlates with severe carditis.

Sign of carditis

Myocarditis: tachycardia, cardiomegaly, heart failure.

Endocarditis: any valve may be involved and cause transient murmurs. A transient mitral diastolic murmur (Carey Coombs) is the most common. Mitral systolic and aortic murmurs also occur.

Percarditis: friction rub or small effusion.

Investigation

The ESR* is raised. The anti-streptolysin (ASO)* titre may be raised or rising (more than 200 units/ml) and haemolytic streptococci* may be isolated from the throat. The white blood cell count* is raised and a hypochromic normocytic anaemia, unresponsive to iron therapy, may develop. The electrocardiogram may show first-degree heart block*. Almost any rhythm disorder may occur. Chest X-ray may demonstrate progressive cardiac enlargement.

Management

- Bed rest.
- Immobilize inflamed joints.
- Acetylsalicylic acid. The oral dose is 6–12 g/day to achieve blood levels of 2.1–2.4 mmol/l (30–35 mg/100 ml). Side effects of nausea, tinnitus and blurring of vision may limit the dosage. The symptomatic response to salicylates is characteristic. Steroids are frequently used with salicylates but there is no evidence that either improves the prognosis.
- Penicillin G is given during the acute stages and oral penicillin (125–250 mg bd) continued in those with cardiac involvement for at least 5 years and preferably until 20 years of age to prevent recurrence. Erythromycin is used for patients sensitive to penicillin.

Postinfectious arthralgia

Low-grade polyarthralgia may follow some infections, e.g. glandular fever, German measles, *Mycoplasma pneumoniae* and viral hepatitis and meningococcal septicaemia and persist for months or years. The association of this with erythema chronicum migrans occurs in Lyme disease (p. 413) following tick-borne infection with the spirochaete *Borrelia burgdorferi*.

Osteoarthritis

A common degenerative disorder of the joint surface. There is damage to hyaline cartilage, with sclerosis and osteophyte formation in underlying subchondral bone. It is related to age, previous joint injury and deformity.

Incidence

It is radiologically universal after the age of 55 years. The commonest joints to be affected are the interphalangeal joints (50%), the thumb carpometacarpal joint (30%), the cervical spine (40%), lumbar spine (40%), knees (30%) and hips (20%).

Clinical features

There is pain which is worse with movement and towards the end of the day. There is also stiffness, immobility, deformity and occasionally nerve root involvement. The joints may be red, warm and tender and even produce an effusion (beware of an infected effusion). Joint involvement is asymmetrical. The stiffness tends to wear off in 10–15 min of exercise (cf. rheumatoid arthritis—1–2 h).

Investigation

Joint X-rays show a loss of space, osteophytes and sclerosis of subchondral bone, sometimes with cyst formation. Synovial aspirates produce <100 WBC/mm^3 and these are chiefly monocytes.

Management

Effective analgesia with or without anti-inflammatory agents including paracetamol and the non-steroidal anti-inflammatory drugs. Obese patients should lose weight if the arthritis affects weight-bearing joints.

A walking stick and special orthopaedic shoes may be very effective in relieving symptoms. Orthopaedic surgery can offer arthrodesis, arthroplasty and joint replacement (hips, knees, fingers, shoulders and elbows).

Endocrine Disease

Diabetes mellitus (p. 221) and disorders of the thyroid gland are the only common forms of endocrine disease.

Thyroid

Enlargement of the thyroid of varying degrees is frequent, especially in women, and large non-toxic goitres are not uncommon. Both hypothyroidism and hyperthyroidism are relatively common. Thyroid cancer is rare.

NON-TOXIC GOITRE
Aetiology

The enlargement of the gland (visible and palpable) is due to an increased secretion of thyroid-stimulating hormone (TSH) secondary to diminished output of thyroid hormones. The causes are:

• *Simple goitre.* Iodine deficiency, especially in areas of endemic goitre. Sporadic goitre is probably due to relative iodine deficiency for that patient. Iodine requirement is increased at puberty in girls and during pregnancy. The gland tends to become nodular as age increases.

• *Goitrogens*, e.g. iodides in large doses, antithyroid drugs such as para-aminosalicylic acid (PAS), phenylbutazone, lithium and many others, are rare as causes (except when used therapeutically, e.g. carbimazole).

• *Inborn errors* of thyroid hormone synthesis (dyshormonogenesis). Six types of enzyme defect are known. All are rare. They are autosomal recessive. The commonest is associated with nerve deafness (Pendred's syndrome) and due to impaired organic binding of iodine.

Clinical presentation

A painless swelling of the thyroid is usually noticed by the patient or relatives. If untreated it may develop into a large nodular goitre and cause pressure on the trachea, oesophagus or veins, especially if there is retrosternal extension.

Differential diagnosis

- Autoimmune thyroiditis (Hashimoto's disease).
- Toxic goitre.
- Cancer of the thyroid.
- Solitary nodule—benign (rare) and carcinoma (very rare).

Investigation

- Serum free triiodothyronine (T_3), free thyroxine (T_4) and TSH if hyper-thyroidism is suspected, or free T_4 and TSH if hypothyroidism.
- Thyroid antibodies for Hashimoto's disease.
- X-ray of neck thoracic inlet if pressure symptoms are present.
- Ultrasound will distinguish solid or cystic masses, whether single or multiple.
- Fine-needle aspiration with cytology may be diagnostic but some surgeons prefer excision.

Prophylaxis

Iodized salt, especially during pregnancy. Seafish in the diet.

Treatment

Thyroxine 100–150 microg. daily for long periods to suppress TSH hypersecretion. Surgery for pressure symptoms (rarely necessary) and removal of nodules.

THYROTOXICOSIS (hyperthyroidism)
Aetiology

The clinical picture results from an excess of thyroid hormones (T_4 and/or T_3). Graves' disease refers to the common form of hyperthyroidism in which eye signs and toxic symptoms accompany diffuse enlargement of the gland (F:M = 5:1) with antibodies and occasional pretibial myxoedema. Thyrotoxicosis is an auto-immune disease associated with thyroid-stimulating immunoglobulins (TSI), against the TSH receptor site on the thyroid follicular cell membrane. There also appears to be a thyroid growth immunoglobulin (TGI), which may independently determine the size of any goitre. An ophthalmopathic immunoglobulin to eye muscle basement membrane may be causative and independent. There is an association with human leukocyte antigen (HLA) B8 and DR3. Rarely a single toxic nodule may produce thyrotoxicosis. There is a strong genetic factor. Self-administered T_4 should not be forgotten as a cause of hyperthyroidism, particularly in doctors and nurses. A gross persistent excess of iodine in health foods and some cough medicines may precipitate hyperthyroidism.

Clinical presentation

The symptoms and signs, except the eye signs, can be deduced from a knowledge of the pharmacological action of T_4 and T_3.

The most helpful symptoms are preference for cold weather, excessive sweating, increased appetite and weight loss, nervousness, tiredness and palpitations.

The most helpful signs are goitre, especially with a murmur, exophthalmos, lid retraction and lid lag, hot moist palms, tremor and excessive movements, tachycardia or atrial fibrillation.

Atypical presentations

- Atrial fibrillation, tachycardia or cardiac failure in middle age or older should always suggest thyrotoxicosis.
- Unexplained weight loss in apparently euthyroid patients.

Very rare. Toxic manic confusion. Severe proximal limb girdle myopathy. Diarrhoea.

Differential diagnosis

Thyrotoxicosis is often difficult to differentiate from an anxiety state, particularly when this is associated with a simple goitre. The palms tend to be moist but cold in anxiety state.

Investigation

Always carry out at least one, and preferably two, tests before starting treatment to confirm and document the diagnosis. Use serum free T_3, free T_4 (raised) and TSH (suppressed) in borderline cases. Computed tomographic (CT) scan of the orbit demonstrates thickened external ocular muscle. The orbit contains excess mucopolysaccharide (and water).

Treatment

Antithyroid drugs

Carbimazole can be given in a titration regime to block thyroid hormone synthesis sufficiently to produce a euthyroid state. For this, give carbimazole 15 mg three times a day for 3 weeks reducing to 5 mg three times a day or more according to the response and maintained for 12–18 months. Review at 6 months, 1 year and 18 months. When the drugs are stopped, relapse occurs in at least two-thirds within 1 or 2 years and either surgery or radioiodine is used (see below).

In the block-replacement regime, enough carbimazole is given to block all thyroid hormone production with 40–60 mg in a single daily dose, plus replacement of normal thyroid requirements with L-thyroxine, 100–150 µg/day. Compliance is improved for some patients and relapse is possibly less common after treatment is stopped. Side effects of carbimazole include skin rashes, loss of hair and neutropenia (sore throat is usually the first symptom). Propylthiouracil is a suitable alternative. In pregnancy, carbimazole in the usual doses remains the treatment of choice, with tests of thyroid function kept at the upper end of the normal range. The baby can be breast-fed if the patient remains on modest doses of the drug.

Propranolol
Propranolol 20 mg three times a day may give rapid improvement in cardiac symptoms and a sense of well-being. It should not be used alone in thyrotoxic heart failure or as the sole therapy.

Radioactive iodine therapy
Radioactive iodine therapy is given after rendering the more toxic patient euthyroid with drugs, stopping them 4 days before administration, and reintroducing them 4 days afterwards while awaiting the 5-week delay before the effects of radiotherapy become apparent.

One strategy is to give an ablation, or near-ablation dose of radioiodine (about 550 MBq = 15 mCi) followed by standard replacement doses of thyroid hormone. Patients given more conventional doses of radioiodine experience an inexorable cumulative incidence of hypothyroidism of about 4% per year. Between 5% and 15% develop hypothyroidism in the first year.

Patients with a single toxic adenoma or a toxic multinodular goitre can have a large dose of radioiodine with relatively little chance of hypothyroidism, because the unaffected parts of the thyroid have been dormant following suppression of TSH by excessive thyroid hormone secretion, and do not take up the radioiodine.

Surgery. This requires adequate preoperative treatment with carbimazole and later potassium iodide. Subtotal thyroidectomy is advised for (i) failure of medical treatment, and drug sensitivity in the young, and (ii) large multinodular goitres, especially with pressure symptoms as they may enlarge with medical therapy, and for cosmetic reasons. One year later about 80% are euthyroid, 15% hypothyroid and 5% have relapsed. Complications include hypothyroidism (eventually 10–15% in those with high antibody titres), recurrence of hyperthyroidism, recurrent laryngeal nerve palsy (rare), hypoparathyroidism (rare).

Treatment of complications
Eye
Lid retraction (sclera visible below the upper lid) usually responds to treatment of the thyrotoxicosis. Exophthalmos (sclera visible above lower lid) results from the swelling of retro-orbital tissues and may not improve and may progress. In malignant exophthalmos there is weakness of the external ocular muscles, often with diplopia, oedema of the conjunctivae and corneal damage from exposure. Treatment is difficult. The strabismus and lid retraction of dysthyroid ophthalmopathy may respond to intramuscular injection of botulinum toxin (neurotoxin A) but the place of this in routine therapy is not yet determined. Local or systemic steroids

may be required with tarsorrhaphy in severe cases. Orbital decompression may be required. The condition remits slowly over years with or without treatment.

Atrial fibrillation

Atrial fibrillation responds poorly to digoxin and larger doses are often needed until the patient is euthyroid. Cardioversion may then be used. Propranolol or other β-blocker may control severe tachycardia. Heart failure is unusual and responds to antithyroid drugs plus conventional treatment.

Thyrotoxic crisis

This is rare but dangerous. Dexamethasone (2 mg qds) inhibits T_4 conversion to T_3 in the tissues. Oral carbimazole (60–120 mg) is followed by potassium iodide (60 mg daily in divided doses). β-Blockade (propranolol 80 mg qds) is usually required. Oxygen should be given and particular attention paid to fluid balance since sweating is marked.

HYPOTHYROIDISM

This results from a low level of circulating thyroid hormone, either free T_4 or T_3. The term 'myxoedema' means that there is a deposition of a mucopolysaccharide beneath the skin, producing a non-pitting swelling of the subcutaneous tissues.

Aetiology

Autoimmune thyroiditis. This may present as Hashimoto's disease when a goitre is present, or as spontaneous or primary hypothyroidism if the gland atrophies without producing a goitre. Circulating thyroid antibodies are present.
•   Destructive therapy for hyperthyroidism or carcinoma by operation or by radioiodine.
•   Primary thyroid agenesis may produce cretinism in infants.
•   Ingestion of goitrogens, usually an antithyroid drug (including very large doses of iodine) in too large doses or for too long.
•   Secondary to hypopituitarism; this is rare.
•   Inborn errors of thyroid metabolism.
•   There may be a family history of thyroid disease or of autoimmune disease, e.g. 10% have pernicious anaemia.

Clinical presentation

The onset is insidious, difficult to distinguish from depression and the condition may be far advanced before it is recognized. All who have had destructive therapy to the thyroid should be followed up at 6-monthly intervals. Many of the symptoms also occur in euthyroid individuals, e.g. tiredness, loss of hair. Those which have the greatest diagnostic value are intolerance of cold, diminished energy, physical tiredness, slow cerebration, increase in weight, hoarseness of voice, diminished sweating, dry and rough skin, dry and unruly hair, deafness, constipation, muscular pains and paraesthesiae (carpal tunnel syndrome).

The physical signs include a typical facial appearance with periorbital puffiness and pallor, coarse and cold skin, slow movements, hoarse voice, slow pulse and a slowing of the recovery phase of the ankle jerk reflexes. Ischaemic heart disease is common. Central nervous system involvement may produce intellectual impairment and dementia (myxoedema madness) and coma (with hypothermia). Only 5% of patients presenting with hypothermia have hypothyroidism.

Investigation

- All suspected cases should be investigated: serum T_4 is reduced and this stimulates pituitary secretions of TSH (raised in primary hypothyroidism).
- Raised serum cholesterol (p. 231) is present, though not important in the diagnosis.
- Anaemia (normochromic or macrocytic).
- ECG shows slow rate and low voltage with flattened or inverted T waves.
- Rise in titre of thyroid antibodies.

Treatment

T_4 is given in doses of 25–50 μg/day, starting with a low dose and raising it every month to achieve normal levels of TSH. The average maintenance daily dose is 150 μg. Free T_4 levels are above the normal range given for the untreated patient. If ischaemic heart disease is present, the lowest dose should be used initially. Patients should be warned that treatment is for life. Osteoporosis is a long-term risk of over-treatment.

AUTOIMMUNE THYROIDITIS

This term usually refers to disorders of the thyroid gland in which circulating thyroid antibodies are present in the plasma; in addition lymphoid and plasma cells are found in excess in the thyroid gland. The patients may be hypothyroid, euthyroid or hyperthyroid. Hashimoto's disease refers to the condition in which autoimmune thyroiditis has produced a hard nodular goitre. Destruction of thyroid hormone-producing tissue causes a rise in TSH which leads to thyroid enlargement. At this stage, the level of the circulating thyroid hormones, although reduced for that person, may be within the normal limits and there is no evidence of hypothyroidism. However, thyroid reserve is diminished, and later the free T_4 falls further and symptoms of hypothyroidism occur in about 2% per annum. By then the patient has a goitre which is often hard and sometimes nodular. In some patients the development of autoimmune hypothyroidism is associated with progressive fibrosis of the gland without the production of a goitre. These patients present with hypothyroidism without a goitre.

Clinical presentation

Hashimoto's disease presents as a patient with a goitre who is either euthyroid or hypothyroid. The goitre must be distinguished from other types of non-toxic goitre and from carcinoma of the thyroid.

Investigation

Thyroid antibodies may be directed against thyroglobulin or the microsomal fraction of thyroid cells. The former include the highly specific but relatively insensitive precipitin test, and the sensitive but less specific tanned red cell agglutination test. The complement fixation test against microsomal antibodies is not very specific. The gland usually takes up a normal amount of iodine, i.e. the radio-iodine uptake is within normal limits but there is faulty utilization of iodine, and the iodine is discharged from the gland by potassium perchlorate in about half the cases. The free T_4 is in the lower range of normal or in the hypothyroid free range.

Management

T_4 in full doses will suppress TSH, cause the gland to diminish in size and relieve any symptoms of hypothyroidism if present.

ACUTE THYROIDITIS

Although relatively uncommon, acute thyroiditis may often follow an upper respiratory tract infection or other microbial infection (e.g. measles, infections mononucleosis, mumps, Coxsackie). There is fever and malaise, usually with some local swelling and tenderness of the gland and sometimes dysphagia. Initially there may be some hyperthyroidism. The serum T_4 may be normal or raised but the radioiodine uptake is suppressed. The differential diagnosis includes carcinoma (less tender but harder), haemorrhage into a cyst or Hashimoto's thyroiditis. Pyogenic infection in the thyroid causes a more severe illness.

Management

Simple analgesia may suffice. Prednisolone 30 mg daily may be necessary and can usually be tailed off rapidly.

AMIODARONE

Amiodarone is rich in iodine and also inhibits peripheral conversion of T_4 to T_3, making thyroid investigations difficult to interpret. Basal T_3, T_4 and TSH levels should be checked before starting amiodarone to identify any underlying thyroid disease.

THYROID CANCER (p. 41)

All types are rare and some carry a relatively good prognosis. Ionizing radiation during childhood is a predisposing factor. The main types and their clinical features are:

Papillary

Commonest type. It occurs in the relatively young and may present with lymph gland enlargement (lateral aberrant thyroid). It is often TSH-dependent and regresses if thyroxine is given. The prognosis is relatively good.

Follicular

Often produces functioning secondaries which are sensitive to radioiodine. It has a relatively good prognosis and is relatively common.

Anaplastic

Usually presents with gland enlargement in the elderly and is highly malignant.

Medullary

Rare. It secretes calcitonin and may produce ectopic corticotrophin and other substances. It may be associated with a phaeochromocytoma in multiple endocrine neoplasia (MEN; p. 219). The prognosis is poor, though relatively better than anaplastic cancers. Relatives should be screened.

Thyroid nodules

A thyroid nodule which appears to be single is usually not single. Even if it is, the likelihood of malignancy is low. Ultrasound may distinguish solid from cystic lesions, but this does not distinguish between the presence and absence of thyroid carcinoma. Fine-needle biopsy and aspiration of fluid for cytology may miss a carcinoma and single cysts tend to refill. Surgical removal is preferred.

Pituitary

The hypothalamus controls the secretion of the anterior and posterior pituitary hormones. Hypothalamic nerve fibres liberate releasing factors which are carried in the portal blood stream to the pituitary gland and there cause release, synthesis or inhibition of pituitary hormones. At least nine factors have been suggested and three, corticotrophic-releasing hormone (CRH), thyrotrophin-releasing hormone (TRH) and gonadotrophin-releasing hormone (GnRH), have been isolated and their chemical structure determined. GnRH causes release of both luteinizing hormone (LH) and follicle-stimulating hormone (FSH). Prolactin (PRL) release is inhibited by dopamine.

The anterior lobe produces at least six types of hormone—growth hormone (GH), FSH, LH, TSH, adrenocorticotrophic hormone (ACTH) and PRL. The posterior lobe secretes two hormones, antidiuretic hormone (ADH) and oxytocin. The gland has a close anatomical and physiological relationship to the hypothalamus. The anatomical relationship to the optic chiasma is important and all patients with suspected pituitary tumours should have their visual fields plotted. X-ray of the pituitary fossa and CT or MRI scan will accurately define the pituitary fossa.

The clinical features of pituitary disease differ according to the type of lesion and the region of the gland which is predominantly affected. All are rare and in examinations will have received some treatment. Failure of secretion is more common than increased secretion. Non-functional (chromophobe) adenoma is the commonest cause of hypopituitarism. It also gives rise to increased intracranial pressure and to local pressure effects. Prolactinomas are the commonest secreting tumours of the pituitary. They cause infertility and galactorrhoea in women, and impotence with gynaecomastia in men. The commonest tumour in childhood is the craniopharyngioma which often calcifies. Classically eosinophilic tumours (rare) give giantism in the child or acromegaly in the adult; and basophil hyperplasia or adenoma produce Cushing's syndrome. However, acromegaly may be associated with eosinophil, chromophobe or mixed-cell tumours.

HYPOPITUITARISM

The pattern of deficiency depends on the nature of the lesion and its rate of progress. In general, deficiencies of GH, FSH and LH secretions occur early, TSH and ACTH next. Last of all, ADH secretion fails if the posterior lobe is involved by surgical intervention or suprasellar disease. Deficiency of each hormone is measured by suitable blood hormone assay and the integrity of the target organs assessed by applying the appropriate physiological stimulus, e.g. ACTH.

Aetiology

- Iatrogenic from hypophysectomy or irradiation — adequate replacement therapy prevents symptoms occurring.
- Non-functional (chromophobe) adenoma.
- Postpartum pituitary necrosis in the female (Sheehan's syndrome). This is now extremely rare with improved standards of midwifery.
- Other tumours (including secondary tumours), granulomas (sarcoid and tuberculosis) and head injury—all rare.

Clinical presentation

In children hypopituitarism produces pituitary infantilism (Peter Pan dwarfs — small but well-formed and in proportion). In adults the presentation depends upon the pattern of deficiency of the various hormones and associated pressure symptoms. The symptoms and signs can be worked out from a knowledge of the functions of the target organs involved.

Hormone deficiency

Loss of sexual function occurs, both primary with amenorrhoea and loss of libido, and secondary with loss of body hair (male patients may find shaving unnecessary).

Adrenal insufficiency (p. 217) from failure of ACTH occurs but there is little change in electrolyte metabolism since aldosterone is still secreted.

Pallor and skin depigmentation occur.

Symptoms of hypothyroidism (p. 205) from lack of TSH appear but there is no myxoedema—the face is not coarsened.

Coma may occur from low cortisol levels, spontaneous hypoglycaemia or hypothermia.

Pressure effects

Compression of the optic chiasma produces bitemporal hemianopia and optic atrophy.

Pressure on the hypothalamus may cause somnolence and weight gain.

NB   In the male, hypopituitarism is usually due to a non-functional adenoma or large prolactinoma. In Sheehan's syndrome, there is a history of postpartum haemorrhage, failure of lactation with atrophy of breast tissue, and amenorrhoea in addition to the other effects described.

Investigation

Assessment of pituitary function involves:

- measurement of pituitary hormones (TSH, ACTH, FSH, LH, GH and PRL);
- measurement of target organ secretion (thyroid and adrenal, and sex hormones); and
- dynamic tests of hypothalamic pituitary function:
    (a) insulin hypoglycaemia test (now rarely performed as it is potentially lethal in inexperienced hands);
    (b) Synacthen (tetracosactrin) tests (p. 218);
    (c) metyrapone test (p. 215);
    (d) TRH stimulation test; and
    (e) LH-releasing hormone test.

Treatment

The pituitary is removed if there are pressure symptoms, particularly visual loss, unless a prolactinoma is present, when bromocriptine usually shrinks the tumour without surgery.

Replacement therapy by:

- cyclical oestrogen–progesterone therapy in women or intramuscular depot testosterone esters every 2–4 weeks (e.g. Sustanon 250) in men;
- hydrocortisone 20 mg in the morning and 10 mg at night. Fludrocortisone is not usually required;
- T_4 0.1–0.3 mg (100–300 µg) daily;
- coma is treated as in Addisonian crisis (p. 217).

ACROMEGALY

Excess GH gives acromegaly in the adult (after the epiphyses have fused) and giantism in earlier life. The onset is between 20 and 40 years.

Giantism is almost always the result of the action of excessive secretion of GH before the epiphyses have united. Later in life pituitary failure tends to occur and giants are therefore not usually strong, aggressive or virile.

Aetiology

Excessive secretion of GH from an adenoma of the pituitary, often of eosinophil cells. GH causes overgrowth of soft tissues, including the skin, tongue and viscera and of bones. It has an anti-insulin action.

Clinical presentation

The onset is insidious, often with early changes (look at old photographs). Headache occurs early due to stretching of the dura mater. Pressure effects with bitemporal hemianopia are rarer. Excessive secretion of GH causes:

• Face. Increase in size of skull, supraorbital ridges, lower jaw (separation of teeth) and the sinuses.

• The tongue is enlarged.

• Vertebral enlargement, and kyphosis from osteoporosis.

• Hands and feet are spade-shaped and carpal tunnel syndrome may be present.

• Enlarged heart, liver and thyroid.

• Hypertension (15%).

• Diabetes mellitus (10%) and reduced glucose tolerance (30%).

• Arthropathy (50%).

The following also occur:

• acne, hirsutes, excessive sweating;

• gynaecomastia and galactorrhoea (prolactin excess); and

• hypogonadism, oligomenorrhoea.

Investigation

• Assay of GH by radioimmunoassay; the levels are raised only in active disease and are not suppressed by glucose in a standard glucose tolerance test.

• Perimetry for bitemporal visual field defects (50%).

• X-ray of skull for enlargement of the sella, erosion of the clinoid processes, supraorbital ridges and lower jaw. The floor of the pituitary fossa may appear eroded or double in lateral-view tomograms.

• CT scan to show suprasellar extension.

• X-ray of hands for tufting of the terminal phalanges and increased joint spaces due to hypertrophy of the cartilage. The heel pad is usually thickened. These tests are interesting rather than diagnostic.

• The glucose tolerance curve may be diabetic.

• Fasting serum phosphate may be raised but is of no diagnostic value.

• Chest X-ray and ECG may show left ventricular hypertrophy from hypertension.

Prognosis and treatment

Life expectancy is halved due to cardiorespiratory complications. Successful management means destruction of the tissue producing excess GH. Surgery is indicated for progressive visual deterioration (regular perimetry is obligatory) and some would recommend it for all acromegalics who are fit for surgery. Transsphenoidal hypophysectomy is the treatment of choice. Craniotomy is sometimes

used in those with suprasellar extension. Yttrium-90 implants or external irradiation are alternatives to surgical removal in active disease, but may cause further
damage to the optic tracts, diabetes insipidus and aseptic bone necrosis, and have
much lower cure rates. Cerebrospinal rhinorrhoea may result from yttrium
implantation. Bromocriptine reduces GH and PRL levels and may be a useful
adjunct to conventional therapy or used as sole therapy. Unlike destructive therapies, diabetes insipidus is not produced. Somatostatin analogues (octreotide)
may be used, particularly for young patients, male or female, who wish to retain
fertility.

DIABETES INSIPIDUS

A very rare disease due to deficiency of ADH (vasopressin).

Aetiology

- Idiopathic, often familial and the commonest form.
- Tumours: craniopharyngioma or secondary tumour.
- Surgery or radiation to pituitary gland.
- Head injury — usually mild and short-lived. Rarely complete and permanent
with transaction of the pituitary stalk with frontal vault fractures.
- Granulomas, e.g. sarcoid; or infections, e.g. basal meningitis.

Clinical presentation

Polyuria and polydipsia—5–20 litres of urine/24 h.

Investigation

The specific gravity of the urine is very low and fails to increase with water deprivation. Fluids are allowed overnight and stopped in the morning. It is dangerous to
lose more than 2–3% of the body weight. In normal people plasma osmolality does
not rise above 300 mosmol/kg and urine osmolality rises to 600 mosmol/kg during
8 h of water deprivation. In diabetes insipidus the former rises and the latter does
not, or remains at about plasma level. Vasopressin corrects the abnormality in
ADH-deficient diabetes insipidus but not in the nephrogenic type.

Differential diagnosis

Psychogenic polydipsia. Thirst dominates the picture. The patient resents the water
deprivation test, and surreptitious drinking is common. Renal concentrating
power may be moderately reduced due to the prolonged polyuria and consequent
low medullary osmolality.

Nephrogenic diabetes insipidus. This refers to a vasopressin (ADH)-resistant
polyuria. This is a rare sex-linked recessive inherited disorder with a primary renal
tubular defect of water reabsorption. Secondary nephrogenic diabetes insipidus
occurs with:
- diabetes mellitus (glycosuria);

- chronic renal failure;
- postobstructive uropathy;
- hypercalcaemia;
- hypokalaemia; and
- lithium toxicity.

Treatment

Desmopressin (DDAVP or arginine vasopressin) nasal spray 10–20 μg bd has replaced lysine vasopressin in the treatment of ADH deficiency.

Carbamazepine 200–800 mg daily may increase the renal response to ADH. Chlorpropamide (100–300 mg daily) acts similarly but is obsolescent due to the risk of hypoglycaemia.

Thiazide diuretics probably act by reducing glomerular filtration rate and are also used in nephrogenic diabetes insipidus.

PROLACTINOMA

These tumours cause galactorrhoea in both sexes and gonadal dysfunction — infertility in the female and impotence in the male. Measurement of PRL levels suggests the diagnosis, usually before pressure symptoms occur. The tumours vary in size from pinhead (microadenoma) to very large (rare) and may necrose. Hyperprolactinaemia may be caused by a variety of physiological stimuli such as pregnancy and stress and by certain drugs such as oestrogens and tranquillizers. Bromocriptine (1.25–10 mg or more daily) inhibits PRL secretion and is usually tried before surgery or radiotherapy. Visual fields need checking periodically because pituitary tumours may press on the optic chiasma to cause a bitemporal field loss. If the patient becomes pregnant, a small tumour may enlarge rapidly.

Adrenal

ADRENAL GLANDS

The medulla secretes adrenaline and noradrenaline. The cortex produces steroid hormones, of which the most important are cortisol (hydrocortisone) and aldosterone. The secretion of most of the steroids is controlled by pituitary corticotrophin (ACTH) which itself is released by the hypothalamic hormone — corticotrophin-releasing hormone factor (CRF). The secretion of aldosterone is independent of the pituitary and controlled by the renin–aldosterone system. The adrenals also produce androgens and oestrogens. The effects of the three main groups of adrenocortical hormones differ. In summary they are:

Glucocorticoids (e.g. cortisol)

Raise the blood sugar and antagonize insulin. They have a permissive effect on the action of catecholamines on the heart and blood vessels and are essential for the body's response to shock. They suppress the reaction to injury, infection and inflammation. In excess they have a protein catabolic effect, atrophy skin and weaken capillaries. They reduce the circulating eosinophil and lymphocyte counts. They cause sodium retention and potassium depletion and alkalosis when given in large doses or over long periods.

Mineralocorticoids (e.g. aldosterone)

Cause sodium retention and potassium depletion, with hypertension, alkalosis and oedema. The synthetic steroids, fludrocortisone and deoxycorticosterone acetate, have similar actions.

Sex hormones

Produce effects depending on the dominance of male hormone, e.g. andros-terone, or female hormone, e.g. oestrogens and progesterone. Hence they may be virilizing or feminizing. Androgens antagonize some of the metabolic effects of the glucocorticoids.

CUSHING'S SYNDROME
Aetiology

The syndrome is the result of excess corticosteroids and by far the commonest cause is *prolonged treatment with relatively large doses*. Most of the synthetic ana-logues of cortisone produce these side effects but they are less liable to give rise to sodium retention. Apart from iatrogenic disease, this disorder is very rare.

The other causes are:
• Basophil or chromophobe hyperplasia or adenoma of the pituitary gland, with excess production of corticotrophin (60%). This produces bilateral adrenal hyper-plasia and is called pituitary-dependent Cushing's syndrome and is properly called Cushing's disease
• Primary tumours of the adrenals, either adenoma (20%) or carcinoma (10%)
• Secondary to carcinoma elsewhere — usually an oat cell carcinoma of the bronchus causing the ectopic ACTH syndrome. Other sites are the thymus, pancreas, thyroid or ovary. Pigmentation may occur in this condition.

Clinical presentation

The onset is insidious.
• Alteration in appearance with redistribution of body fat, 'mooning' of the face and truncal or 'buffalo' obesity (about 90%). The limbs are often spared but the obesity may be generalized. Growth is retarded in children.
• Protein breakdown leads to muscle weakness which may present as a proximal myopathy, wide purple striae (50%) on the abdomen, thighs and buttocks, and easy bruising (30%). The striae of obesity are pink.
• Osteoporosis with backache and vertebral collapse (50%).
• Disturbance of carbohydrate tolerance which may amount to diabetes (10%).
• Electrolyte disturbance with sodium retention, potassium loss and hypokalaemic alkalosis, especially in the ectopic ACTH syndrome, where ACTH levels are very high. Renal stones may occur (20%).

- Hypertension, probably related to sodium retention (60%).
- Masculinization due to adrenal androgens — amenorrhoea, hirsutism, deep voice, greasy skin with acne in the female (80%).
- Mental disturbance—depression or mania and sometimes exaggeration of previous psychiatric abnormalities.

NB   Almost all of these can be produced by large doses of corticosteroids.

Investigation

Screening tests for cortisol excess

Cortisol levels. Measuring random plasma cortisol levels is of little value. Loss of the normal circadian rhythm is commonly found. Twenty-four-hour urinary free cortisol reflects total cortisol production and is the most useful screening test.

Dexamethasone suppression test. Dexamethasone 2 mg at midnight normally suppresses plasma cortisol to less than 200 nmol/l 8 h later.

If these tests suggest excess cortisol production the following will confirm the diagnosis and establish the aetiology.

- ACTH levels are high in pituitary-dependent Cushing's syndrome (Cushing's disease) or ectopic production. ACTH levels are low in patients with adrenal adenomas.
- Dexamethasone 2 mg 6-hourly for 3 days suppresses urinary cortisol levels in Cushing's syndrome, but not adrenal lesions, which are usually autonomous.
- Patients with Cushing's disease demonstrate an exaggerated rise in ACTH and cortisol in response to CRH, whereas patients with ectopic ACTH secretion or adrenal adenomas fail to respond.
- CT or magnetic resonance imaging scanning of the pituitary may demonstrate an adenoma, or abdominal CT scanning may reveal an adrenal lesion.

Management

Hypophysectomy is the treatment of choice for pituitary-dependent Cushing's syndrome. In some centres metyrapone and aminoglutethimide which block adrenal cortisol production are used to control the plasma cortisol and produce regression of symptoms in all patients with Cushing's syndrome of adrenal or pituitary origin before definitive surgical therapy. Others use mitotane (o.p.'-DDD). When bilateral adrenalectomy is performed to treat Cushing's syndrome due to a pituitary basophil or chromophobe adenoma, Nelson's syndrome may result with hyperpigmentation from excess β-lipotrophin activity (melanocyte-stimulating hormone (MSH) and ACTH) which is now not suppressed by high blood cortisol.

If the disease is primarily adrenal (yet to be called 'adrenal-dependent Cushing's syndrome'), unilateral or bilateral adrenalectomy is performed and the latter is followed by replacement therapy with cortisol 20–40 mg daily and fludrocortisone 0.1 mg daily.

Removal of ectopic ACTH sources is rarely possible (bronchial carcinoma).

CONN'S SYNDROME (primary hyperaldosteronism)

This is a very rare condition caused by a solitary benign adenoma or hyperplasia of the zona glomerulosa producing excess aldosterone.

Clinical presentation

Hypokalaemia and muscle weakness often in attacks. Polyuria and polydipsia are secondary to the hypokalaemia.

Sodium retention often leading to hypertension, but there is usually no oedema.

It may mimic hypertension from other causes, especially when potassium-losing diuretics are being given, or Cushing's syndrome.

Investigation

The condition is marked by renal potassium wasting, i.e. serum potassium reduced often <3 mmol and urinary potassium increased for serum blood level. It is usually associated with a metabolic alkalosis. The serum sodium is usually over 140 mmol.

Stop diuretics for 3 days and if potassium is still <3.2 mmol check the urinary output of potassium: if it is <20 mmol this is appropriate to the blood concentration and is probably normal: if it is >30 mmol further investigation for primary hyperaldosteronism is required.

The serum renin is low and this differentiates it from secondary aldosteronism (which occurs in the nephrotic syndrome, cirrhosis of the liver with ascites and, rarely, in congestive cardiac failure and bronchial carcinoma).

The best screening test is a 24-h urinary aldosterone. If this is raised, take a 7 am plasma specimen from a rested and recumbent patient for renin and aldosterone.

Management

Surgical resection should be considered because some tumours are malignant. Spironolactone is an antagonist to aldosterone and may be given in primary or secondary aldosteronism.

ADRENOGENITAL SYNDROME

A very rare condition of infancy or childhood due to a congenital enzyme defect (usually of 21-hydroxylase) affecting cortisol synthesis. The resulting decrease in circulating cortisol stimulates overproduction of ACTH, which in turn stimulates the adrenals to produce excess of androgenic steroids. Females show virilization early in life and are treated with cortisol. Males are less often diagnosed and may die in acute adrenal insufficiency, but if the infant survives, growth is excessive though precocious puberty results in a short final height. Treat with corticosteroids sufficient to suppress excess ACTH.

ADRENAL INSUFFICIENCY (Addison's disease)

Acute

Adrenal crisis. There is apathy, coma and epigastric pain. The blood sugar is low. It occurs after trauma, severe hypotension and sepsis.

Less commonly it may occur in patients previously (within 1–1½ years) or currently being treated with corticosteroids when there is trauma, surgery or acute infection or withdrawal of steroids. It may follow surgical removal of the adrenals for Cushing's syndrome or in the treatment of breast carcinoma unless there is adequate replacement therapy.

NB The Waterhouse–Friderichsen syndrome of severe acute meningococcal septicaemia, associated with purpura, is usually associated with raised levels of circulating corticosteroids despite the massive bilateral adrenal haemorrhage. It appears to be a special form of vascular rather than adrenal collapse. Adrenal haemorrhage is frequently found at postmortem as a non-specific finding.

Chronic

Insidious onset of weakness and fatigue with gastrointestinal symptoms of anorexia, weight loss, nausea, vomiting, intermittent abdominal pain and diarrhoea. Hypotension, often postural, and tachycardia occur late in the disease. Hyperpigmentation occurs in exposed areas, friction areas, hand creases and buccal mucosa.

Chronic adrenal insufficiency (Addison's disease) is rare (4/100 000 prevalence in UK) and causes include: autoimmune adrenal destruction; adrenal infiltration with secondary carcinoma, Hodgkin's or leukaemic tissue; destruction in tuberculosis, haemochromatosis, amyloidosis and histoplasmosis where prevalent. It may be associated with other organ-specific autoimmune disease, especially Hashimoto's thyroiditis (Schmidt's syndrome).

It may occur secondary to hypopituitarism (p. 209) during treatment of adrenal (or renal) tuberculosis and in the adrenogenital syndrome (p. 216).

Investigation

Plasma cortisol levels are usually low and show no diurnal variation.

No increase in output after tetracosactrin (Synacthen). Serum electrolytes are usually normal but in impending crisis the sodium may be low, the potassium high and the blood urea raised.

There is a high plasma ACTH.

Screening of basal function

Both 24-h urinary free cortisol and 8 am cortisols may be well in the normal range, even in strongly suspected cases.

A single basal plasma ACTH assay shows high levels in primary adrenal disease and undetectable values in pituitary disease.

Dynamic tests

Synacthen (tetracosactrin) tests

• *Short Synacthen test.* Take blood at 0, 30 and 60 min. In normal subjects, the initial level should be >170 nmol/l (6 μg/dl), and rise by at least 190 nmol/l (7 μg/dl) to >580 nmol/l (21 μg/dl). If the response is flat, proceed to a long Synacthen test.

• *Five-hour test* to 1 mg of depot tetracosactrin. In normal patients the serum cortisol more than doubles in the first hour.

Treatment

Maintenance therapy—hydrocortisone 20 mg am and 10 mg pm and fludrocortisone 0.1 mg daily. The doses are adjusted according to response as judged by lying and standing blood pressure, plasma urea and electrolytes and clinically.

In acute crisis — intravenous hydrocortisone 100 mg 6-hourly, intravenous saline and glucose are required. Underlying infection must be treated.

PHAEOCHROMOCYTOMA

This is usually a benign tumour of the adrenal medulla. It can arise from other chromaffin tissues of the sympathetic nervous system, e.g. the para-aortic ganglia, and it may be associated with neurofibromatosis. Medullary thyroid carcinoma (calcitonin-producing) and parathyroid adenoma are associated with it. Very rarely is it malignant.

It is a very rare cause of hypertension (<1 in 200) but it is important to recognize, since it is treatable. It can be familial and bilateral.

Clinical presentation

The clinical features depend on the activity of the tumour and the relative amounts of adrenaline (β- and some α-effects) and noradrenaline (α-effects). Usually α-effects predominate. Some tumours secrete intermittently.

The β-effects include a rise in systolic blood pressure with an increase in heart rate, increase in the cardiac output and dilatation of muscle vessels. The α-effects include a rise in both systolic and diastolic blood pressure with reflex slowing of the heart rate and constriction of blood vessels.

A few patients have normal blood pressure between attacks of paroxysmal hypertension, but most are hypertensive all the time. In a typical attack there is pallor, palpitation, anxiety and sometimes angina, headache, sweating and nausea. The blood pressure may be very high and death may occur from myocardial infarction or a cerebrovascular accident. Hyperglycaemia may occur if adrenaline is secreted.

NB   Paroxysmal bradycardia (an α-effect) may occur.

Investigation

Estimation of catecholamines (adrenaline and noradrenaline) in the blood or urine or the urinary metabolite vanillylmandelic acid (VMA) or hydroxymethylmandelic acid (HMMA).

Abdominal CT scan will usually show the tumour. This has superseded aortography, which may precipitate an attack. The patient must be fully α- and β-blocked before any interventional investigation or surgery.

Treatment

The tumour is removed under cover of α- and β-blocking agents given 3–4 days previously to prevent the effects of the release of catecholamines during operation. Plasma volume must be monitored throughout the period of sympathetic blockade and during surgery the central venous pressure should be monitored because changes in pulse and blood pressure are blocked.

In emergencies, α-effects may be antagonized by phenotolamine and β-effects by propranolol.

MULTIPLE ENDOCRINE NEOPLASIA   (MEN syndrome)

There are two main autosomal dominant syndromes type I (chromosome 11) and type II (chromosome 10). These are tumours originating from two or more endocrine (or neural) tissues which produce peptide hormones. They are very rare.

MEN type I refers to benign adenomas of parathyroid, pancreatic islets (hypo- or hyperglycaemia, watery diarrhoea, hypokalaemia, achlorhydria or Zollinger–Ellison syndrome), pituitary (PRL), adrenal cortex and thyroid (in that order of frequency).

MEN type II refers to the association of a phaeochromocytoma, commonly bilateral, and occasionally malignant, calcitonin-producing medullary carcinoma of the thyroid and, less commonly, parathyroid adenoma or hyperplasia. Over 90% have a defect in the proto-oncogene which encodes a tyrosine kinase receptor.

Families tend to run true. Patients with any one of the above tumours should be screened for others within the type and, if these are discovered, all other members of the family too. In type II there are provocative tests for calcitonin excretion (e.g. pentagastrin). Assays of both calcitonin and catecholamines are used to assess complete removal of tumour and for early recognition of recurrence.

Shortness of stature

The term 'dwarf' is better avoided. The common cause is short parents. Other causes are:
- Deficiency of GH — sometimes familial (see *Hypopituitarism*, p. 209), often associated with delayed or failure of sexual development. Bone age is retarded.
- Bone diseases, e.g. achondroplasia and rickets.

- Malnutrition, including the malabsorption syndrome.
- Renal (relatively common), liver or heart failure in early childhood.
- Large doses of steroids in childhood.
- Cretinism and childhood hypothyroidism.

Metabolic Disease

Diabetes mellitus

The World Health Organization criteria for diagnosis are:
- fasting venous glucose >8 mmol/l; and/or
- glucose of >11 mmol/l 2 h after 75 g of oral glucose.

Classification (Table 14.1)

Type I diabetes mellitus (insulin-dependent diabetes mellitus; IDDM) is an auto-immune disorder in which the insulin-producing β cells of the pancreas are destroyed. Patients are dependent upon insulin therapy and prone to ketosis.

Type II diabetes mellitus is the commoner form, accounting for 90% of patients with diabetes, and affecting 5% of the world's population. Patients are typically obese adults. Insensitivity of the tissues to insulin (insulin resistance) and inadequate pancreatic β-cell response to blood glucose are characteristic, leading to overproduction of glucose by the liver and underutilization by the tissues. Ketosis is unusual as patients have sufficient insulin to prevent lipolysis. Although initially controlled with diet and oral hypoglycaemics, many patients eventually need supplemental insulin, making them insulin-requiring type II diabetics.

Secondary diabetes
Secondary diabetes results from:
- hormonal antagonism of insulin: Cushing's syndrome, acromegaly, phaeochromocytoma;

TYPES OF DIABETES MELLITUS

Clinical classes	Distinguishing characteristics
Type I insulin-dependent diabetes mellitus (IDDM)	Patients may be of any age, are usually thin or have lost weight and usually have abrupt onset of signs and symptoms with insulinopenia before age 40. These patients often have strongly positive ketonuria and are dependent upon insulin to prevent ketoacidosis and to sustain life
Type II non-insulin-dependent diabetes mellitus (NIDDM; obese or non-obese)	Patients usually are older than 40 years at diagnosis, obese, and have relatively few classic symptoms. They are not prone to ketoacidosis except during periods of stress. Although not dependent upon exogenous insulin for survival, they may require it for stress-induced hyperglycaemia, and hyperglycaemia that persists in spite of other therapy
Other types of IGT IGT (obese or non-obese)	Patients with IGT have plasma glucose levels that are higher than normal but not diagnostic for diabetes mellitus
GDM	Patients with GDM have onset or discovery of glucose intolerance during pregnancy
———	
IGT, impaired glucose tolerance; GDM, gestational diabetes mellitus	

Table 14.1 Types of diabetes mellitus and other categories of glucose intolerance. From *Weight Concern* (1985). No. 3 (special issue). *Diabetics and the Overweight*.

- pancreatic destruction: carcinoma of the pancreas, pancreatitis, pancreatectomy, cystic fibrosis, haemochromatosis; and
- other causes of glucose intolerance: thiazide diuretics, pregnancy.

Genetics

Type I diabetes mellitus

The identical twin of a patient with type I diabetes has a 30–50% chance of developing the disease, implying that both genetic and environmental factors are involved.

Two chromosome regions have been established as being associated with, and linked to, IDDM: the major histocompatibility complex (MHC) class II region (designated IDDM1; 6p21) and the insulin gene region (IDDM2; 11p15). The recent construction of high-resolution human genetic linkage maps has allowed a total genome screen in sibling pairs with type I diabetes to identify susceptibility genes. This tremendous achievement has allowed identification of 18 other regions showing positive evidence of linkage to type I diabetes. These included regions on 15q (IDDM3), 11q (IDDM4) and 6q (IDDM5). The major locus is IDDM1, but the inheritance of diabetes is clearly complex and polygenic.

Type II diabetes mellitus

There is usually a family history, although inheritance is likely to involve interaction between multiple genes involved in both insulin secretion and insulin action. Mutations in the insulin gene, the insulin receptor gene and the glucagon receptor gene have all been reported. Mutations in the glucokinase gene cause maturity-onset disease of the young (MODY), a rare type of early-onset diabetes mellitus that is inherited as an autosomal dominant.

Complications

Long-term complications occur in all forms of diabetes. Although the development of complications is unpredictable, good glycaemic control has been shown conclusively to prevent or ameliorate diabetic microvascular complications in patients with insulin-dependent diabetes.

Vascular complications

Vascular complications account for 75% of deaths. The incidence of coronary artery occlusion at postmortem is five times higher in diabetics than non-diabetics, regardless of age or sex. Peripheral artery occlusion is 40 times more common in diabetics, leading to claudication, rest pain, ulcer formation and gangrene.

Small-vessel disease (diabetic microangiopathy) is associated with homogeneous thickening of vascular basement membrane. It produces renal failure, invariably associated with retinopathy, and gangrene of the skin and feet with wedge-shaped infarcts — arterial pulses are usually present and the skin is warm.

Eye

Fifty per cent of patients have *background retinopathy* after 10 years of diabetes. It is characterized by:
- microaneurysms — focal dilatations of capillary walls, not visible with the ophthalmoscope;
- dot or blot intraretinal haemorrhages;
- soft (cotton-wool) exudates due to microinfarction of superficial nerve fibres;
- hard exudates due to leakage of plasma into the retina; and
- retinal oedema.

In *proliferative retinopathy* new vessels proliferate in response to ischaemia, mainly near the disc margins. These fragile vessels are prone to haemorrhage into the retina and vitreous. Vitreous haemorrhage is followed by fibrosis and contraction leading to retinal detachment and thrombotic glaucoma. Laser photocoagulation destroys new vessels and reduces oxygen requirements throughout the retina, thereby retarding new vessel proliferation.

Kidney

Thirty per cent of patients with type I diabetes develop end-stage renal failure.

Hyperfiltration and increased creatinine clearance occur early after the onset of diabetes.

After several years microvascular changes (basement membrane thickening, hyaline degeneration of afferent and efferent arterioles) are associated with increased glomerular permeability and proteinuria. Kimmelstiel–Wilson nodules (nodular glomerulosclerosis) are pathognomonic of diabetic nephropathy.

Microalbuminuria heralds the onset of diabetic renal disease. Normal 24-h urinary albumin excretion is less than 15 mg. Microalbuminuria is defined as a 24-h urinary albumin excretion of 30–300 mg. Once persistent proteinuria occurs (>300 mg in 24 h), renal failure usually develops within 5 years.

The progression of microalbuminuria is closely associated with changes in blood pressure, and control of blood pressure may be more important than glycaemic control in preventing renal disease.

Angiotensin-converting enzyme inhibitors prevent progression of microalbuminuria to proteinuria in non-hypertensive patients with IDDM. They are generally favoured, alone or in combination with other agents, in the treatment of hypertension in diabetics.

Pyelonephritis is commoner in diabetics. Renal papillary necrosis can occur as a result of ischaemia of the papillae, which may slough and cause obstruction.

Neuromuscular complications

Neuromuscular complications affect up to 50% of patients with long-standing diabetes.
- Peripheral neuropathy is the commonest, initially causing loss of ankle jerks and absent vibration sense in the lower limbs. Later there is loss of touch and pain sensation. Patients often complain of numbness, and a burning sensation that is worse at night. Chronic painless ulcers develop in areas of repeated trauma (e.g. pressure points with ill-fitting footwear). Painless neuropathic arthropathy (Charcot's joints) most commonly affects the tarsometatarsal joints.
- Mononeuritis is thought to result from ischaemia following occlusion of a vasa nervorum. The third cranial nerve, ulnar nerve or lateral popliteal nerve are most commonly affected. More than one nerve can be involved. They are often transient, and spontaneous recovery of function usually occurs over a period of months.
- Diabetic amyotrophy usually occurs in middle-aged diabetics who develop painful, asymmetrical weakness and wasting of the quadriceps muscles. Improving diabetic control is often associated with recovery.
- Autonomic neuropathy (Table 14.2) produces impotence (25% of male patients), nocturnal diarrhoea, gastroparesis, postural hypotension and hypotonic bladder.

AUTONOMIC FUNCTION TESTS

Parasympathetic
Heart rate response to deep breathing
Heart rate response to standing
Heart rate response to the Valsalva manoeuvre

Sympathetic
Blood pressure response to standing
Blood pressure response to muscle exercise such as sustained hand grip

Table 14.2 Tests of autonomic function.

Skin

- Insulin sensitivity may occur in the first month of insulin therapy with production of tender lumps after each injection. Spontaneous recovery occurs, and no change of therapy is indicated.
- Lipodystrophy is painless atrophy or hypertrophy at injection sites. It is uncommon since the introduction of recombinant human insulins.
- Necrobiosis lipoidica diabeticorum is rare but pathognomonic of diabetes and may precede it. It is characterized by atrophy of subcutaneous collagen, usually over the shins. The lesions are violet rings with yellow masses at the periphery and scarring and atrophy at the centre.
- Photosensitivity may occur with chlorpropamide.

Intercurrent infection

Intercurrent infection is common in diabetics, particularly of the urinary tract and skin. Tuberculosis and candidiasis (vulvitis and balanitis) are more common in diabetes.

Management

Diabetics are best managed in diabetic clinics (where there is close liaison between expert physicians, special experienced nursing staff, ophthalmologist, dietician and chiropodist), in combination with mini-clinics in general practice.

Annual review should include:
- assessment of diabetic control from home blood glucose estimation and glycosylated haemoglobin;
- blood pressure;
- visual acuity by Snellen chart; examination of dilated optic fundi;
- examination of the feet for neuropathy (sensation, ankle jerks), arteriopathy (pulses, temperature), and for infection and care of nails — regular expert chiropody may prevent serious complications, particularly in the elderly;
- inspection of injection sites;
- urine for albuminuria and microalbuminuria; and
- blood urea and creatinine.

TRIALS

The **Diabetes Control and Complications Trial Research Group** compared intensive and standard treatment in 1441 patients (mean age 27) over a 6½-year period. In all, 726 patients had no retinopathy (primary prevention), whereas 715 had mild retinopathy (secondary prevention). Intensive treatment involved insulin given by a pump, or by three or more injections daily, with dosages adjusted according to blood glucose measured at least four times daily. Standard treatment involved insulin given once or twice daily, with once-daily monitoring of blood or urinary glucose. Intensive treatment reduced the risk of developing retinopathy by 76% in the primary prevention group, and reduced the risk of worsening retinopathy by 54% in the secondary prevention group. In both groups the risk of developing albuminuria was reduced by 54%, and the risk of neuropathy by 60%. *N Engl J Med* 1993; **329**: 977–986.

The **Microalbuminuria Collaborative Study Group, United Kingdom** compared the effects of intensive therapy with continuous subcutaneous infusion or multiple daily injections of insulin with conventional therapy in 70 insulin-dependent diabetics with microalbuminuria. Intensive therapy had no impact on the progression of albuminuria. Blood pressure, rather than glycaemic control, seemed to be the main determinant of progression of microalbuminuria. *Br Med J* 1995; **311**: 973–977.

The **European Microalbuminuria Captopril Study Group** compared the effect of captopril and placebo in 92 non-hypertensive patients with insulin-dependent diabetes and microalbuminuria. Captopril impeded progression to proteinuria and prevented any increase in albumin excretion rate. *JAMA* 1994; **271**: 275–279.

Mathiesen *et al.* studied the effect of captopril in 44 normotensive insulin-dependent diabetics with microalbuminuria. Captopril postponed the development of clinical proteinuria when compared with no treatment. *Br Med J* 1991; **303**: 81–87.

Type I diabetes

Type I diabetics require insulin to control blood glucose. Good control decreases the incidence of coma, intercurrent infection, retinopathy and probably neuropathy and nephropathy (see Trials, above). Hypoglycaemia remains the commonest complication of insulin therapy.

The new patient is instructed about diet, the effects of exercise, insulin therapy, injection technique, urine testing for ketones and home blood glucose monitoring and recording. Insulin regimes need to be individualized according to the patient's lifestyle, motivation and comprehension. A knowledge of insulin preparations and their duration of action (Table 9.1, p. 110) is essential. Premixed insulins are convenient for patients with poor sight or problems with dexterity.

The normal pancreas secretes about half its insulin at a continuous basal level, and the other half as boluses in response to food. Most diabetic patients are managed with twice-daily medium-acting preparations to provide continuous basal insulin levels, and two or three injections of short-acting insulin (often using a pen device) before main meals. Dietary caloric intake (unless excessive) is best chosen by the individual patient with professional dietetic advice, according to personal needs, and insulin therapy adjusted for the chosen diet. After pancreatectomy patients usually need 0.6 U/kg per day.

Control is best monitored by home blood glucose estimations, with periodic HbA$_{1c}$ at the clinic.

Type II diabetes

Reduction of dietary calorie intake to roughly 1200–1500 kcal with weight loss may be sufficient to reduce the blood sugar to normal. If not, use an oral hypoglycaemic agent in the form of a sulphonylurea or metformin, alone or in combination.

Sulphonylureas augment any residual pancreatic insulin secretion. Chlorpropamide has a long duration of action and is thus more likely to cause hypoglycaemia. It can also cause facial flushing after alcohol. Glibenclamide is usually given as a single dose before breakfast, whereas the short-acting tolbutamide is given in divided doses. Tolbutamide may be used in renal impairment, as may gliclazide, which is principally metabolized in the liver.

Thirty per cent of patients have a poor response to sulphonylureas, and the failure rate in the remaining 70% is 5% per year.

Metformin inhibits hepatic glucose production, mainly by inhibiting gluconeogenesis. It also promotes weight loss and has beneficial effects on plasma lipid levels, reducing total and low-density lipoprotein (LDL) cholesterol and triglycerides. It is generally well-tolerated and improves glucose control as either monotherapy or in combination with a sulphonylurea. Gastrointestinal side effects are initially common, but usually subside. It should be avoided in patients with renal impairment because of the risk of lactic acidosis. Vitamin B$_{12}$ deficiency may occasionally occur as a result of decreased absorption.

The use of *insulin* is complicated by the invariable insulin resistance that is associated with type II diabetes. In addition insulin stimulates appetite and can lead to weight gain in already obese patients. However, many patients with type II diabetes eventually require insulin therapy to control blood glucose.

Insulin should be given to patients at times of stress (e.g. infection, surgery, myocardial infarction).

Diabetic coma

There are two common types:

- hypoglycaemia; and
- hyperglycaemic ketoacidosis.

There is rarely any difficulty in differentiating between these two situations. If in doubt, blood sugar can easily be estimated at the bedside with 'stix'.

Hypoglycaemia. Patients are usually known diabetics on insulin or, less commonly, sulphonylurea therapy, and very rarely have insulinoma or Addison's disease. In diabetics it is caused by excess therapy, excess exercise, decreased food intake or an alcoholic binge. The rate of onset of symptoms is rapid. Most patients are aware of impending coma and may prevent it by taking sugar. Patients present either in pre-coma with agitated, often aggressive confusion, or in coma when marked sweating is usually present.

The differential diagnosis of hypoglycaemia involves the following considerations:

- excess insulin, which may be exogenous, endogenous (usually from insulinoma) or sulphonylurea therapy (frequently chlorpropamide or glibenclamide, because of their long duration of action);
- after excess alcohol;
- postgastrectomy;
- hypopituitarism and hypoadrenalism; and
- 'hungry neoplasm', e.g. hepatic carcinoma.

Oral glucose or, if necessary, intravenous glucose (20–40 ml of 50%) will reverse symptoms within minutes. Glucagon 1 mg intramuscularly acts as rapidly and can be given by relatives.

NB Hypoglycaemia must be treated rapidly since it may produce irreversible brain damage. Fluid replacement and corticosteroids are required in addition to glucose if Addison's disease is present.

The hypoglycaemia of chlorpropamide therapy may require continued glucose administration for several days (the drugs effects last up to 60 h).

Rarely, warning symptoms of hypoglycaemia may be absent on human insulin, or in those on β-blockers.

Hyperglycaemic ketoacidotic coma. This appears to be occurring less frequently, perhaps due to better education of patients.

Onset is gradual over hours or days. There is often evidence of infection (25–35%), particularly of the renal, respiratory or gastrointestinal tracts. Septicaemia and meningitis are uncommon but important causes. The patient may not have been eating properly, and has often stopped taking insulin.

Symptoms include thirst and dry mouth, polyuria, air hunger, nausea and vomiting, weakness, myalgia, headache and abdominal pain. Drowsiness may progress to confusion and coma.

Signs are those of confusion and dehydration, with hyperventilation (Kussmaul respiration) and the characteristic smell of ketones. There is fever, hypotension and tachycardia.

Management

- Replace fluids.
- Correct electrolytes.
- Give insulin.
- Look for and treat any underlying cause.

Fluid replacement

Venous blood should be taken for glucose, urea and electrolytes, and haemoglobin and intravenous fluid therapy started immediately. No fixed regime can be given, and therapy depends upon an assessment of the degree of dehydration. (The average deficit is 6–8 l, to be replaced in the first 24 h in addition to the daily requirement.)

Ketoacidotic patients are water, sodium and potassium-depleted and acidotic. For moderate to severe cases, in young people, 1 litre of normal (0.9%) saline may be given in the first half-hour and repeated in the following hour and continued at a rate of 0.5–2 l/h for the first 2 h.

Electrolytes

Nearly all patients have a low total body potassium with a deficit of 200–400 mmol on admission. Treatment will tend to exacerbate the dangers of this situation (acidosis will have caused a shift of intracellular potassium into the blood, and treatment causes it to move back into the cells again).

If the serum potassium is >5.5 mmol/l, then no potassium chloride is added to the initial intravenous fluids, but serum potassium is measured at least every 2 h.

If the serum potassium is normal then 20–40 mmol of potassium chloride is given hourly.

If the serum potassium <3.5 mmol/l then 40–80 mmol of potassium chloride is given hourly.

The potassium may be monitored by electrocardiogram (ECG), though this is not fully reliable — if signs of hyperkalaemia are present on the ECG, potassium is withheld until plasma results are known. Aim to keep plasma potassium between 4 and 5 mmol/l.

The use of bicarbonate to correct acidosis is controversial. Rapid correction of the acidosis leads to a rise in arterial $P\text{CO}_2$ and a paradoxical fall in cerebrospinal fluid pH, exacerbating central nervous system depression. In addition a shift of the haemoglobin oxygen dissociation curve to the left increases tissue hypoxia. If the pH is <7.1 some physicians infuse sodium bicarbonate until the pH reaches 7.2. A rough guide to the infusion of sodium bicarbonate in adults is 50 mmol of bicarbonate for every 0.1 units of pH below 7.1 given at a rate of 50 mmol/30 min + 10 mmol of extra KCl.

Insulin

Soluble insulin must be given immediately. A low-dose regime, given as an intravenous infusion or as hourly intramuscular injections, is preferred. The subcutaneous route is avoided as reduced skin blood flow in shocked patients leads to unpredictable absorption. A suggested regime is a loading dose of 8 U followed by an infusion of 6 U per hour until the blood sugar falls below 15 mmol/l (monitor glucose hourly), when the amount of insulin infused is reduced. The patient is not returned to the normal insulin regime until awake and able to eat and drink.

Underlying cause

Intercurrent infection must always be considered and treated. In the absence of obvious infection, it is advisable to perform urine microscopy and culture, chest X-ray and blood culture.

Special measures

Aspiration. There is usually gastric dilatation, and death can occur from aspiration pneumonia. If the conscious level is depressed, a nasogastric tube should be inserted and the gastric contents aspirated.

Catheterization. Urinary catheterization should be avoided in mild cases where confusion is minimal, but is required in those who are in a coma. Urine is sent to the laboratory for culture.

Hyperosmolar non-ketotic coma. This occurs in the elderly obese diabetic, often previously undiagnosed. There is often a precipitating factor such as myocardial infarction, stroke or infection. The onset is slow with polyuria over 2–3 weeks and progressive dehydration. Blood glucose levels are very high (often above 45.0 mmol/l), plasma osmolality is increased (often above 400 mosmol/l). Plasma bicarbonate is usually normal with no ketonuria. If plasma bicarbonate is low, think of lactic acidosis.

These patients need large quantities of fluid (up to 10 litres) given as normal saline.

Monitoring of central venous pressure or pulmonary wedge pressure is usually required. Insulin is required over the acute episode, often in small doses (10–20 U may suffice). The mortality is high (50%) and cerebral oedema from overhydration is a real risk. Prophylactic heparin may reduce the increased risk of thrombosis, arterial and venous. Unlike in patients with ketoacidosis, subsequent insulin therapy is not mandatory — survivors may do well on diet and oral hypoglycaemics.

Lactic acidosis. This usually occurs in the elderly diabetic, precipitated by alcohol or metformin. It may occur in shocked patients or with uraemia. Patients are very acidotic and hyperventilating. Blood lactic acid levels are raised. Blood glucose may be normal and there is little or no ketonuria.

There is an increased anion gap in which the cation total (predominantly Na^+ plus K^+) exceeds the anion total (predominantly Cl^- plus HCO_3^-) by up to 25 mmol/l, the difference being lactate.

These patients require insulin, glucose, bicarbonate (upto 2500 mmol in 24 h), and fluid replacement. The mortality is very high (over 50%).

NB   Cerebrovascular accidents and aspirin overdosage may both produce the combination of coma plus glycosuria.

Diabetics also have strokes, take overdoses and become concussed.

Hyperlipidaemia

Cholesterol and triglycerides are absorbed from dietary fat, and also synthesized by the liver. Both cholesterol and triglycerides are insoluble in water, and are transported from the gut and liver as water-soluble lipoproteins, in which they are surrounded by a coat of phospholipid, free cholesterol and specific proteins known as apoproteins. In addition to stabilizing the lipoprotein complex, apoproteins act as enzyme cofactors and interact with cell-surface receptors. The density of lipoproteins decreases as the triglyceride content increases.

Dietary lipids

In the intestinal mucosa triglycerides are coated with cholesterol, lipoprotein and phospholipid to form *chylomicrons* which are secreted into mesenteric lymphatics. Chylomicrons in the circulation are gradually depleted of triglyceride by lipoprotein lipase, an enzyme found on vascular endothelium in both muscle and fat. Triglyceride-depleted chylomicron remnants are taken up by the liver. Chylomicrons are normally absent after a 10-h fast. Apolipoprotein CII (apo-CII) in chylomicrons activates lipoprotein lipase, whereas apolipoprotein E mediates hepatic uptake of chylomicron remnants.

Hepatic synthesis of lipids

Cholesterol is synthesized in the liver from acetyl-coenzyme A. The enzyme 3-hydroxy-3-methylglutaryl coenzyme A (HMG CoA) reductase catalyses an early step in cholesterol synthesis. Triglycerides are formed by binding three fatty acids to glycerol.

Triglyceride-rich *very-low-density lipoproteins* (VLDL) are synthesized in the liver and depleted of triglyceride in the circulation to form *intermediate-density lipoproteins* (IDL). IDL have a short half-life (less than 30 min) in the circulation. They are either taken up by the liver, or further depleted of triglyceride to form *LDL* which have a half-life of several days. LDL can deliver cholesterol to the tissues, in part by interacting with the LDL receptor on the surface of cells. Lipoprotein a resembles LDL, but contains apoprotein a, which is structurally similar to plasminogen. In addition to being a source of cholesterol, lipoprotein a may also interfere with fibrinolysis.

High-density lipoprotein (HDL) is synthesized in gut and liver, and has a relatively high apoprotein content. HDL accept cholesterol from other lipoproteins and cells.

Hence, LDL is the chief form of cholesterol in the blood, and VLDL the chief form of fasting serum triglyceride.

Classification

The commonest problem is an elevated cholesterol. Although this is usually polygenic, or secondary to other diseases, rarer familial causes of hyperlipidaemia should be considered so that screening of family members can be performed. The Fredrickson WHO classification (Table 14.3) is still referred to.

Polygenic hypercholesterolaemia

This is the commonest cause of raised cholesterol. Triglycerides may be normal (WHO type IIa) or raised (type IIb). Coronary heart disease risk is increased, and can be reduced by lowering cholesterol levels (see Trials, pp. 234–235).

HYPERLIPIDAEMIAS

Type of hyperlipidaemia	Prevalence	Fredrickson/ WHO lipoprotein phenotype	Typical lipid levels (mmol/l)	Lipoproteins	Chronic heart disease risk	Pan-creatitis risk	Clinical signs
Polygenic hyper-cholesterolaemia	—	IIa	Cholesterol: 6.5–9.0 Triglyceride: normal	LDL↑ HDL→↓	+	—	Xanthelasma, corneal arcus
Familial combined hyperlipidaemia	1 : 200	IIb (IIa or IV)	Cholesterol: 6.5–10.0 Triglyceride: 2.5–12.0	VLDL↑→ LDL↑→ HDL→↓	+ +	—	Corneal arcus, xanthelasma
Familial hyper-cholesterolaemia (heterozygous)	1 : 500	IIa (or IIb)	Cholesterol: 7.5–16.0 Triglyceride: <5.0	LDL↑ VLDL→↑ HDL→↑	+ + +	—	Tendon xanthomata, corneal arcus, xanthelasma
Remnant particle disease	1 : 10 000	III	Cholesterol: 9.0–14.0 Triglyceride: 9.0–14.0	IDL↑ HDL→↑	+ + +	+	Palmar tuberous and occasional tendon xanthomata
Chylomicronaemia syndrome	—	I	Cholesterol: <6.5 Triglyceride: 10.0–30.0	Chylomicrons ↑	—	+ + +	Eruptive xanthomata, lipaemia retinalis, hepato-splenomegaly
Familial hyper-triglyceridaemia	—	IV (or V)	Cholesterol: 6.5–12.0 Triglyceride: 10.0–30.0	VLDL↑ Chylomicrons→↑	?	+ +	Eruptive xanthomata, lipaemia retinalis, hepato-splenomegaly

Table 14.3 Classification of hyperlipidaemias. Modified from *Mims* (Supplement) 1989, by permission of Haymarket Medical Publications, London.

Familial hypercholesterolaemia
In familial hypercholesterolaemia a deficiency of the receptor for LDL results in hypercholesterolaemia (severe in the homozygous form, less marked in hetero-zygotes) leading to atherosclerosis. Corneal arcus, xanthelasma and tendon xanthomata are characteristic. Patients die prematurely, usually from myocardial infarction. Prevalence is estimated at 1:500.

Familial defective apolipoprotein B-100
This is due to a single amino-acid substitution in apolipoprotein B, resulting in defective binding of LDL to its receptor. It is clinically indistinguishable from familial hypercholesterolaemia.

Familial hypertriglyceridaemia
This may be due to increased hepatic VLDL production or a failure of triglycerides to be cleared from chylomicrons by lipoprotein lipase. Marked hypertriglyceridaemia (>10 mmol/l) is associated with eruptive xanthomata, lipaemia retinalis and acute pancreatitis.

Familial combined hyperlipidaemia
This condition is inherited as an autosomal dominant. Cholesterol and triglycerides are both increased. Corneal arcus and xanthelasma (but not tendon xanthomata) are frequently present, and the risk of atherosclerosis is increased.

Dysbetalipoproteinaemia
This is a rare disorder in which mutations in the apolipoprotein E gene lead to elevations in triglycerides and total cholesterol.

Secondary hyperlipidaemia
This may occur in hypothyroidism, nephrotic syndrome, oral oestrogen or thiazide diuretic therapy, alcohol abuse and liver disease. These conditions should be excluded when investigating lipid abnormalities.

Associations between lipids and vascular disease
There is a strong association between plasma total cholesterol or LDL cholesterol and coronary heart disease, whereas there is an inverse relationship between HDL cholesterol and risk of coronary heart disease. As 60–70% of plasma cholesterol is present in LDL, total cholesterol is often used as a surrogate measure of LDL cholesterol. Raised levels of lipoprotein a also predict the risk of coronary heart disease.

Raised plasma triglyceride levels are associated with coronary heart disease. However, increased triglyceride levels are commonly found with hypercholesterolaemia, and it is less clear whether triglyceride levels are independent predictors of coronary heart disease risk. Xanthelasma and corneal arcus usually indicate hypercholesterolaemia, although they can occur with normal cholesterol levels. Tendon and palmar xanthomata only occur in hypercholesterolaemia, whereas eruptive xanthomata and lipaemia retinalis are found in hyper-triglyceridaemia.

Management of hyperlipidaemia

There is good evidence that lowering raised cholesterol in patients with coronary heart disease improves morbidity and mortality. Some primary prevention studies have also shown a benefit in lowering cholesterol in asymptomatic individuals (see Trials, below).

Cholesterol levels of 5.2, 6.5 and 7.8 mmol/l (corresponding to 200, 250 and 300 mg/dl) are frequently used to evaluate management. Levels below 5.2 mmol/l are desirable, whereas levels below 6.5 mmol/l are often considered acceptable, particularly in the absence of other atherosclerosis risk factors. Many physicians would treat levels above 7.8 mmol/l, even in the absence of other risk.

Diet typically lowers cholesterol by 5–10%. Saturated fatty acids raise, and mono- and polyunsaturated fatty acids lower, LDL cholesterol. Alcohol tends to increase plasma HDL cholesterol, reduce platelet aggregation and promote the effects of fibrinolytic factors.

TRIALS

Fibrates

The **Helsinki Heart Study** compared the effect of gemfibrozil on cardiac end-points in 4081 asymptomatic middle-aged men with non-HDL cholesterol >5.2 mmol/l. The incidence of coronary heart disease was 34% lower in patients treated with gemfibrozil than those receiving placebo. *N Engl J Med* 1987; **317**: 1237–1245.

Resins

The **Lipid Research Clinics Coronary Primary Prevention Trial (LRC-CPPT)** compared the incidence of coronary heart disease in 3806 middle-aged hypercholesterolaemic (cholesterol >265 mg/dl) men treated with cholestyramine and diet, with that in similar men treated with placebo and diet. The incidence of coronary heart disease was 19% lower in those receiving cholestyramine. *JAMA* 1984; **251**: 351–364.

Statins

The **Scandinavian Simvastatin Survival Study (4S)** studied 4444 patients (mostly men) aged 35–70 years with serum cholesterol above 5.5 mmol/l, despite 2 months' dietary advice, and angina or previous myocardial infarction. Patients were randomized to receive simvastatin (20–40 mg/day) or placebo. Simvastatin

continued

TRIALS (continued)

reduced total cholesterol by 25% and total mortality by 30%. Major coronary events (non-fatal myocardial infarction, resuscitated cardiac arrest, death) were reduced by 44%. Risks of developing unstable angina or needing coronary artery revascularization, or suffering a stroke or transient ischaemic attack were reduced by about 30%. *Lancet* 1994; **344**: 1383–1389.

The **Pravastatin Limitation of Atherosclerosis in the Carotid Arteries (PLAC-I)** trial studied 408 patients with coronary artery disease and a serum LDL cholesterol of 130–190 mg/dl. Fatal and non-fatal myocardial infarctions were reduced in patients receiving pravastatin 40 mg/day compared with placebo. *J Am Coll Cardiol* 1994; **131A**: 1A–484A.

The **Pravastatin, Lipids and Atherosclerosis in the Carotid Arteries (PLAC-II)** trial studied 151 patients with coronary artery disease and a serum LDL cholesterol of 130–190 mg/dl. Coronary events and all deaths, when combined, were lower in patients receiving pravastatin 20–40 mg compared with placebo. *Am J Cardiol* 1995; **75**: 455–459.

The **Regression Growth Evaluation Statin Study (REGRESS)** studied the effect of pravastatin 40 mg daily or placebo in 885 symptomatic men with significant coronary atherosclerosis and serum cholesterol 4–8 mmol/l. There were fewer cardiovascular events, and less progression of atherosclerosis, in patients receiving pravastatin. *Circulation* 1995; **91**: 2528–2540.

The **West of Scotland Coronary Prevention Group** compared the effect of treatment with pravastatin and placebo for an average of 4.9 years in 6595 men aged 45–65 with a mean plasma cholesterol level of 7.0 mmol/l and no history of myocardial infarction. Pravastatin lowered plasma cholesterol and reduced the incidence of myocardial infarction and death from cardiovascular causes without adversely affecting the risk of death from non-cardiovascular causes. *N Engl J Med* 1995; **333**: 1301–1307.

The **CARE (Cholesterol and Recurrent Events) Investigators** studied the effect of pravastatin or placebo in 3583 men and 576 women with myocardial infarction who had plasma total cholesterol levels below 240 mg/dl. Pravastatin reduced the need for coronary bypass surgery and coronary angioplasty over a 5-year period. *N Engl J Med* 1996; **335**: 1001–1009.

Fibrates reduce serum triglyceride levels, principally through increased lipoprotein lipase activity. They tend to reduce LDL cholesterol and raise HDL cholesterol. Clofibrate increases biliary cholesterol secretion, predisposing to gallstones. Gemfibrozil has been shown to be effective in reducing both cholesterol and coronary heart disease (Helsinki Heart Study; see Trials, above). Bezafibrate, ciprofibrate and fenofibrate reduce both lipid and fibrinogen levels. All fibrates can cause myositis.

Resins reduce LDL levels by sequestering bile acids in the small intestine. Cholestyramine and colestipol are both effective in reducing cholesterol, but their use is limited by gastrointerstinal side effects.

Statins are competitive inhibitors of HMG CoA reductase. They are potent in lowering LDL-cholesterol, but less effective than fibrates in reducing triglycerides or increasing HDL-cholesterol. Myositis is a rare but severe complication in patients also receiving cyclosporin. Several studies have shown beneficial effects of statins in secondary prevention of coronary artery disease.

Nicotinic acid derivatives reduce synthesis of both cholesterol and triglyceride. Their use is limited by side effects, particularly vasodilatation leading to flushing.

Porphyrias

There are six main inborn errors of metabolism in which there is increased intermittent excretion of porphyrins in the urine and/or faeces.

Physiology

Porphyrins are intermediates in the biosynthesis of haem. The precursors are glycine and succinyl-CoA, which are converted to δ-aminolaevulinic acid (δ-ALA) by δ-ALA synthetase. Two molecules of δ-ALA condense to form the single pyrrole ring, porphobilinogen. Four porphobilinogen molecules are then cyclized by porphobilinogen deaminase to form the four-pyrrole ring structure which is characteristic of porphyrins. Porphyrins are divided into uro-, copro- and proto-porphyrins according to the structure of side chains around the ring. Porphyrin biosynthesis occurs predominantly in the liver and bone marrow.

Classification

Porphyrias are classified as hepatic or erythropoietic according to the principal site of the enzyme defect and excess precursor production. They can also be classified as acute or non-acute. Porphyrins are colourless, but become coloured on oxidation. Porphyrins in urine darken on standing. Porphobilinogen is detected by Ehrlich's aldehyde reagent, which produces a pink colour with both urobilinogen and porphobilinogen. When chloroform is added, urobilinogen, but not porphobilinogen moves into it. Porphyrins fluoresce in UV light.

ACUTE PORPHYRIAS (all inherited as autosomal dominant)

These are characterized by gastrointestinal, neuropsychiatric and cardiovascular features. Attacks are usually precipitated by drugs (particulary barbiturates, which increase ALA synthase activity) or less commonly, by fasting or infection.

The following drugs precipitate acute porphyria:

- alcohol;
- anticonvulsants and sedatives: carbamazepine, phenytoin, barbiturates, benzodiazepines (although intravenous benzodiazepines have been used in controlling seizures);
- antibiotics: cephalosporins, doxycycline, erythromycin, flucloxacillin, pivampicillin, sulphonamides;
- antidepressants: tricyclic and related, monoamine oxidase inhibitors;
- antidiabetics: sulphonylureas;
- antiemetic: metoclopramide;
- antifungals: econazole, griseofulvin;
- antihistamines (chlorpheniramine may be safe);
- antihypertensives: some angiotensin-converting enzyme (ACE) inhibitors, methyldopa, nifedipine, verapamil;
- antiparkinsonian: orphenadrine;
- antituberculous drugs: pyrazinamide, rifampicin;
- contraceptives, hormone replacement therapy;
- diuretics;
- ergot derivatives;
- gold salts;
- non-steroidal anti-inflammatory drugs; and
- theophyllines.

The patient should carry a complete list, and wear a bracelet.

Clinical features

- Severe abdominal pain, vomiting and constipation.
- Tachycardia and hypertension, or severe postural hypotension.
- Peripheral neuropathy with weakness or paralysis, including respiratory paralysis.
- Confusion with agitation or depression, hallucination and psychosis. Seizures may occur, even in between attacks, and may be difficult to treat as many anticonvulsants are contraindicated.
- Occasionally, inappropriate antidiuretic hormone syndrome with severe hyponatraemia, sweating, pallor and fever.

Attacks are rare before puberty, and in females may be related to the menstrual cycle.

Acute intermittent porphyria (the Swedish type)

This is due to a defect in porphobilinogen deaminase. Onset is usually between 15 and 35 years, and abdominal pain and vomiting are the commonest presenting features. The skin is 'never' affected. There may be a family history. The urine turns red-brown on standing, and the diagnosis is confirmed by detecting excess porphobilinogen in the urine.

Variegate porphyria (the South African type)

This is due to a defect in protoporphyrinogen oxidase. Clinical features are similar to those of acute intermittent porphyria, together with cutaneous features. The skin, photosensitized by porphyrins, is fragile, particularly on the backs of the hands.

Hereditary coproporphyria

This is due to a defect in coproporphyrinogen oxidase. Features are similar to variegate porphyria. It is extremely rare.

Management of acute porphyria

Avoid precipitant drugs and alcohol. During acute attacks a high carbohydrate intake (glucose polymer drinks or intravenous infusion) suppresses ALA synthase activity. Pain is controlled with paracetamol or morphine derivatives; agitation, nausea and vomiting with chlorpromazine; constipation with co-danthramer or neostigmine; tachycardia and hypertension with propranolol, seizures with diazepam or valproate; and respiratory paralysis with assisted ventilation.

NON-ACUTE PORPHYRIAS

Porphyria cutanea tarda

This is due to a defect in hepatic uroporphyrinogen decarboxylase. It may be acquired or, less commonly, inherited. It is usually secondary to liver disease (particularly alcoholic), although in such cases there may be a genetic predisposition. Patients are not usually sensitive to drugs, although they may present after an alcoholic binge. The features are predominantly cutaneous with porphyrin-induced photosensitivity leading to bullae on exposed areas and hyperpigmentation. Urinary uroporphyrin excretion is increased, but urinary porphobilinogen is normal.

Congenital porphyria

This is due to a defect in uroporphyrinogen cosynthase. It is inherited as an autosomal recessive and characterized by extreme skin manifestations plus red staining of the teeth and bones which presents before the age of 5 years. It is extremely rare.

Erythropoietic porphyria

This is relatively common and inherited as an autosomal dominant. It is due to a defect in ferrochetalase activity. It presents in childhood with cutaneous photosensitivity of varying severity. It is distinguished by the presence of free protoporphyrin in the red cells which fluoresce in UV light.

Carcinoid syndrome

Carcinoid tumours originate from argentaffin cells, usually in the small bowel. *Carcinoid syndrome* results from a malignant carcinoid tumour, usually of the ileum, which has metastasized to the liver. Carcinoid of the appendix rarely metastasizes. The majority of bronchial adenomas are carcinoid but only a few produce the syndrome.

Physiology

Carcinoid tumours secrete serotonin (5-hydroxytryptamine) and kinin peptides. These are normally metabolized in the liver, so the syndrome only occurs if they are released from the liver by hepatic metastases. 5-Hydroxytrypamine is metabolized to 5-hydroxyindoleacetic acid (5-HIAA), which is excreted in the urine.

Clinical features

Symptoms of the primary tumour may be present, e.g. episodic diarrhoea or recurrent haemoptysis. The carcinoid syndrome is characterized by episodes of facial flushing, fever, dyspnoea from bronchospasm, nausea, vomiting, colic and diarrhoea. Later valvular stenosis of the pulmonary and tricuspid valves may develop. There may be evidence of malignancy with cachexia and irregular hepatomegaly from metastases.

Investigation

The 24h urinary excretion of 5-HIAA is measured on a low-serotonin diet (excluding bananas, tomatoes, walnuts etc.). Normal range: 2–10mg in 24h.

Management

Cyproheptadine 4mg tds, α-blockade, octreotide (somatostatin analogue) or methysergide 1–2mg qds (serotonin antagonist) and tumour chemotherapy (e.g. streptozocin) may be given, but usually with disappointing results. Surgery is used to remove localized carcinoid, and can be of benefit in reducing bulk of liver tumour. Hepatic arterial embolization is helpful in some. Treat diarrhoea symptomatically.

Metabolic bone disease

Physiology

Bone normally consists of 60% mineral and 40% organic matter (matrix). The former is mostly calcium and the latter mostly collagen. In all, 99% of total body calcium is contained within the skeleton. Cortical (compact) bone comprises 80% of the skeleton and forms the shafts of long bones and the surface of flat bones. Cortical bone is arranged concentrically around channels, known as the Haversian system, containing blood vessels, lymphatics and nerves. Trabecular bone is found at the end of long bones and inside flat bones.

Osteoblasts—derived from bone marrow stromal cells. Synthesize and mineralize bone matrix. About 20% of osteoblasts become calcified into lacunae and differentiate terminally into *osteocytes*.

Osteoclasts — derived from haematopoietic cells. Large, multinucleated cells which resorb bone. Osteoclasts express receptors for calcitonin, but not for vitamin D or parathyroid hormone. However, osteoclast activity is modulated by these agents, probably through signals generated by osteoblasts.

Bone remodelling occurs continuously at the endosteal surface (interface between bone and marrow), and to a lesser extent at the periosteal surface. In the normal young adult the amount of bone resorbed and formed in the skeleton is similar.

Parathyroid hormone (PTH) secretion is predominantly controlled by the concentration of ionized calcium in extracellular fluid. Intact PTH is rapidly cleared from the circulation by the liver and kidney (half-life less than 4 min), but inactive C-terminal fragments persist longer, and account for about 90% of circulating PTH.

Increased PTH levels are associated with bone resorption, which releases calcium.

Osteoclastic cell number and activity are increased. However, intermittent administration of low doses of PTH increases formation of trabecular bone.

PTH decreases renal tubular phosphate reabsorption, and increases renal tubular calcium reabsorption. It indirectly increases intestinal calcium absorption through increased formation of 1,25-dihydroxyvitamin D.

PTH-related protein (PTHrP) is secreted by tumours which are associated with hormonal hypercalcaemia, including squamous, breast and renal carcinoma. It is only homologous to PTH in its amino terminus. PTHrP binds to the same receptor as PTH and shares its biological activities. Circulating levels of PTHrP are normally very low.

Vitamin D is principally synthesized from 7-dehydrocholesterol in the skin on exposure to UV light (Fig. 14.1). Dietary intake is only important when UV irradiation does not occur. Because of this, vitamin D is often regarded as a steroid hormone rather than a vitamin. The major circulating form is 25-hydroxyvitamin D_3, which is converted to either 1,25-dihydroxyvitamin D_3 or 24,25-dihydroxyvitamin D_3 in the kidney. 1,25-Dihydroxyvitamin D_3 is the most potent vitamin D metabolite. 1,25-Dihydroxyvitamin D_3 decreases 1-hydroxylase activity and increases 24-hydroxylase activity, whereas PTH increases 1-hydroxylase activity and decreases 24-hydroxylase activity.

Vitamin D is thought to diffuse across the plasma membrane of target cells and interact with an intracellular receptor. The ligand–receptor complex regulates gene expression by binding to regulatory DNA sequences in the promoter region of genes, thereby acting directly as a transcription factor.

Calcitonin is secreted by C cells of the thyroid. Its principal action is to inhibit osteoclastic bone resorption. It has been used in the treatment of Paget's disease, osteoporosis and hypercalcaemia of malignancy.

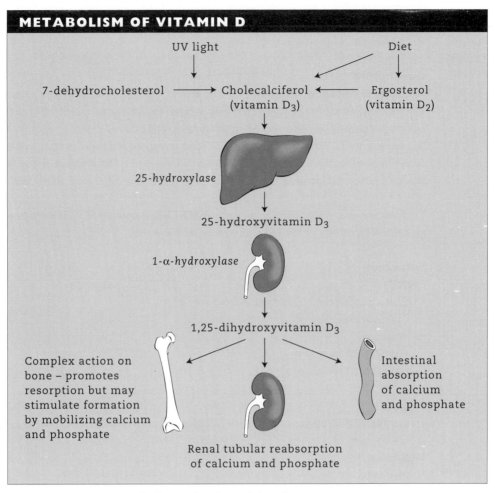

METABOLISM OF VITAMIN D

UV light   Diet

7-dehydrocholesterol ⟶ Cholecalciferol ⟵ Ergosterol
(vitamin D_3)   (vitamin D_2)

25-hydroxylase

25-hydroxyvitamin D_3

1-α-hydroxylase

1,25-dihydroxyvitamin D_3

Complex action on bone – promotes resorption but may stimulate formation by mobilizing calcium and phosphate

Intestinal absorption of calcium and phosphate

Renal tubular reabsorption of calcium and phosphate

Fig. 14.1 Metabolism and actions of vitamin D.

OSTEOPOROSIS

Osteoporosis refers to a loss of bone mass rather than an alteration in its constituents. It is characterized by increased risk of fragility fracture. The commonest fracture sites are the spine, femoral neck and radius.

Aetiology

Pathogenesis is multifactorial. The risk is increased by ageing, female sex, race (white and Asian) and small body build. Oestrogen deficiency is a major factor in postmenopausal women, and women with premenopausal oestrogen deficiency (premature menopause, oophorectomy, anorexia, chronic illness, excessive physical exercise) are at risk. Family history of osteoporosis is a weak risk factor. Immobilization, often due to arthritis, appears to contribute. Some drugs, including steroids, thyroid hormones and alcohol, adversely affect bone mass. The role of calcium intake, calcium absorption and vitamin D is less clear.

Classification

Generalized

Normal ageing, especially in women:

1 *Postmenopausal (type 1)*, with trabecular bone loss giving vertebral lesions of end-plate collapse, wedging and crush fracture, up to about 70 years.

2 *Senile (type 2)*, with additional cortical bone loss giving fractures characteristic of the neck of femur, usually in women over 75 years old. This fracture is partly due to the normal increase in body sway with age and resultant instability with falls.

Idiopathic — any age, but excessive in degree when compared within the age group. It is usually more dramatic, therefore, in the young.

Secondary

Endocrine
- Cushing's syndrome (including steroid therapy).
- Thyrotoxicosis (including thyroid therapy).
- Pregnancy.
- Hypogonadism.
- Hyperparathyroidism.

Drugs
- Corticosteroids, thyroxine, heparin, alcohol, anticonvulsants.

Malignancy
- Myeloma.

Gastrointestinal
- Malabsorption.
- Chronic liver disease.

Localized
- Immobilization and paralysis.
- Rheumatoid arthritis.

Clinical features

Clinical features are related to fracture. Vertebral fractures (wedge or crush) are commonest in the mid dorsal spine and the dorsolumbar junction (T12 and L1). They may be asymptomatic, or cause sudden severe back pain. Spinal cord compression is not a feature, and suggests other causes such as metastases or Paget's disease. Multiple fractures cause loss of height and spinal deformity. Hip fractures invariably follow a fall and are often associated with prolonged hospital admission.

Mortality at 6 months is around 15%. Colles' fracture usually follows a fall on to the outstretched hand.

Investigation

Biochemistry

Serum calcium, phosphate and alkaline phosphatase and urinary calcium are normal. (Alkaline phosphatase may be elevated following a fracture.)

Radiology

Lateral X-rays of lumbar and dorsal spine. There may be wedging or concave deformities (codfishing) of the vertebral bodies. Discs may rupture into the vertebral bodies (Schmorl's nodes). Loss of bone density may be evident but radiological evaluation of bone mass is unreliable. Unequivocal osteopenia on X-ray signifies advanced bone loss.

Bone densitometry

Quantitative computed tomography (CT), single- and dual-photon absorptiometry to dual-energy X-ray absorptiometry (DXA) assesses bone density by measuring the absorption of γ- or X-rays at clinically relevant sites such as the radius, hip or spine. Where available, DXA is the preferred method, providing a rapid method of assessment which is associated with low radiation exposure.

Histology

This is not indicated routinely, but shows a diminished number of normally calcified trabeculae.

Prevention and treatment

A number of agents have been shown to have beneficial effects on bone density or fracture rates in postmenopausal women. Efforts should be directed towards prevention in those with identifiable risk factors. These include late menarche, early menopause, oophorectomy before age 50, slimness, long-term corticosteroid therapy, alcoholism and smoking.

Hormone replacement therapy

Oestrogen therapy slows bone loss and reduces the occurrence of fractures when started at menopause. The increased risk of endometrial carcinoma is countered by cyclical progestogen for 10–12 days each month in women who have not undergone hysterectomy. Prolonged use ($>$10 years), which is probably necessary to prevent bone loss, appears to increase risk of breast cancer. Oestrogen therapy also protects against ischaemic heart disease and stroke, although this effect may be blunted by cyclical progestogen. There is a small (2–3%) increased risk of venous thromboembolism, which disappears after hormone replacement therapy is stopped. Absolute contraindications to hormone replacement therapy are breast cancer, endometrial cancer, malignant melanoma and pregnancy.

Bisphosphonates

Bisphosphonates are synthetic analogues of inorganic pyrophosphate. They have a high affinity for hydroxyapatite, and inhibit bone resorption, but are also capable of inhibiting bone mineralization with prolonged usage. Cyclical administration is

---

TRIALS

Oestrogens

Many prospective and retrospective studies have shown beneficial effects of oestrogens, alone or in combination with other agents, on postmenopausal osteoporosis. Examples include:

Nordin et al. studied the effects of various treatments prospectively in 95 postmenopausal women with vertebral fracture. Calcium, hormonal treatment (ethinyoestradiol or, where contraindicated, norethisterone) and vitamin D with hormonal treatment appeared to be useful in reducing cortical bone loss. Vitamin D alone was of no value. *Br Med J* 1980; **280**: 451–455.

Genant et al. prospectively studied 37 premenopausal women for 24 months following hysterectomy and oophorectomy for benign conditions. Spinal quantitative CT demonstrated bone mineral loss after oophorectomy which was prevented by conjugated oestrogens (Premarin up to 0.6 mg daily). *Ann Intern Med* 1982; **97**: 699–705.

Ettinger et al. measured spinal bone mass prospectively in 73 women immediately after the menopause. Bone loss was reduced by treatment with conjugated oestrogens (Premarin 0.3 mg daily) with calcium supplements, but not calcium supplements alone. *Ann Intern Med* 1987; **106**: 40–45.

Felson et al. performed a cross-sectional study of bone density in 670 postmenopausal women. Bone density was higher in women who had taken oestrogen therapy, but this effect was only apparent in women who had received treatment for 7 or more years. *N Engl J Med* 1993; **329**: 1141–1146.

Bisphosphanates

Storm et al. compared the effect of intermittent cyclical etidronate (400 mg daily for 2 weeks followed by 13 weeks with no drugs repeated 10 times over 150 weeks) and placebo on bone mass and fracture rate in 66 women with postmenopausal osteoporosis. All

continued

TRIALS (continued)

patients received calcium and vitamin D supplements. Etidronate significantly increased vertebral bone mineral content, and after the first year reduced the risk of vertebral fracture. *N Engl J Med* 1990; **332**: 1265–1271.

Watts *et al.* compared cyclical etidronate (400 mg daily for 14 days within a 91-day cycle, which was repeated eight times) with placebo in 429 postmenopausal women with osteoporosis. All patients received calcium supplements, and some received supplemental phosphate. Etidronate increased spinal bone mass and reduced the incidence of new vertebral bone fractures. There were no additional benefits from phosphate. *N Engl J Med* 1990; **323**: 73–79.

The **Alendronate Phase III Osteoporosis Treatment Study Group** studied the effect of oral alendronate, an aminobisphosphanate that inhibits bone resorption without impairing mineralization, in 994 women with postmenopausal osteoporosis. Daily alendronate with calcium supplementation increased bone mass and reduced vertebral fractures over a 3-year period. *N Engl J Med* 1995; **333**: 1437–1443.

Calcium and vitamin D
Dawson-Hughes *et al.* studied the effect of calcium supplementation (500 mg daily) on bone loss in 301 postmenopausal women. Calcium supplementation was only of benefit in reducing bone loss in older women (>6 years postmenopausal) with a daily dietary calcium intake of less than 400 mg. *N Engl J Med* 1990; **323**: 878–883.

Chapuy *et al.* studied the effect of vitamin D_3 (20 μg daily) and calcium (1.2 g daily) on the frequency of hip fractures and other non-vertebral fractures in 3270 healthy elderly women (mean age 84 years). Vitamin D_3 and calcium supplementation reduced the risk of hip fracture by 43% and other non-vertebral fractures by 32%. *N Engl J Med* 1992; **327**: 1637–1642.

Tilyard *et al.* compared the effect of 1,25-dihydroxyvitamin D_3 (0.25 μg twice daily) or supplemental calcium (1 g daily) for 3 years in 622 postmenopausal women who had one or more vertebral compression fractures. Calcitriol reduced the number of new vertebral fractures. *N Engl J Med* 1992; **326**: 357–362.

therefore recommended for etidronate which has been shown to increase verte-bral bone density, and may reduce vertebral fracture rate (see Trials, above). The newer aminobisphosphanate aledronate has less effect on mineralization and can be given continuously.

Calcium

A daily calcium intake of 1–1.5 g is recommended ($^1/_2$ litre of milk contains about $^3/_4$ g). Those who are unable to achieve this through diet should receive calcium supplements.

Vitamin D

Studies suggest that small doses of vitamin D can reduce bone loss and prevent fractures in women with postmenopausal osteoporosis.

Calcitonin

Calcitonin prevents bone resorption. Although it may prevent postmenopausal bone loss, it is often used to treat bone pain following fracture. Its use is limited by side effects (nausea, flushing, tingling, unpleasant taste), the need for parenteral administration and cost.

Fluoride

Sodium fluoride stimulates osteoblast proliferation. It increases bone mass, but bone formation may be abnormal and the effect on fracture rate is unclear.

OSTEOMALACIA

In osteomalacia (soft bones) there is inadequate mineralization of bone. In child-hood, osteomalacia presents as rickets.

The commonest cause is:
- vitamin D deficiency.

It may also result from:
- vitamin D resistance or abnormal vitamin D metabolism;
- phosphate depletion; and
- chronic metabolic acidosis.

Clinical features

Adult osteomalacia may present with:
- bone pain and tenderness;
- pathological fracture;
- weakness, most marked in the quadriceps and glutei, which results in a wad-dling gait and difficulty rising from a chair; and
- the signs of underlying disease, e.g. malabsorption — the osteomalacia being diagnosed in the course of investigation.

Rickets presents differently, because the reduced mineralization affects growing bones, causing:

- deformities in the legs (bow-legs, knock-knees);
- deformities in the chest (prominent costochondral junctions — ricketic rosary);
- deformities in the skull (craniotabes, open fontanelles and delayed eruption of the teeth); and
- hypotonia, weakness, tetany.

NB   Rickets in the UK occurs chiefly in Asian immigrants due to a combination of poor sunlight and a diet poor in vitamin D.

Aetiology

- *Reduced intake of vitamin D*—either dietary calciferol or cutaneous cholecalciferol (from 7-dehydrocholesterol), but usually both (dark skin, northern climate, poor diet).
- *Malabsorption*, especially gluten-sensitive enteropathy and postgastrectomy states.
- *Abnormal vitamin D metabolism*. Failure of 1-hydroxylation by the kidney is common in chronic renal failure. In type I vitamin D-dependent rickets there is a recessively inherited defect in the 1-hydroxylase enzyme. Hepatic enzyme induction with long-term anticonvulsant therapy can increase vitamin D metabolism and inactivation.
- *End-organ resistance to vitamin D*. Vitamin D-dependent rickets type II is an autosomal recessive disorder of the vitamin D receptor. 1,25-Vitamin D levels are markedly elevated.
- *Phosphate depletion*. X-linked hypophosphataemic rickets (familial vitamin D-resistant rickets) is a dominant disorder in which there is a renal phosphate leak and abnormal 1,25-vitamin D production. In Fanconi's syndrome the phosphate leak is accompanied by aminoaciduria and glycosuria.
- *Chronic metabolic acidosis*. Usually as a result of chronic renal failure or renal tubular defects.

Investigation

Biochemistry

Reduced serum phosphate with increased alkaline phosphatase. Plasma calcium is usually low normal (maintained by secondary hyperparathyroidism).

X-ray

Rickets. In addition to bone deformities there are widened and irregular metaphyses ('cupping, splaying and fraying').

Pseudofractures (Looser's zones) are translucent bands (≈ 2 mm) perpendicular to the surface of the bone, extending from the surface inwards, best seen in the pubic rami, the necks of the humeri and femurs and in the outer borders of the scapulae which are points of stress.

Generalized osteopenia with cortical thinning may be associated with multiple fractures, particularly in the ribs.

Bone scan

There is a generalized diffuse increase in uptake. Occasionally Looser's zones show multiple areas of increased uptake. In osteoporosis bone scanning is normal, whereas in Paget's there is strong focal uptake.

Histology

The number of bone seams is normal. There is excess volume of osteoid tissue. Calcification fronts (identified by tetracycline labelling) are absent. There is usually some evidence of hyperparathyroidism.

Investigation of underlying disease (malabsorption, uraemia) may be required.

Treatment

Vitamin D (calciferol). The dose and formulation depend on the aetiology. Serum calcium must always be monitored.

NB   Calciferol $10\,\mu g = 400$ units.

• Deficiency states: 1000 units/day. Maintenance requirements in the normal individual, including children, are around 500 units/day.

• Malabsorption states: water-soluble hydroxylated metabolites can be absorbed by the small intestine, e.g. 1α-hydroxycholecalciferol (alfacalcidol) or 1,25-dihydroxyvitamin D (calcitriol).

• Vitamin D-resistant states: in familial vitamin-resistant (hypophosphataemic) rickets treatment is with oral phosphate supplements with calcitriol. Type II vitamin D-dependent rickets (end-organ resistance) responds poorly to treatment, although huge doses of calcitriol ($20–60\,\mu g$ daily) with calcium supplements are sometimes effective.

• In uraemia there is failure of 1α-hydroxylation. Treatment is with alfacalcidol or calcitriol.

Calcium supplements are not usually required unless there is severe osteomalacia or poor dietary intake. In these circumstances calcium uptake into bone may precipitate hypocalcaemia.

NB   About 1 g of calcium is contained in 850 ml ($1\,^{1}/_{2}$ pints) of milk or 1 tablet of Sandocal 1000.

PAGET'S DISEASE (osteitis deformans)

James Paget, 1814–1899, Great Yarmouth.

Increased bone remodelling, in which both resorption and production of bone are accelerated, leads to deformity and fragility. It is a disease of the elderly, affecting 1% of 50-year-olds and 10% of 95-year-olds. In only about 5–10% is the disease clinically important.

Aetiology

Familial clustering and the finding of viral inclusions in osteoclastic nuclei suggest the disease may be triggered by slow viral infection of osteoclasts in genetically predisposed individuals.

Histology

Initially bone resorption is associated with increased numbers of large osteoclasts which contain up to 100 nuclei. Numerous osteoblasts are then recruited to the site of bone resorption, and produce abnormal new bone. This consists of woven bone in which collagen fibres are laid down in an irregular fashion, and patches of mature lamellar bone which lack the normal Haversian systems. The overall appearance gives a characteristic mosaic pattern.

Biochemistry

Increased bone resorption leads to increased urinary hydroxyproline. Increased osteoblastic activity is reflected in increased levels of serum alkaline phosphatase. Involvement of 10% of the skeleton is associated with a doubling in alkaline phosphatase.

Serum calcium levels are usually normal. In immobilized patients the stimulus to new bone formation may be lost, and hypercalcaemia may result from uncoupled resorption if there is extensive Paget's disease.

Radiology

Expansion and disorganization of bone with both lytic and sclerotic lesions are characteristic. There is cortical thickening and coarsening of trabeculae. The pelvis and lumbar spine are most frequently affected, followed by sacrum, thoracic spine, skull, lower limbs and upper limbs. Bowing deformity occurs in long bones, and osteoarthritis is common in adjacent joints.

Bone scintigrams show increased uptake at affected sites.

Clinical features

Many patients are asymptomatic, the diagnosis being made by an incidental finding on X-ray. Pain is the commonest symptom, sometimes with a rise in temperature over the site of the lesion. Pain may result from arthritis in adjacent joints. Bone deformity is most obvious when there is enlargement of the skull or bowing of the legs.

Complications

• Fractures: up to 15% of patients suffer pathological fractures in abnormal bone. Fissure fractures are small fractures on the convex surface of long bones. They may be asymptomatic, but can cause pain or progress to clinical fractures. Compression of affected vertebrae is common.

• Deafness is common in patients with skull involvement. It may result from involvement of the ossicles or compression of the cochlea or internal auditory canal. Occlusion of other foramina of the skull leading to compression of other cranial nerves occurs less often. Platybasia or flattening of the base of the skull may rarely lead to brainstem compression or obstructive hydrocephalus.

• Spinal involvement may cause cord compression, particularly in the cervical and thoracic regions where the canal is narrower, and paraparesis may result.

- Less than 1% of patients develop osteosarcoma in Pagetic bone. The pelvis and femur are the commonest sites. It may be heralded by increasing pain. Lesions are typically osteolytic and X-rays may reveal a soft-tissue mass. Diagnosis is confirmed by open or needle biopsy.
- High-output cardiac failure is a rare complication of extensive disease.

Treatment

Pain may be controlled with analgesics and non-steroidal anti-inflammatory drugs. Physiotherapy maintains mobility.

A number of specific treatments are now available. These agents are effective in relieving symptoms. They may also be of benefit in preventing complications in asymptomatic patients.

Calcitonin

Salmon calcitonin (salcatonin) given subcutaneously is the most widely used. It inhibits osteoclastic activity and is of use in relieving pain. It may also be of benefit in relieving complications such as deafness. Calcitonin is safe, but side effects, including nausea, flushing, unpleasant taste and pain at the injection site, are common.

Bisphosphanates

Bisphosphanates reduce bone turnover in Paget's disease, probably by binding to hydroxyapatite crystals on the surface of newly deposited bone. Administration of high doses for long periods inhibits new bone formation as well as bone resorption. Periods without treatment are therefore important in prolonged usage.

Etidronate is usually given as a single oral dose of 5 mg/kg daily for 6 months, followed by 6 months without treatment. Pamidronate is often given as a single intravenous infusion of up to 60 mg; this can induce remission for many months.

Plicamycin

Plicamycin (mithramycin) is now rarely used in the treatment of Paget's disease because of hepatic, renal and bone marrow toxicity.

Serum alkaline phosphatase and urinary hydroxyproline measurement can be used to monitor response to treatment. Urinary hydroxyproline levels reflect bone resorption and give a more rapid indication of response and an earlier warning of relapse.

URAEMIC BONE DISEASE (renal osteodystrophy)

In renal failure, there is reduced 1,25-dihydroxyvitamin D_3 ($1,25\text{-}(OH)_2D_3$) with increased PTH. In addition there is reduced renal phosphate excretion. The mechanisms of renal osteodystrophy are:

Phosphate retention

This has two secondary effects:
- reciprocal depression of serum calcium level (mediated at the bone surface); and
- rise in the calcium $\times$ phosphorus product (despite the serum calcium depression), which may lead to ectopic calcification.

Lack of vitamin D

The diseased kidneys fail to hydroxylate 25-hydroxycholecalciferol to 1,25-$(OH)_2D_3$. This failure is expressed at two important sites:
- the gut, where there is reduced calcium absorption; and
- the bone, to produce osteomalacia and hypocalcaemia.

Hypocalcaemia produced by these mechanisms is a stimulus to the parathyroid glands which are thus in a state of continuous hypersecretion, tending to return the serum calcium levels towards normal. This (secondary) hyperparathyroidism (p. 253) may be demonstrated on bone X-rays (p. 254), and the serum level of parathyroid hormone is elevated.

The hypocalcaemia only rarely leads to tetany because acidosis reduces the protein binding of calcium, and thus increases the level of ionized calcium.

The clinical consequences of renal failure on calcium metabolism are thus:
- Osteoporosis produced by hyperparathyroidism;
- Osteomalacia due to lack of vitamin D; and
- Ectopic calcification.

Management

There are five chief therapeutic manoeuvres:
- *Restriction of dietary phosphate.* Aluminium or calcium-containing antacids (aluminium hydroxide or calcium carbonate) are used as phosphate-binding agents to prevent intestinal absorption. Aluminium-containing agents are now rarely used because of concerns about aluminium toxicity. Calcium-containing agents are contraindicated if hypercalcaemia is present.
- *Dialysis* against a suitable ionized calcium concentration (about 1.5 mmol/l) and no phosphate should return the calcium and phosphate levels towards normal.
- *Vitamin D* increases calcium levels, and reduces hyperparathyroidism. It may be used to treat muscular weakness, bone pain and biochemical or radiological osteomalacia. Unwanted effects are increased absorption of phosphate from the gut, and hypercalcaemia. 1α-Hydroxylated forms (alfacalcidol or calcitriol) are used.
- *Parathyroidectomy* should reduce calcium and phosphate levels and permit vitamin D therapy without the risk of metastatic calcification.
- *Renal transplantation*, if successful, returns renal function to normal and corrects deficient $1,25(OH)_2D_3$ production. Persistent hyperparathyroidism can lead to marked hypercalcaemia. In the long-term, the side effects of immunosuppressive drugs may influence the skeleton adversely.

Hypercalcaemia

Physiology

The physiologically relevant measurement is of ionized calcium, but this is seldom performed. The normal total serum calcium level is 2.2–2.6 mmol/l (varying slightly according to laboratory). Approximately half of this is bound to plasma proteins, predominantly albumin, and half circulates as free ionized calcium. Changes in serum albumin may alter total calcium without changing ionized calcium concentrations. A simple correction for hypoalbuminaemia involves adding 0.02 mmol/l to the total serum calcium concentration for every 1 g/l by which the serum albumin concentration is below 40 g/l. Acidosis increases ionized calcium by decreasing binding of calcium ions to albumin, whereas alkalosis has the reverse effect.

Aetiology

• Malignant disease — PTH-related protein (p. 240), lytic bone metastases (myeloma, carcinoma), ectopic vitamin D production (lymphoma).
• Primary hyperparathyroidism (p. 253).
• Drug-induced—vitamin D, thiazide diuretics, lithium, milk-alkali syndrome.
• Granulomatous disease — sarcoidosis, rarely others, such as tuberculosis, leprosy, histoplasmosis.
• Endocrine—thyrotoxicosis, phaeochromocytoma, Addison's disease.
• Renal failure (p. 250).
• Immobilization.
• Total parenteral nutrition.
• Familial hypocalciuric hypercalcaemia.

Clinical features

• Neurological—depression, confusion, muscle weakness.
• Gastrointestinal—anorexia, nausea and vomiting, constipation.
• Renal—polyuria (impaired distal tubular function), stones, nephrocalcinosis.
• Cardiovascular — cardiac repolarization is increased, leading to shortening of the QT interval. Bradycardia and atrioventricular block can occur.

Investigation

A detailed history and examination should eliminate most of the differential diagnoses.

Malignancy and hyperparathyroidism account for 90% of patients. Malignancy can often be detected clinically or radiologically. Protein electrophoresis should be performed to exclude myeloma. Normal or elevated levels of parathyroid hormone in the presence of hypercalcaemia are inappropriate, and imply hyper-parathyroidism. Sarcoid should not be overlooked.

The hydrocortisone suppression test is not often required or diagnostically conclusive (hyperparathyroidism does not suppress in response to 40 mg 8-hourly for 10 days, whereas sarcoid and most malignancies do).

Treatment

Emergency

Rehydrate with intravenous saline and give frusemide. Loop diuretics inhibit sodium and calcium reabsorption from the thick ascending limb of the loop of Henle. Dialysis (haemo- or peritoneal) against a low calcium dialysate is reserved for severe hypercalcaemia or those with renal impairment.

Intravenous or oral bisphosphanates inhibit osteoclast-mediated bone resorption and can be used with rehydration to treat hypercalcaemia of malignancy. Corticosteroids are of particular value in haematological malignancies (myeloma, lymphoma) and sarcoid. They are ineffective in parathyroid disease.

Parenteral calcitonin (4 units/kg every 6–8 h) is usually effective in lowering serum calcium levels, but the effect is transient.

Long term

Remove the cause by specific therapy.

Endocrine bone disease

OSTEOGENESIS IMPERFECTA

A hereditary connective tissue abnormality with involvement of collagen-containing tissues such as the skeleton (fragile), sclerae (blue), skin (thin), teeth (thin dentine), tendons (hypermobile joints), heart (valve disorders) and ear (deafness).

Osteogenesis imperfecta tarda is a commoner, mild, autosomal dominant disease and fractures are rare.

Osteogenesis imperfecta congenita is a rare, severe, autosomal recessive disease with the above features plus scoliosis, bowed legs and multiple fractures.

HYPERPARATHYROIDISM

PTH increases serum calcium by:

- increasing calcium absorption from the gut;
- increasing mobilization of calcium from bone; and
- reducing renal calcium clearance.

It also increases renal phosphate clearance and this may also indirectly increase mobilization of calcium from bone.

Primary hyperparathyroidism results from an adenoma (85%) or hyperplasia of the parathyroid glands. Very rarely a functioning carcinoma may occur. Ectopic PTH may be produced by carcinoma elsewhere, particularly of the lung and kidney. It may be part of a multiple endocrine neoplasia (MEN) syndrome (p. 219).

Secondary hyperparathyroidism is a physiological response to hypocalcaemia produced by another disease, e.g. chronic renal failure and hypovitaminosis D (dietary deficiency or malabsorption). Hypocalcaemia persists.

Tertiary hyperparathyroidism refers to the situation where chronic secondary hyperparathyroidism has resulted in an autonomous adenoma. This, as in primary hyperparathyroidism, is characterized by hypercalcaemia, though the hyperphosphataemia of renal failure may persist.

Clinical presentation

- 'Bones, stones, groans (peptic ulcer) and moans (psychiatric disease).' Hypercalcaemia may be found on routine screening (0.1% of the general population; higher in hospital admissions: up to 8%).
- Hypercalciuria produces renal calculi, nephrocalcinosis and later renal failure.
- X-ray changes (see below).
- Severe hypercalcaemia may produce anorexia, nausea, vomiting, thirst, polyuria, constipation, muscle fatigue and hypotonicity and calcium deposition in the conjunctiva, usually at the medial limbus of the eye (3%). Dyspepsia and peptic ulceration may occur (5%).
- Psychiatric disorders (3%) include depression and confusion.

Differential diagnosis

This is from other causes of hypercalcaemia (pp. 252 and 290) and hypercalciuria.

Investigation

Biochemistry

In primary hyperparathyroidism the serum calcium is raised and the phosphate reduced. A raised serum alkaline phosphatase indicates increased bone activity. There is a high renal clearance of phosphate and a mild renal tubular acidosis (with a high serum chloride level). The serum calcium level is not reduced by corticosteroids. The serum PTH is raised. In the secondary hyperparathyroidism of renal failure, the serum phosphate is high and the serum calcium tends to be low.

Radiology

More specific changes include loss of the lamina dura of the teeth (25%) and small subperiosteal bone resorption cysts most marked in the middle phalanges of the hands (and feet). Osteitis fibrosa cystica with bone cysts is relatively rare. CT scan and isotopic subtraction scan of the neck and mediastinum (up to 20% are ectopic) seldom helps to localize the abnormal gland.

Treatment

Surgical resection of the diseased parathyroid glands is indicated for a serum calcium persistently over 3.0 mmol/l (after correction for serum albumin level) or for patients with lower levels plus any of the clinical presenting features given above if more than minor. It is important to visualize and probably biopsy all four parathyroid glands to determine whether they are normal or hyperplastic. A single enlarged gland is removed or, if all are enlarged, three and a half, the remaining half either being left *in situ* or implanted in the forearm. Some advocate the removal of all hyperplastic glands and subsequent treatment with alfacalcidol. A postoperative 'hungry bones syndrome' can develop with tetany and hypomagnesaemia.

HYPOPARATHYROIDISM
Aetiology

Secondary to thyroid surgery.

Primary idiopathic. This appears to be an organ-specific autoimmune disease and is associated with an increased incidence of Addison's (hypoadrenal) disease, pernicious anaemia and malabsorption. Parathyroid agenesis occurs in DiGeorge's syndrome with thymic hypopolasia as a result of maldevelopment of the third and fourth pharyngeal pouches. There is T-cell deficiency and children die from infection in infancy.

Pseudohypoparathyroidism (very rare) is due to a failure of end-organ response in bone and kidney to endogenous PTH which is thus present in excess amounts. Unlike patients with true idiopathic hypoparathyroidism, there is no increase in urinary cyclic adenine monophosphate when PTH is injected.

Clinical presentation

This depends upon its speed of onset and its degree. Acute hypocalcaemia gives paraesthesia around the mouth and in the extremities followed by cramps, tetany, stridor, convulsions, and death if untreated.

Trousseau's (twitching of the angle of the mouth on tapping over the 7th nerve) and Chvostek's (carpopedal spasm) signs may be present.

Ectodermal changes: teeth, nails, skin and hair. There is an excessive incidence of cutaneous moniliasis in primary hypoparathyroidism.

Ocular changes: cataract and occasionally papilloedema.

Calcification in the basal ganglia and, less commonly, other soft tissues.
NB   The hereditary syndrome of pseudohypoparathyroidism is caused by tissue resistance to PTH and usually presents in childhood. The patients have a moon face, are short, mentally retarded, have calcification of the basal ganglia and often have short fourth or fifth metacarpals. The biochemistry is similar to idiopathic hypoparathyroidism. Pseudopseudohypoparathyroidism refers to patients who have the somatic manifestations of pseudohypoparathyroidism but normal biochemistry.

Tetany may also occur rarely in rickets, the malabsorption syndrome, alkalosis, especially hyperventilation (p. 354) and, very rarely, in osteomalacia and uraemia.

Investigation

There is a low serum calcium and a high serum phosphate level with normal alkaline phosphatase. There is no common diagnostic radiological skeletal abnormality. X-ray of the skull may show calcification of the basal ganglia. If the patient is thought to have idiopathic hypoparathyroidism investigate for the associated pathologies.

The differential diagnosis of hypocalcaemia is that of the causes of PTH deficiency (p. 255) and of hypovitaminosis D — reduced intake or absorption, and resistance (p. 248).

Treatment

Emergency
Treat tetany with 10–20 ml of 10% calcium gluconate intravenously.

NB   Rebreathing from a bag if there is hyperventilation.

Intravenous magnesium chloride may also be required if there is also hypomagnesaemia.

Long-term therapy involves the use of vitamin D analogues, alfacalcidol or calcitriol supplements to raise the serum calcium towards normal (p. 248).

Gout and hyperuricaemia

A disease characterized by episodes of acute arthritis, at first affecting only one joint and associated with hyperuricaemia. Hyperuricaemia is 10 times commoner without clinical gout than with it.

Primary gout
An error of purine metabolism which occurs in men and postmenopausal women (10:1) with a prevalence in the UK of 3/1000. The hyperuricaemia is familial and there is a family history of gout in 30%. Hyperuricaemia can also result from increased consumption of purine-containing foods and excess alcohol, especially in predisposed individuals who are often also obese.

Secondary gout
This occurs at all ages in both sexes.

Ten per cent of all gout is associated with myeloproliferative disease which causes increased purine turnover and release, and hence a rise in serum uric acid (e.g. myeloid leukaemia, myelofibrosis, polycythaemia rubra vera, multiple myeloma and in Hodgkin's disease). This occurs particularly after treatment with antimetabolite drugs when the serum uric acid and urea rise as a result of tissue destruction.

Drug-induced hyperuricaemia may follow treatment with diuretics, particularly thiazides, and salicylates in small doses.

Chronic renal failure may be associated with hyperuricaemia and rarely clinical gout, secondary to reduced renal uric acid excretion.

Clinical features
In the first attack, the big toe is affected in 75% of cases, the ankle or tarsus in 35%,

and knee in 20%. In 40% it involves more than one joint. The onset is usually sudden and the joint is red, hot, shiny and exquisitely tender. The patient is febrile, irritable and anorexic. Attacks, at first monarticular in most patients, tend to be recurrent and to become polyarticular. They may be precipitated by trauma (including surgery), exercise, dietary excess, alcohol and starvation. Chronic gouty arthritis remains asymmetrical and tophi appear, especially on the cartilages of the ears and close to joints in 20% of untreated patients.

Complications

Renal disease. Uric acid stones occur in 10% of patients in the UK and may produce renal colic. Chronic renal failure may follow long-standing hyperuricaemia (chronic urate nephropathy).

Hypertension, obesity and coronary artery disease are more common in patients with hyperuricaemia. Secondary pyogenic infection of gouty joints is uncommon.

Investigation

The serum uric acid is raised.

NB   Five per cent of men have levels of 0.42 mmol/l or more but only 0.6% have clinical gout.

Leukocytosis is common and the erythrocyte sedimentation rate (ESR) is raised.

Radiology: asymmetrical soft-tissue swelling may be the only abnormality in acute gout. Chronic disease produces irregular punched-out bony erosions near but not usually involving the articular margins. Tophi may be seen if calcified. Osteoarthritic changes are common in gouty joints. Uric acid renal stones are radiolucent.

Aspirates of joint fluid contain negatively birefringent needle crystals of monosodium urate when viewed by polarized light.

Differential diagnosis

Acute gout must be distinguished from other causes of acute arthritis, particularly septic staphylococcal arthritis and rheumatic fever. Pseudogout may occur in chronic renal failure.

Chronic gout, particularly if widespread, may resemble rheumatoid or osteoarthritis.

Hyperuricaemia may be secondary to diuretic therapy.

Acute episodes

Indomethacin 100 mg followed by 25 mg tds or naproxen 750 mg followed by 250 mg tds. Hydrocortisone 100 mg intramuscularly repeated as required, may be given in resistant cases and may relieve pain almost instantaneously.

Colchicine (0.5–1 mg 2-hourly until pain is relieved, vomiting and diarrhoea begin or a total of 8 mg) may be given if non-steroidal anti-inflammatory drugs are contraindicated. Allopurinol may be started a fortnight after the acute attack has subsided but must be covered by continuation of non-steroidal anti-inflammatory drug therapy or colchicine 0.5 mg bd until at least one month after hyperuricaemia is corrected, because acute gout may otherwise be precipitated.

Chronic recurrent gout and hyperuricaemia

Probenecid 0.5 g two or three times a day and sulphinpyrazone 100 mg tds act by increasing renal clearance of uric acid and urates.

Allopurinol 300 mg daily is of particular value in the treatment of chronic tophaceous gout or chronic hyperuricaemia and when renal disease is present. It blocks the metabolic pathway at xanthine and hypoxanthine (by inhibiting xanthine oxidase), both of which are more soluble than uric acid and less liable to form stones. The dose is adjusted between 200 and 900 mg daily to keep the serum uric acid normal. It should be given well before starting cytotoxic chemotherapy otherwise the release of uric acid in the tumour lysis syndrome can precipitate acute renal failure.

These drugs may precipitate an acute attack and 3 months' cover with colchicine or anti-inflammatory agent (steroidal or non-steroidal) is advised.

Indications for long-term therapy are the presence of clinical gout, urate nephropathy, tophaceous gout, myeloproliferative disorders under therapy, or non-symptomatic but persistent plasma uric acid levels over 0.8 mmol/l.

Overeating and overdrinking (of alcohol) should be corrected (not only for gout), the obese should lose weight, and drug therapy, particularly thiazides and aspirin-containing drugs, assessed and modified where necessary.

PSEUDOGOUT (articular chondrocalcinosis or calcium pyrophosphate gout)

This is rare and sometimes familial. It is less uncommon in females (M/F 2:1) than gout. The patients are usually elderly. It is associated with diabetes mellitus (40%), hyperparathyroidism (p. 253) and haemochromatosis (p. 302). It may occur in chronic renal failure. Chondrocalcinosis is frequently found by chance on X-ray of the knees and may be symptom-free. It may present as osteoarthritis. However, there may be episodic pain and effusions into large joints and it may thus mimic gout, though the big toe is seldom affected and the symptoms are usually less acute, less severe and more prolonged. The effusions contain calcium pyrophosphate crystals which are rod- or brick-shaped and positively birefringent (whereas crystals in gout are negatively birefringent). The disease is associated with radiological calcification of the joint capsule and cartilage. The cartilages of the knee are characteristically outlined by calcium but calcification may occur in any cartilaginous joint. The patient may develop osteoarthritis secondary to the destruction of joint cartilage. Intra-articular steroids have been used. Indomethacin may be needed in acute episodes.

Diagnosis is established by calcification on X-ray of the joint, a normal serum uric acid and the characteristic crystals in the aspiration of joint fluid.

Nutrition

OBESITY

Excess body fat can be measured only indirectly and weight in relation to height and age is used as a measure. The body mass index (BMI = weight in kg/height^2 in m^2) is increasingly used. The normal range is 20–25 kg/m^2.

Aetiology

It is impossible to differentiate between genetic, environmental and socioeconomic factors. Most fat people have at least one fat parent. There are likely to be controlling endocrine factors yet to be determined—fat people have high plasma insulin and cortisol with low levels of growth hormone. The presence of less brown fat in the obese remains of uncertain significance.

Ultimately obesity is perpetuated by ingestion of calories in excess of needs and reduced by lowering the calorie intake and maintaining this reduced level.

Differential diagnosis

Weight gain is a feature of myxoedema and Cushing's syndrome and a rapid weight gain occurs with fluid retention in heart failure, renal failure and hypoalbuminaemia of chronic liver disease.

Prognosis

Mortality is increased in obesity. Actuarial figures suggest that weight reduction to normal reduces the increased mortality to normal.

Common complications include hypertension, myocardial infarction, diabetes mellitus, risk from surgery, osteoarthritis, herniae, gallstones, hiatus hernia and varicose veins. In women there is also an increased incidence of hirsutism and breast and endometrial carcinoma. Perhaps the saddest complications are psychological.

Treatment

The principle is simple: eat less. Therapy is aimed at encouraging and supporting patients during the period when they readjust to a redued calorie intake. Many patients lose 5–10% weight after starting a diet, and this is mainly water. Losing more weight is often very difficult but the initial weight loss is always encouraging. Exercise is of limited benefit in using calories, but improves general fitness and morale (walking at normal speed for 1 h uses the energy equivalent of about three chocolate biscuits).

The embarrassment and sometimes depression felt by the patient and the irritation of many clinicians based on poor results and poor patient compliance make successful treatment very difficult. Self-care groups (e.g. Weight Watchers) are usually more successful in the short term. If depression is a feature this will invariably prevent successful attempts at weight reduction unless the cause disappears or it responds to therapy. There is probably no role for anorectic drugs or thyroxine.

MALNUTRITION

Malnutrition is a major problem of the developing world. *Marasmus* refers to severe protein-energy malnutrition. Children are grossly underweight with muscle wasting and no fat. There is no oedema. In kwashiorkor there is protein deficiency with adequate calorie intake. There is oedema from hypoproteinaemia, and lipids accumulate in the liver, causing hepatomegaly.

In developed countries, malnutrition occurs during any acute illness, but particularly of the gastrointestinal tract, e.g. carcinoma of the stomach, ulcerative colitis, Crohn's disease, malabsorption. Protein loss is marked following burns from cutaneous loss, and also postoperatively from reduced intake and increased catabolism.

Enteral or intravenous feeding may be indicated.

Vitamin deficiencies

Vitamins (vital amines) are organic substances with specific biochemical functions. They are found in food, and are only required in small amounts.

Fat-soluble vitamins

Vitamin A (retinol) is found in liver, fish and dairy products. It is also produced in the intestine by cleavage of β-carotene which is found in carrots and other vegetables. Vitamin A is required for night vision (11-*cis*-retinaldehyde combines with rhodopsin in retinal rods). It is also important for epithelial keratinization.

Deficiency is rarely seen in developed countries. It causes night blindness and xerophthalmia (metaplasia of the cornea), a common cause of blindness in the developing world. Overdosage reduces keratinization of skin and sebum production. It causes rough, dry skin and hair, and liver enlargement. The recommended daily intake for adults is 750 μg.

Vitamin D: see p. 240.

Vitamin E (α-Tocopherol and related compounds) is found in vegetable oils. It is antioxidant, and present in all cell membranes. Severe deficiency causes haemolytic anaemia, and muscle and neurological disorders. The recommended daily intake for adults is 10 mg.

Vitamin K is found in green vegetables. It is a cofactor for the synthesis of clotting factors (II, VII, IX and X), and deficiency causes prolonged prothrombin time and bleeding. The recommended daily intake for adults is 100 μg.

Water-soluble vitamins

Vitamin B₁ (thiamine) is found in many foods, including wheat, cereals and meat. Deficiency rapidly occurs if intake is low as body stores are small. It is a cofactor of many metabolic pathways. The recommended daily intake for adults is 1 mg.

Deficiency causes:

- *Wernicke–Korsakoff* syndrome occurs in chronic alcoholics. There is ataxia, nystagmus and ophthalmoplegia, and confusion. The inability to retain new memories is accompanied by confabulation (Korsakoff's psychosis). Ischaemia and capillary haemorrhages occur in the mamillary bodies and around the aqueduct in the midbrain. Red cell transketolase levels are reduced. The disorder usually responds to parenteral thiamine (50–100 mg), although the memory defect often persists.

- *Beriberi* is now rare outside Asia. In addition to Wernicke's encephalopathy there is cardiomyopathy and peripheral neuropathy.

Vitamin B$_2$ (riboflavin) is found in most foods. Rich sources are dairy products, liver and cereals. It is a cofactor for cellular oxidation. Deficiency causes angular stomatitis, atrophic glossitis and seborrhoeic dermatitis. It usually occurs with other B vitamin deficiencies. The recommended daily intake for adults is 1 mg.

Nicotinamide forms part of the coenzymes nicotinamide adenine dinucleotide (NAD) and nicotinamide dinucleotide phosphate (NADP). It is found in many foods, including liver, meat, fish and cereals. It can also be synthesized from the amino acid tryptophan. Deficiency causes pellagra with dermatitis, diarrhoea and dementia. The adult daily requirement of nicotinamide is 20 mg, although this can partly be supplied by tryptophan (60 mg tryptophan is converted to 1 mg nicotinamide). *Nicotinic acid* can also be given, although its use is limited by vasodilatation.

Vitamin B$_6$ (pyridoxine) is found in many foods, including liver, meat, fish and cereals. Dietary deficiency is rare, but a number of drugs, including isonizid, penicillamine and hydralazine, antagonize its effects. Isoniazid peripheral neuropathy is prevented by pyridoxine. It may also be of benefit in hyperoxaluria and sideroblastic anaemia. The normal adult daily requirement is 3 mg daily.

Vitamin B$_{12}$ and *folic acid*: see p. 420.

Vitamin C (ascorbic acid) is an antioxidant. The main sources are fresh fruits and vegetables. One of its many roles is the reduction of proline to hydroxyproline, which is necessary for collagen formation. Impaired collagen production is the principal defect in scurvy, which is characterized by:

- Swollen, spongy gums;
- Spontaneous bleeding—bruising, bleeding gums, perifollicular haemorrhages, subperiosteal haemorrhages;
- Anaemia; and
- Hair follicle keratosis with 'corkscrew hairs'.

   The normal adult daily requirement is 30–60 mg daily.

ENTERAL FEEDING

Indications

Patients who cannot eat sufficient food, but have a functioning gut.

- Unconsciousness.
- Dysphagia—neurological, oesophageal obstruction, head and neck surgery.
- Loss of nutrients from fistulas or stomas.

- Any major illness, e.g. postoperatively, following radiotherapy or chemo-therapy, burns.

Administration

A fine-bore nasogastric tube is usually well-tolerated. If there is oesophageal obstruction, or prolonged feeding is necessary, a tube can be inserted directly into the stomach across the abdominal wall.

Requirements

An average patient needs:
- 2000–3000 kcal, of which 30–40% should be provided by fat; and
- 10–15 g nitrogen (60–90 g protein).

A number of commercial preparations are available. Most contain milk or soya proteins. Protein hydrolysates or free amino acids are only necessary if the ability to break down protein is limited by pancreatic or bowel disease. The mixture should contain vitamins and trace elements.

Complications

- Vomiting.
- Aspiration.
- Diarrhoea.
- Electrolyte and metabolic disturbances.

PARENTERAL NUTRITION

Parenteral nutrition is indicated when feeding via the gut is not possible because of:
- a reduction in functioning gut mass, either due to parenchymal disease or loss of small intestine—short-bowel syndrome;
- ileus—usually postoperatively; or
- loss of intestinal contents via fistulas.

It may supplement oral or enteral feeding, or be the only source of nutrition—total parenteral nutrition.

Requirements

Protein is provided as essential and non-essential L-amino acids. Energy is given as 150–250 kcal/g nitrogen. Glucose is the usual source of carbohydrate. Insulin may be necessary, particularly if more than 180 g of glucose is given daily. Some 30–40% of required energy is provided as fat. Fat emulsions provide essential fatty acids, and have a high energy to volume ratio.

The mixture of amino acids, glucose and fat together with trace elements and vitamins is prepared under sterile conditions by pharmacy, usually in a 3-l bag.

Administration

The tendency for peripheral veins to thrombose makes administration through a central venous catheter necessary. The catheter is inserted under full aseptic conditions. Tunnelling reduces the risk of infection. Patients requiring long-term parenteral nutrition can be taught to administer infusions overnight at home.

Complications
- Catheter-related—infection, blockage, venous thrombosis.
- Air embolism.
- Metabolic problems—hyperglycaemia, electrolyte imbalance, trace element or vitamin deficiencies.
- Fluid overload if renal insufficiency or cardiac problems.

ANOREXIA NERVOSA

This is a relatively common disorder of young women (incidence 1/250 schoolgirls aged 16 or under in the UK) who fast, vomit and/or purge to maintain a markedly low weight. Bulimia nervosa is habitual vomiting or purging, with eating binges between.

Anorexia nervosa is associated with extreme thinness, anovular amenorrhoea and fine hairs on the arms and legs (lanugo). Such patients have a markedly altered body image, and a craving to be very thin after considering themselves overweight. The cause is not known.

There is evidence of hypothalamopituitary dysfunction with low levels of lutenizing hormone (LH), follicle-stimulating hormone (FSH) and oestradiol. LH and FSH levels respond to gonadotrophin-releasing hormone injections, indicating an intact anterior pituitary. The levels of circulating hormones return to normal with recovery.

Treatment requires expert psychiatric advice and often periods of hospitalization with the aim of readjusting abnormal psychopathology, and increasing weight. Improvement of varying degrees, and often complete, occurs in most patients, though treatment may be necessary for many years. The mortality is 5–15%, often from suicide.

Renal Disease

Disease of the renal tract presents in only a few ways. Urinary tract infection is the commonest, especially in females. In males it is prostatic hypertrophy and its consequences. Proteinuria, haematuria and disorders of excretory function often cause no symptoms if mild, being picked up during routine screening (e.g. insurance medical).

Urinary tract infection

There are two main clinical syndromes:

1 *Cystitis*, which is characterized by suprapubic tenderness, dysuria and frequency. NB These symptoms can occur without infection (the urethral syndrome). Other causes include non-specific urethritis, gonococcus, interstitial cystitis, drug-induced cystitis (e.g. cyclophosphamide), bladder stones or tumours, vaginitis (infections or senile).

2 *Acute pyelonephritis* presents with dysuria, frequency, loin tenderness and fever, often with rigors and vomiting. Fever may be the only feature in children, in whom recurrent infection may be associated with vesicoureteric reflux which tends to diminish with age.

Bacteriuria is confirmed by finding a urinary excretion of more than 100 000 organisms/ml urine (counts <10 000/ml are usually due to contamination). Infection may be symptom-free. *Escherichia coli* is the most frequent organism (70–80%

of cases). Other organisms (*Proteus, Staphylococcus, Streptococcus, Klebsiella* and *Pseudomonas*) are usually associated with structural abnormality or catheterization, and reinfection. Tuberculosis classically causes a sterile pyuria.

Pyuria can almost always be detected by careful microscopic examination of fresh unspun urine. Microscopic haematuria is common.

Management

Uncomplicated cases are treated with oral antibiotics such as trimethoprim or ampicillin (3-day course for cystitis, at least 7 days for pyelonephritis) after obtaining urine for culture and antibiotic sensitivity. Resistant organisms can be treated with Augmentin or ciprofloxacin. Patients with acute pyelonephritis who are vomiting, pregnant or have evidence of septicaemia (blood cultures are positive in 20%) require intravenous antibiotics.

There may be an obvious predisposing cause, e.g. pregnancy, urinary obstruction or catheterization. Diabetes mellitus must be excluded. Acute pyelonephritis or more than two episodes of cystitis in a woman, or any infection in a man, suggest a structural abnormality. Ultrasound of the renal tract is performed to look for perinephric abscess, renal scarring, stone, tumours or obstruction. Intravenous urography (IVU) and possibly cystoscopy may be necessary (frequent infections, persistent haematuria, dysuria or loin pain) to exclude small stones/tumours or bladder diverticula.

Women prone to recurrent infections should be given advice about complete emptying of the bladder (double micturition), and voiding soon after intercourse. Low-dose antibiotic prophylaxis (e.g. trimethoprim 100 mg daily or nitrofurantoin 100 mg daily) reduces the incidence of infection, and can be used safely for long periods.

Children always require investigation as infection in the presence of ureteric reflux leads to permanent kidney damage.

Imaging the kidneys

A *plain abdominal film* usually shows the renal outlines, and identifies any calcification in the renal tract.

Renal ultrasound is useful in determining renal size and contour, and defining the size, location and consistency (solid or cystic) of any renal mass, and looking for pelvicalyceal dilatation of obstruction.

IVU has the advantage of demonstrating the whole urinary tract, but its usefulness has been replaced in many cases by ultrasound, computed tomographic (CT) scanning and radionuclide scanning. Ultrasound and CT are particularly useful for anatomical studies, and radionuclide scanning for providing functional information.

It should not be performed if there is a history of sensitivity to contrast media. Dehydration prior to the examination should be avoided in renal failure, diabetes or myeloma.

The patient fasts for 6 h. A supine plain abdominal film is taken and inspected to identify the renal areas and look for opacities. Contrast medium is injected as an intravenous bolus and images of the renal areas obtained. A compression band is applied to the lower abdomen to compress the ureters and distend the pelvicalyceal system. The compression is then released and further films taken.

Timed serial X-rays should be available. First inspect the plain film for renal tract calcification. Contrast is normally visible in the parenchyma as a nephrogram after 1 min (delayed in renal artery stenosis), and in the pelvicalyceal system by 5 min. Measure the size (Table 15.1; normal adult kidneys are 11–15 cm, or three vertebrae in length), and look for the normally smooth outline. An irregular outline due to renal scarring is a feature of *chronic pyelonephritis*, *tuberculosis* and *analgesic nephropathy*. The calyces are usually cupped, but become dilated and clubbed (Fig. 15.1) in *urinary tract obstruction* and *papillary necrosis*. Look for filling defects due to *carcinoma*. After 10–20 min the compression bands are removed and contrast should fill the ureters and bladder. Look for dilatation due to *obstruction*, or filling defects due to *calculi* or *carcinoma*. Look at the postmicturition film to assess emptying of the bladder and urinary tracts.

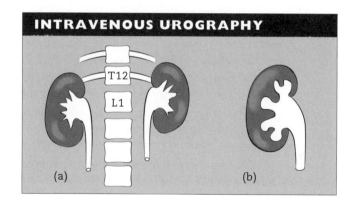

Fig. 15.1 Radiological appearance of intravenous urography (IVU). (a) Normal; (b) calyceal clubbing.

SMALL AND LARGE KIDNEYS

Causes of small kidneys	
Unilateral	Hypoplasia, chronic pyelonephritis, obstructive atrophy, tuberculosis, renal artery stenosis
Bilateral	All of the above plus chronic glomerulonephritis, hypertension, diabetes, analgesic nephropathy
Causes of enlarged kidney	
Unilateral	Compensatory hypertrophy, bifid collecting system, renal mass, hydronephrosis, renal vein thrombosis
Bilateral	Polycystic kidneys, amyloid, acute glomerulonephritis

Table 15.1 Causes of small and large kidneys.

Isotope scanning (most commonly ^{99m}Tc-diethylenetriaminepentacetic acid (DTPA) or ^{99m}Tc-dimercaptosuccinate (DMSA) can be used to assess renal blood flow, renal function and transit time of filtrate across the parenchyma into the collecting system. It is useful in the diagnosis of renal artery stenosis and obstruction. In addition the renal parenchyma can be visualized for evidence of scarring.

Chronic interstitial nephritis

The term *chronic pyelonephritis*, which implies infection, has been replaced by *chronic interstitial nephritis*, which is characterized by a chronic tubulointerstitial inflammatory infiltrate. Interstitial involvement is usually secondary to papillary or tubular damage by infection, ischaemia, radiation, toxins or metabolic disease. The commonest cause is reflux nephropathy (see below). Other causes include obstructive uropathy, drugs (cyclosporin, lithium, chronic analgesic ingestion), renovascular disease, sickle-cell disease, long-standing hypokalaemia, hypercalcaemia or hyperuricaema, tuberculosis, sarcoid, heavy metal poisoning (lead, cadmium), radiation nephritis, Sjögren's syndrome and hereditary nephritides (e.g. Alport's syndrome).

Clinical features

There is usually altered tubular function (glycosuria, aminoaciduria, renal tubular acidosis and tubular proteinuria) with a variable degree of renal failure. Ultrasound and radionuclide scans may show obstruction, and the kidneys are often small and scarred.

Management

Treat any underlying cause. Antibiotics (prophylactic if necessary) for infection. Patients are commonly unable to concentrate their urine, and need a high fluid intake.

REFLUX NEPHROPATHY

Reflux of urine through a congenitally abnormal vesicoureteric junction occurs in about 1% of infants. Reflux of sterile urine into the kidney may cause renal damage through hydrostatic injury, but there is clear evidence that reflux of infected urine leads to renal scarring. Reflux is present in 50% of infants who develop urinary infection during their first year, and a third of children who have infection before the age of 12. Reflux can also present with enuresis, hypertension and proteinuria. There is a familial incidence.

Management

Children with urinary infections (and possibly those with affected siblings or parents) should be screened with an ultrasound of the renal tract followed by a micturating cystourethrogram. In some centres radionuclide cystography is used. Ureteric reimplantation and conservative treatment with antibiotics to prevent infection are equally effective in preventing scarring. Without surgery reflux generally resolves as the child grows older.

Proteinuria

Small amounts of low-molecular-weight proteins are normally filtered by the glomerulus, and reabsorbed or catabolized by proximal tubular cells. The kidneys normally excrete 50–80 mg of protein daily, of which 30–50 mg is Tamm–Horsfall protein, a mucoprotein secreted by tubular cells. Proteinuria >150 mg daily is abnormal. Proteinuria detected by dipstick should be quantified on a 24-h collection. Dipsticks primarily detect albumin, and are relatively insensitive at detecting immunoglobulins or Bence-Jones protein (immunoglobulin light chains). Micro-albuminuria (urinary albumin excretion of 30–300 mg/day) is an early sign of diabetic nephropathy (p. 224).

Causes of proteinuria

- Glomerular disease: glomerulonephritis, glomerulosclerosis (diabetic and hypertensive), glomerular amyloid deposition.
- Tubular disease (due to impaired reabsorption of filtered proteins): chronic interstitial nephritis, polyuric phase of acute tubular necrosis, Fanconi's syndrome, tubular toxins (aminoglycosides, lead, cadmium).
- Non-renal disease: fever, heavy exercise, heart failure. Orthostatic proteinuria, a benign condition in 2% of adolescents who have proteinuria when upright but not when recumbent.
- Urinary tract disease: infection, tumours, calculi.
- Increased production of filterable proteins: immunoglobulin light chains (Bence-Jones protein) in myeloma, myoglobinuria, haemoglobinuria.
   Renal vein thrombosis is both a cause and consequence of proteinuria.

Clinical presentation

Often asymptomatic (routine screening). Nephrotic syndrome (p. 269) if severe. There may be evidence of underlying cause (e.g. urinary infection, diabetes, hypertension).

Assessment

The history should include enquiries about recent infections (urinary or as a cause of glomerulonephritis), renal disease (including any family history), drugs and occupation. Examination may be normal but there may be oedema, hypertension, heart failure or evidence of renal failure.

Investigation

Serum creatinine, urea and electrolytes and 24-h urine collection for protein content and creatinine clearance.

Serum proteins for albumin and protein electrophoresis (serum and urine) for monoclonal gammopathy. Blood glucose for diabetes.

Serum complement (may be low in glomerulonephritis; p. 282), antinuclear antibodies (systemic lupus erythematosis; SLE), antineutrophil cytoplasmic antibodies (systemic vasculitis), cryoglobulin levels.

Plain abdominal X-ray and ultrasound of renal tract for stones, structural abnormalities and renal size.

In the majority of cases these investigations fail to define the underlying cause, and renal biopsy may be necessary, particularly if proteinuria exceeds 2 g/day or there is impaired excretory function. This usually establishes the diagnosis, and may identify a treatable cause (particularly some forms of glomerulonephritis).

In the absence of oedema, treatment should be directed towards any underlying cause or associated conditions (e.g. hypertension).

Nephrotic syndrome

The triad of:
- proteinuria;
- hypoalbuminaemia; and
- oedema.

Aetiology

Any cause of severe proteinuria. Usually it is a consequence of glomerular disease — commonly glomerulonephritis (p. 279), diabetic glomerulosclerosis, renal amyloid. More than 75% of childhood and 25% of adult nephrotic syndrome is due to minimal-change disease (p. 282). Tubular proteinuria is usually less than 2 g/day and does not cause nephrotic syndrome.

It is associated with thrombosis (loss of anticoagulant proteins such as antithrombin III, protein S, protein C), infection (loss of immunoglobulins) and hyperlipidaemia.

Management

Identify and treat any underlying cause.

Diabetic glomerulosclerosis — angiotensin-converting enzyme inhibitors reduce proteinuria by lowering glomerular capillary pressure, and slow progression of diabetic nephropathy.

General management is aimed at:
- Reducing oedema with salt restriction and diuretics. Salt-free albumin (to restore intravascular volume) with diuretics is sometimes used in resistant cases.
- Angiotensin-converting enzyme inhibitors reduce proteinuria, probably by lowering glomerular capillary pressure. Non-steroidal anti-inflammatory drugs also reduce proteinuria, but these agents reduce renal blood flow and glomerular filtration rate and cause salt retention.

- Treatment of hypertension: angiotensin-converting enzyme inhibitors and diuretics in the first instance, but additional agents may be required.
- The optimum dietary protein intake is controversial. Most physicians recommend a normal protein intake. Any protein restriction should allow for urinary protein loss.
- Anticoagulate if immobile or thrombotic episode. Look for and treat intercurrent infection.
- Hyperlipidaemia may be severe. Very-low-density lipoprotein cholesterol, low-density lipoprotein cholesterol and total plasma cholesterol are elevated, as are triglyceride levels. Although this pattern is associated with increased cardiovascular risk, the value of treatment with diet or lipid-lowering agents (3-hydroxy-3-methyl glutaryl coenzyme A (HMG CoA) reductase inhibitors are usually effective; p. 236) has not been fully assessed.

Haematuria

Isolated haematuria on dipstick testing of urine can occur in normal individuals.

Microscopic haematuria is confirmed by finding more than three red cells per high-power-field of spun urine. Macroscopic haematuria is always abnormal.

Aetiology

Common
- Renal tract infection.
- Renal tract stones (calcium oxalate 80%, triple phosphate 10%, urate 10%, cystine <1%).
- Tumours of the bladder, kidneys and prostate.
- Glomerulonephritis.
- Schistosomiasis is common worldwide.

Uncommon
- Hypertension.
- Renal trauma.
- Papillary necrosis.
- Renal infarction.
- Drugs—cyclophosphamide (haemorrhagic cystitis), anticoagulants.
- Medullary sponge kidney (usually benign developmental abnormality with medullary cysts which may be complicated by infection or calculi).

Familial causes
- Polycystic kidneys (p. 275).
- Alport's syndrome (p. 275).
- Thin basement membrane disease (a benign condition in which haematuria is usually the only clinical feature).

- Medullary cystic disease (tubulointerstitial nephritis with medullary cysts that usually progresses to renal failure).

The causes vary with age. Glomerular causes predominate in children and young adults, whereas tumours and calculi are common in the elderly.

Investigation

The likely source may be suspected from the history and examination.

Microscopy of a fresh urine sample is performed in all patients to confirm the presence of red cells. The presence of red-cell casts or dysmorphic (abnormally shaped) red cells indicates glomerular bleeding (red cells are deformed by mechanical and osmotic stress as they pass through the tubules). Heavy proteinuria suggest a glomerular lesion, whilst white cell casts indicate renal inflammation. Bacteria may be seen and culture should be performed. Urine should also be sent for cytology.

Plasma urea and *creatinine* to assess renal function

Plain abdominal film and *ultrasound of the renal tract* to assess renal size and look for structural lesions (calculi, tumours, cysts)

If glomerular bleeding is suspected (young age, hypertension, proteinuria, renal impairment, absence of structural lesion), consider *renal biopsy*.

If a lesion of the renal tract is suspected (older age, no evidence of intrinsic renal disease) proceed to *cystoscopy* with *IVU* if the upper renal tract has not been clearly identified by ultrasound.

NB   Normal urine (centrifuged deposit) contains:
- Red cells 1×10^6 cells/24h (3 per high-power-field).
- White cells 2×10^6 cells/24h (6 per high-power-field).
- Hyaline casts are composed of uromucoid (Tamm–Horsfall protein which is excreted by normal tubular cells).
- Cellular casts result from adherence of either red cells (implying glomerular bleeding) or white cells (implying tubular inflammation) to the surface of hyaline casts.
- Epithelial cells may be found in normal urine due to contamination by cells from the vulva or prepuce.

Acute renal failure

Characterized by a rapid rise in serum creatinine, usually with a decrease in urine output. The causes can be divided into prerenal, renal and postrenal.

Prerenal
Aetiology

- Sepsis—the commonest cause, usually complicating surgery or pneumonia.
- Hypovolaemia from any cause (e.g. haemorrhage, burns, severe diarrhoea or vomiting).
- Cardiogenic shock.

- Drug-induced hypotension (e.g. following drug overdose).

NB   Angiotensin-converting enzyme inhibitors may reduce glomerular perfusion sufficiently to cause renal failure if given in the presence of bilateral renal artery stenosis (p. 381). In accelerated (malignant) hypertension acute, severe hypertension is associated with marked renal abnormalities. The most striking of these is gross intimal hyperplasia, leading to occlusion of the lumen in small arteries and arterioles. Renal failure is a rapid consequence of this condition if the blood pressure is not controlled.

Renal failure commonly complicates advanced liver disease. Plasma urea and creatinine may be normal because of reduced hepatic urea synthesis, low dietary protein intake and loss of muscle mass. There is often a precipitating cause (e.g. hypovolaemia following diuretic therapy, paracentesis or gastrointestinal bleeding, sepsis). Unexplained renal failure complicating liver disease is the *hepatorenal syndrome*. The prognosis is poor. Reinfusion of ascites into the internal jugular vein via a peritoneo-venous shunt can expand plasma volume and improve renal function, but does not improve survival.

Pathophysiology

Despite high blood flow (20% of cardiac output) the kidneys are particularly susceptible to ischaemia. Factors contributing to ischaemic or toxin-induced renal cell injury include cellular adenosine triphosphate depletion (due to hypoxia and mitochondrial injury), and free radical generation.

The medulla receives less than 10% of renal blood flow, and is at greatest risk of injury. The common response to severe injury (regardless of cause) is *acute tubular necrosis* (ATN). The necrosis of tubular epithelial cells is most prominent in the proximal tubules and thick ascending limb of the loop of Henle. The tubular lumen may be obstructed by cell debris and casts. Regeneration of tubular cells leading to recovery can take weeks. Severe prolonged ischaemia can cause acute cortical necrosis from which there is little chance of recovery.

The distinction between prerenal failure (in which concentrating powers are retained) and ATN (in which concentrating powers are lost) can be made on urinalysis. In prerenal failure urine osmolality is high (>500 mosmol/kg), urine sodium is low (<20 mmol/l) and urine:plasma urea ratio is >10:1. In ATN urine is isotonic with plasma (<400 mosmol/kg), urine sodium is >40 mmol/l and urine:plasma urea ratio is <10:1.

Renal Causes

- Glomerulonephritis (pp. 279–286).
- Nephrotoxic drugs (e.g. aminoglycosides, cyclosporin A, amphotericin B).
- Poisoning (e.g. heavy metals).
- Myoglobinuria—following rabdomyolysis myoglobin may cause tubular toxicity or form tubular casts. Creatine kinase is markedly elevated.
- Acute tubular (or cortical) necrosis complicating prerenal disease.

- Acute interstitial nephritis (usually drug-induced hypersensitivity reaction which responds to withdrawal of the drug and a short course of corticosteroids. Eosinophils may be present within the predominantly mononuclear cell interstitial infiltrate).
- Intrarenal obstruction (e.g. urate or oxalate crystals, calcium precipitation, tubular casts in myeloma).

NB   Hypercalcaemia causes renal failure through renal vasoconstriction, direct tubular cell toxicity and distal tubular calcium phosphate precipitation.

Haemolytic–uraemic syndrome (HUS) is characterized by thrombocytopenia (platelet consumption), microangiopathic haemolytic anaemia (red cell fragments on film) and acute renal failure. Commonly follows a diarrhoeal illness in infants infected with a verotoxin-producing strain of *Escherichia coli*. In adults it may follow an upper respiratory tract infection or be associated with cyclosporin A, the oral contraceptive pill or cytotoxic agents. Familial forms occur. Renal biopsy shows occlusion of glomerular capillaries with fibrin and thrombi, without evidence of complement or immunoglobulin deposition. Recovery usually occurs over a few weeks in children, but the prognosis for adults is poor. Responses to plasma exchange with fresh frozen plasma have been reported. *Thrombotic thrombocytopenic purpura* (TTP; p. 106) is closely related to HUS, but is commonest in women and central nervous system involvement and fever are typical additional features.

Postrenal

Acute urinary tract obstruction from:
- prostatic hypertrophy;
- renal and ureteric stones;
- tumour of renal pelvis, ureters or bladder;
- blood clot;
- sloughed papillae;
- external compression from retroperitoneal fibrosis or tumours; and
- surgical mishap (e.g. ureteric involvement in hysterectomy).

NB   Lesions above the bladder must involve both urinary tracts.

Investigation

Where there is no obvious cause following careful history and examination, and preliminary biochemical and haematological assessment:
- Check that there is no obstruction. Rectal examination is obligatory to exclude prostatic disease in men, or a pelvic mass. The bladder is enlarged in urethral obstruction. Ultrasound to look for urinary tract dilatation is the simplest method of excluding obstruction. This will also give information about renal size (small kidneys indicate chronic renal disease; scarring usually indicates chronic interstitial nephritis or ischaemia).
- If renal size is normal and there are no clues on investigations, including urinalysis (exclude infection; heavy proteinuria, granular or red cell casts indicate

intrinsic renal disease), calcium, uric acid, protein electrophoresis (myeloma), antineutrophil cytoplasm antibodies (vasculitis), antiglomerular basement membrane antibodies (Goodpasture's disease), antinuclear antibodies (SLE), platelet, eosinophil count and coagulation (disseminated intravascular coagulation (DIC), TTP, HUS, drug-induced hypersensitivity):

• Proceed to renal biopsy providing there are no contraindications.

Management

Should be undertaken in a specialized unit where facilities for dialysis are available.

Identify and correct underlying causes — often multiple (e.g. hypotension, sepsis, DIC and aminoglycoside toxicity).

Rapid correction of prerenal causes (intravenous fluids or blood for hypovolaemia, antibiotics for sepsis, inotropes, avoidance of nephrotoxic drugs) may prevent ATN and restore renal function. Loop diuretics (e.g. frusemide) are often given, and may prevent tubular cell ischaemia through inhibition of active sodium chloride reabsorption, thereby reducing oxygen requirements.

Relieve urinary tract obstruction from below (urethral catheterization with or without ureteric stents) or above (nephrostomy). Prostatic obstruction in elderly men is the commonest cause.

Initiate treatment for any intrinsic renal disease (e.g. immunosuppression for certain forms of glomerulonephritis; p. 279).

Continuing assessment of fluid status through input–output records, physical examination, daily weight, lying and standing blood pressure. Fluids should be restricted if there is oliguria or anuria, but patients are usually catabolic and nutrition should not be neglected. A protein intake of 0.6–0.8 g/kg per day with 30 kcal/kg per day should be maintained. In severely ill patients parenteral nutrition may be necessary.

Careful monitoring of electrolytes, urea, creatinine and acid–base status.

If renal failure persists, renal replacement therapy with haemodialysis, peritoneal dialysis or haemofiltration will be required. Absolute indications include hyperkalaemia (potassium above 6–7 mmol/l), markedly elevated plasma creatinine (>1000 μmol/l, but absolute level must take clinical state into account), severe acidosis (bicarbonate below 10–15 mmol/l) and fluid overload with pulmonary oedema.

Chronic renal failure

Common causes

• *Chronic glomerulonephritis* (p. 279).
• *Diabetic nephropathy* (p. 267).
• *Chronic interstitial nephritis* (p. 224).
• *Hypertension*: estimates of the prevalence of chronic renal failure due to essential hypertension vary widely from 0.002% to 20% of all cases of renal failure, reflecting the fact that the diagnosis of renal disease due to hypertension depends

on the exclusion of other causes. Many cases may have undiagnosed renal disease. Renal failure due to hypertension is much commoner in blacks than whites, and within the black population there appears to be familial clustering of renal disease caused by hypertension, suggesting a genetic susceptibility to hypertensive renal damage.

- *Renovascular disease* (p. 380).
- *Hereditary renal disease.*

Polycystic kidney disease

Autosomal dominant condition in which renal failure results from progressive cystic degeneration of the kidneys. Patients present with hypertension, abdominal pain, haematuria or chronic renal failure. The diagnosis is confirmed by ultrasound, and family members should be screened. Progression to renal failure with hypertension is usual, although the age at which renal replacement therapy becomes necessary varies. Approximately 85% of cases are due to a defect in PKD1 which maps to 16p13.3. The PKD2 gene, responsible for most non-16p-linked polycystic kidney disease, has been localized to 4q13–q23.

The disease should be considered a multisystem disease in which cysts occur in other organs (liver, pancreas, testes). There is an increased incidence of cardiac valve disease, cerebral aneurysms, hernias and diverticular disease. The underlying cellular defect is at present unknown. Analysis of the DNA sequence available so far has not revealed homologies to other known proteins. Characterization of the protein should help clarify the molecular pathology.

Alport's syndrome

X-linked hereditary nephritis — associated with sensorineural deafness and eye lesions. Characterized by thinning and splitting of glomerular basement membrane (GBM). There is an abnormality of type IV collagen (α5 chain; gene locus Xq22).

- Long-standing urinary tract obstruction.

NB   About 20% of patients with chronic renal failure present with bilaterally small kidneys and no diagnosis is reached. Under these circumstances renal biopsy is hazardous and unlikely to show reversible changes.

Clinical features

Screening for renal disease and the availability of dialysis mean that the classical manifestations of *uraemia* (literally *urine in the blood*) are now seen infrequently. Chronic renal failure is, by definition, slow to progress and usually presents with lethargy, general malaise, anorexia and nausea. Generalized pruritus is common. Impotence, menstrual irregularities and loss of fertility are common complaints in younger patients. In severe uraemia there is a characteristic fishy fetor, hiccups, vomiting, severe pruritus with skin excoriations, skin pigmentation, peripheral neuropathy and CNS derangements leading to lethargy, stupor and coma with fitting. Pericarditis may be associated with effusion and tamponade.

Investigations

Biochemical

Plasma urea and creatinine provide a guide to the severity of renal failure.

Urea. Although there is little evidence that urea (H_2N-CO-NH_2; molecular mass 60 Da) is toxic, it is the most abundant nitrogenous compound to accumulate in renal failure. It is the end-product of protein metabolism and is synthesized primarily in the liver. It is freely filtered by the glomerulus, but approximately 50% is reabsorbed so urea clearance is less than glomerular filtration rate (GFR). Urea production increases with cellular catabolism (infection, trauma, steroid therapy) or following protein load (dietary or following gastrointestinal haemorrhage). It is reduced in liver failure.

Creatinine is derived from metabolism of creatine in muscle. The rate of production correlates with muscle mass, and depends little on protein intake. Fifty per cent loss of renal function is needed before the serum creatinine rises above the normal range; it is therefore not a sensitive indicator of mild to moderate renal injury.

Creatinine clearance provides a more accurate assessment (if performed correctly). The patient performs a 24-h collection of urine (the first urine passed on waking is discarded, and all urine passed up until and including emptying the bladder the following morning is collected). A single measurement of plasma creatinine is made during this time. Creatinine clearance is measured as:

(urine creatinine concentration ÷ plasma creatinine) × urine volume per minute

In addition to being filtered by the glomerulus, small quantities of creatinine are excreted by the tubules. The creatinine clearance therefore slightly overestimates the GFR. Cr^{51} *ethylene diaminetetra-acetic acid (EDTA) clearance* more accurately reflects the GFR. It is calculated from the rate of disappearance of a bolus injection of Cr^{51} EDTA from the blood. The normal GFR is 110–130 ml/min per 1.73 m².

Hyperkalaemia (p. 288) is common.

A number of abnormalities of *calcium* and *phosphate* homeostasis occur.

Phosphate retention leads to:
• reciprocal depression of serum calcium level; and
• rise in the calcium × phosphate product which may lead to ectopic calcification.

The diseased kidneys fail to hydroxylate *25-hydroxycholecalciferol* (25-HCC) to the more active form 1-25-dihydroxycholecalciferol (1-25-DHCC). This results in:
• reduced calcium absorption from gut; and
• osteomalacia.

Hypocalcaemia stimulates the parathyroid glands which are thus in a state of chronic hypersecretion, tending to return the serum calcium level to normal.

Thus, dihydroxycholecalciferol is reduced (because of reduced 1α-

hydroxylase activity in the kidney) with increased parathyroid hormone (PTH). The increased PTH may result from phosphate retention which leads to a decrease in ionized calcium. The clinical consequences are:
- osteoporosis produced by hyperparathyroidism;
- osteomalacia due to lack of vitamin D; and
- ectopic calcification.

Hypocalcaemia rarely leads to tetany because acidosis and hypoproteinaemia reduce protein binding and increase ionized levels of calcium.

Plasma *uric acid* is often raised (but clinical gout is rare).

Haematological investigations usually reveal a *normochromic normocytic anaemia* which responds to parenteral erythropoietin. Gastrointestinal blood loss, iron, vitamin B_{12} or folate deficiency, decreased red cell survival, hyperparathyroidism and aluminium toxicity may also contribute to anaemia, and should be considered if there is a failed response to erythropoietin.

Urinalysis should be performed to exclude urinary infection and look for cellular casts indicating active renal inflammation.

Renal ultrasound identifies obstruction or renal scars, and defines renal size. *Plain abdominal X-ray* also defines the renal outline, and excludes renal tract calcification. If renal size is normal, and the cause of renal disease unknown, *renal biopsy* should be considered.

Management

There are two main aims:
1 slowing the decline in renal function; and
2 preventing or treating complications (bone disease, cardiovascular disease, endocrine effects, anaemia, socio-economic).

Regardless of the cause of renal disease, once renal function is compromised, a steady progressive fall in GFR is usually observed.

Risk factors for progression of renal disease are:
- persistent activity of underlying disease;
- uncontrolled hypertension;
- infection; and
- nephrotoxins (drugs).

Pathophysiology

Possible mechanisms of progression of renal failure include:
- increased glomerular pressure (as a result of increased systemic blood pressure, or efferent arteriolar constriction as a consequence of increased angiotensin II levels);
- glomerular protein leakage; and
- lipid abnormalities.

Hypertension in chronic renal failure
Progression in chronic renal failure is attenuated by treatment of hypertension.

Thiazide diuretics, β-blockers, angiotensin-converting enzyme inhibitors and calcium antagonists are all effective in patients with early renal damage. Angiotensin-converting enzyme inhibitors and calcium channel blockers do not modify glucose or lipid metabolism, have a favourable effect on left ventricular hypertrophy and have a potentially nephroprotective effect by reducing increased renal vascular resistance. Angiotensin-converting enzyme inhibitors have the additional advantage of producing a fall in proteinuria in patients with both diabetic and non-diabetic renal disease. They should be introduced with caution as they can reduce renal blood flow and precipitate acute renal failure, particularly in the presence of renal artery stenosis (p. 381).

Dietary protein restriction

Protein is often restricted to 0.6 g/kg per day once GFR falls below 50 ml/min, although there is little evidence that this retards progression of renal failure.

Complications

Bone disease

Hypocalcaemia from decreased renal $1,25\text{-(OH)}_2D_3$ synthesis, hyperphosphataemia and resistance to peripheral actions of PTH all contribute to renal bone disease. Treatment is by dietary phosphate restriction with or without phosphate binders (calcium carbonate providing calcium has not become elevated as a result of tertiary hyperparathyroidism; p. 254), and early use of low-dose 1α-hydroxylated vitamin D derivatives.

Cardiovascular disease

Cardiovascular disease is the commonest cause of mortality in patients with chronic renal failure. It is likely to reflect an increased incidence of hypertension, lipid abnormalities, glucose intolerance and haemodynamic abnormalities, including left ventricular hypertrophy. Of these, hypertension is probably the most susceptible to treatment.

Anaemia

Circulating erythropoietin levels are inappropriately low. Parenteral recombinant erythropoietin increases haemoglobin, improves exercise tolerance and reduces the need for blood transfusion. In patients with pre-dialysis advanced renal failure erythropoietin corrects anaemia and improves well-being, without affecting the rate of decline in renal function. Dose-dependent hypertension occurs in 35% of patients and can usually be controlled with hypotensive agents, although hypertensive encephalopathy can develop suddenly.

Sexual dysfunction

Decreased libido and impotence are common. Hyperprolactinaemia is present in at least one-third of patients, resulting in an inhibitory effect on gonadotrophin secretion. Prolactin levels may be reduced by bromocriptine, although side effects are common (nausea, headache, drowsiness, postural hypotension).

End-stage renal disease requires replacement of renal function by

- *Haemodialysis.* Diffusion of solutes occurs between blood and dialysate which flow in opposite directions, separated by a semipermeable membrane. The commonest problems are cardiovascular instability during dialysis, and difficulty establishing vascular access. This is achieved by:

    (a) arteriovenous fistula, typically at the wrist with arterialization of the cephalic vein;

    (b) double-lumen jugular, subclavian or femoral line;

    (c) synthetic graft (usually Goretex) looping subcutaneously between an artery and vein in the forearm or leg; or

    (d) Scribner shunt — arteriovenous Teflon shunt between artery and vein, usually at the wrist or ankle (rarely used now).

- Continuous ambulatory peritoneal dialysis. Patients instil up to 2 litres of isotonic or hypertonic glucose solution into the peritoneal cavity via a permanent indwelling Silastic catheter. The fluid equilibrates, across the $2\,m^2$ of peritoneal membrane, with blood in peritoneal capillaries. After several hours the fluid containing toxic waste products is drained out. This procedure is repeated three or four times daily. Excess fluid is removed by hypertonic solutions. The major complication is peritonitis, usually due to *Staphylococcus epidermidis* or *S. aureus*.

- *Renal transplantation* is the treatment of choice in most patients, but is limited by supply of donor organs.

Assessment of dialysis adequacy

Plasma urea and creatinine are poor predictors of outcome in dialysis patients — low pre-dialysis urea, not high, has been found to be associated with increased mortality. This is because when protein intake is deficient or muscle mass is reduced, pre-dialysis urea and creatinine may remain low even in the presence of inadequate dialysis. Assessment of dialysis adequacy is now achieved by the use of kinetic measurements — often referred to as *urea kinetic modelling*. Two parameters, *urea clearance* corrected for volume of distribution (Kt/V urea, where $Kt =$ urea clearance and $V =$ volume of distribution) and *protein catabolic rate* have been found in several studies to be useful predictors of outcome.

Glomerulonephritis

This describes a number of disorders which affect one or more of the glomerular components in both kidneys (Fig. 15.2). Patients present with one or more features of renal disease — hypertension, haematuria, proteinuria, nephrotic syndrome and various degrees of renal failure.

The classification of glomerulonephritis is based on histology and immunofluorescence of renal tissue. Contraindications to renal biopsy include:

- one functioning kidney
- small kidneys

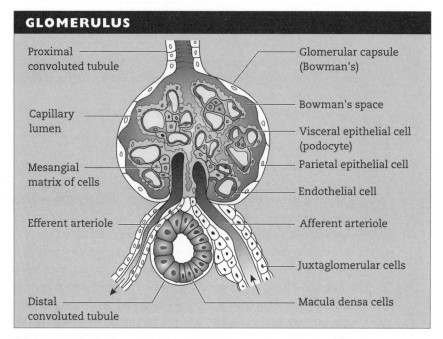

Fig. 15.2 Glomerulus.

- hypertension
- bleeding disorders.

Confusion arises because renal biopsy findings do not necessarily correlate with clinical features, although they are sometimes useful in guiding management and predicting outcome.

Histological changes are described as:

- *focal*—affecting <50% of glomeruli;
- *diffuse*—affecting >50% of glomeruli;
- *segmental*—affecting part of the glomerulus;
- *global*—affecting all of the glomerular tuft;
- *proliferative*—an increase in glomerular cells (mesangial, epithelial and endothelial) with leukocytic infiltration;
- *crescent*—a crescentic-shaped proliferation of epithelial cells and mononuclear cells in Bowman's capsule. It occurs in any severe form of glomerular injury;
- *membranous*—thickening of the glomerular capillary wall; and
- *sclerosis*—capillary collapse with loss of the lumen.

IgA-RELATED GLOMERULONEPHRITIS

Granular mesangial deposition of immunoglobulin A (IgA; and usually C3) with variable segmental mesangial proliferation (measurement of serum immunoglobulins is usually unhelpful—20–50% have raised IgA).

Clinically

Usually presents with haematuria (often provoked by infection).

Aetiology

Unknown. It is associated with liver disease (particularly alcoholic cirrhosis), coeliac disease, seronegative arthritis, neoplasia, infection.

Prognosis

It is probably the commonest form of glomerulonephritis. Approximately 20% progress to renal failure. There is no specific treatment, but control of hypertension which is commonly present slows the decline in renal function.

HENOCH–SCHÖNLEIN PURPURA

Renal lesion is virtually identical to IgA nephropathy.

Clinical features

Abdominal pain, arthralgia and palpable purpura due to an associated vasculitis (Henoch–Schönlein purpura = IgA nephropathy with systemic vasculitis), usually in children or adolescents.

Prognosis

Often self-limiting, but relapsing or chronic cases occur. Immunosuppressive therapy may help the vasculitis but is of unproven value in treating the renal lesion.

MEMBRANOUS NEPHROPATHY

Diffuse uniform thickening of glomerular capillary wall, usually without cellular proliferation.

Classification

- Stage I: small subepithelial electron-dense deposits (diffuse granular IgG staining)
- Stage II: outgrowth of basement membrane between subepithelial deposits (seen as 'spikes' on silver stain)
- Stage III: deposits incorporated into basement membrane which becomes less electron-dense
- Stage IV: thickened vacuolated membrane, sclerosis.

Clinical manifestations

Proteinuria (often nephrotic), hypertension, haematuria, deteriorating renal function.

Aetiology

Idiopathic, drugs (penicillamine, gold), neoplasia, SLE, infections (hepatitis B, malaria), diabetes.

Prognosis

The course of idiopathic membranous nephropathy is highly variable. Approximately 25% undergo complete spontaneous remission, 25% have a partial remission with stable impaired renal function 25% have persistent nephrotic syndrome with stable renal function and 25% progress to end-stage renal disease. Poor prognosis is suggested by heavy proteinuria, hypertension, elevated creatinine at presentation, and stage IV lesion. Deterioration in renal function can be halted or reversed by a regime of alternating steroids and chlorambucil (Ponticelli regime, *N Engl J Med* 1992; **327**: 599–603).

MEMBRANOPROLIFERATIVE (MESANGIOCAPILLARY) GLOMERULONEPHRITIS

Mesangial expansion (due to increased matrix and mesangial cells), and thickened capillary loops (due to extension of matrix and mesangial cells between GBM and endothelium giving the characteristic double contour).

Classification

- Type I: subendothelial immune deposits (stain for C3 and Ig — commonest type).
- Type II: linear dense deposits along GBM (linear C3, occasional Ig).

Aetiology

Secondary causes include:

- infection, whether bacterial (infective endocarditis, 'shunt nephritis', leprosy), viral (hepatitis B) or protozoal (schistosomiasis);
- neoplasia;
- SLE; and
- cryoglobulinaemia.

Nephritic factor occurs in >60% type I, and 10–20% type II mesangiocapillary glomerulonephritis. It is an IgG autoantibody which binds to and stabilizes C3 convertase (C3bBb), permanently activating the alternative pathway and depleting C3. It is associated with partial lipodystrophy.

Clinical features

Proteinuria and haematuria, with variable degree of renal failure.

Prognosis

There is no evidence to support the use of immunosuppressive therapy. Half progress to renal failure in 10 years.

MINIMAL-CHANGE NEPHROPATHY

Normal light microscopy, with negative immunofluorescence. There is podocyte foot process fusion on electron microscopy (a relative non-specific consequence of proteinuria).

Clinical features

Accounts for over 75% of childhood and 30% of adult cases of nephrotic syndrome.

Aetiology

It is associated with allergy and malignancy (Hodgkin's).

Prognosis

The majority respond to steroids. Cyclophosphamide is beneficial if relapsing.

FOCAL GLOMERULOSCLEROSIS

Segmental sclerosis affecting some glomeruli (focal). Granular IgM and C3 may be present in areas of sclerosis.

Aetiology

Idiopathic—focal glomerulosclerosis accounts for 10–20% of adult and childhood nephrotic syndrome. It is also associated with reflux nephropathy, focal proliferative glomerulonephritis, drugs (heroin, analgesic abuse), diabetes mellitus, hyperfiltration in a remnant kidney, human immunodeficiency virus (HIV) infection, sickle-cell disease, malignancy, Alport's syndrome.

Clinical features

Proteinuria, often with hypertension and renal impairment.

Prognosis

There is a poor response to treatment—cyclosporin may be of benefit.

SYSTEMIC VASCULITIS

There is necrotizing inflammation of blood-vessel walls. Any organ system can be involved.

Renal involvement is usually seen in Wegener's granulomatosis and microscopic polyangiitis. Typically there is a focal proliferative glomerulonephritis, often with necrosis and crescent formation. Granulomatous inflammation of upper and lower airway is usually present in Wegener's granulomatosis.

Vasculitis has been classified according to clinical features, size of vessel, and the presence of antibodies against neutrophil cytoplasm antigens (ANCA—most commonly directed against neutrophil proteases, including proteinase-3 and myeloperoxidase; Table 15.2).

Renal lesion

Focal proliferation with necrosis and epithelial cell crescent formation. Immunofluorescence usually negative or sparse granular Ig and C3. Presents with rapidly progressive glomerulonephritis.

CLASSIFICATION OF VASCULITIS

	ANCA+	ANCA±	ANCA–
Small vessel	Wegener's granulomatosis Microscopic polyangiitis	Henoch– Schönlein purpura	
Medium vessel	Churg Strauss	Polyarteritis nodosa	
Large vessel			Takayasu's arteritis Giant-cell arteritis

ANCA, antibodies against neutrophil cytoplasm antigens.

Table 15.2 Classification of vasculitis.

Prognosis

Remission occurs in over 90% of patients using oral cyclophosphamide (2 mg/kg per day) and prednisolone (60 mg/day). Steroids can be reduced and cyclophosphamide changed to azathioprine once remission has been induced. Relapse occurs in one-third of patients during the first year. Intravenous immunoglobulin and monoclonal anti-T-cell antibody therapy may be effective in patients with vasculitis refractory to further increases in immunosuppression.

ANTIGLOMERULAR BASEMENT MEMBRANE DISEASE
(Goodpasture's disease)

Proliferative glomerulonephritis — usually severe glomerular inflammation with crescents and necrosis. Immunofluorescence reveals linear IgG along GBM (may also occur in SLE and diabetes).

Aetiology

Anti-GBM antibodies recognize a restricted epitope on type IV collagen. They bind with high affinity to basement membrane in glomeruli, alveoli, the eye and ear.
NB   Anti-GMB antibodies do not bind to Alport's GBM in which type IV collagen is abnormal (p. 275), but may develop following transplantation of a normal kidney into a patient with Alport's syndrome.

Clinical features

Acute renal failure due to a rapidly progressive glomerulonephritis. Pulmonary haemorrhage (in smokers) causes breathlessness and haemoptysis. Chest X-ray shows pulmonary shadowing and transfer factor (T_{LCO}) is increased by the presence of haemoglobin in alveoli. The combination is known as Goodpasture's syndrome, and anti-GBM disease (Goodpasture's disease) is a common cause. The other major cause is systemic vasculitis (see above).

Prognosis

The disease usually responds to plasma exchange (to remove the autoantibody) combined with steroids and cytotoxic therapy (usually cyclophosphamide). Recovery of renal function is rare once anuria or dialysis dependence has occurred.

SYSTEMIC LUPUS ERYTHEMATOSUS

Renal involvement is common in SLE—over 90% of patients have abnormalities on renal biopsy. The World Health Organization (WHO) classification is shown in Table 15.3.

Clinical features

Almost any manifestation of renal disease, including hypertension, haematuria, proteinuria, nephrotic syndrome, acute renal failure and end-stage renal disease.

Prognosis

Varies according to WHO classification. It is good in class II, but poor in classes III and IV. The significance of membranous change (class V) is unclear. Steroids in combination with azathioprine or cyclophosphamide can slow progressive renal damage. Plasma exchange may provide additional benefits.

POST-STREPTOCOCCAL GLOMERULONEPHRITIS

Diffuse proliferative glomerulonephritis with granular deposits of C3 and IgG.

Clinical features

Oliguria, oedema, hypertension, haematuria and renal impairment follow 2–3 weeks after infection with a nephritogenic strain of group A β-haemolytic streptococci.

Investigations

Throat or skin cultures may show group A streptococci if penicillin has not been

CLASSIFICATION OF SLE	
Class	Description
I	Normal (extremely rare)
II	Mesangial changes
	IIa Deposits by immunofluorescence and electron microscopy
	IIb Hypercellularity as well
III	Proliferative glomerulonephritis (<50%)
IV	Proliferative glomerulonephritis (>50%)
V	Membranous glomerulonephritis

Table 15.3 WHO classification of systemic lupus erythematosus (SLE).

given. Antibodies against streptococcal antigens provide evidence of recent infection, e.g. antistreptolysin (ASO), antideoxyribonuclease-B (ADNase B). Hypocomplementaemia occurs with low C3 and CH_{50}.

Prognosis

Spontaneous recovery is usual. The disease is now very rare.

Fluid and electrolytes

SALT AND WATER

Plasma sodium concentration and extracellular fluid volume vary independently of each other so alterations in plasma sodium reflect alterations in either sodium or water.

Serum sodium decreased (hyponatraemia = plasma sodium <130 mmol/l)
Aetiology

Too little sodium or too much water or both.

Clinical features

In salt depletion there is thirst, dry tongue, reduced tissue turgor and postural hypotension. In severe depletion mental confusion, hypotension and shock occur. None of these features are present if water excess due to inappropriate antidiuretic hormone (ADH) or psychogenic polydypsia is the cause.

Investigation

Check serum osmolality and urine sodium.
    If:
1 Serum osmolality is decreased and urine sodium is increased:
  • excess renal sodium loss (renal failure, Addison's disease; p. 217);
  • inappropriate ADH secretion (NB some drugs such as chlorpropamide and carbamazepine can have an ADH-like action on the kidney);
2 Serum osmolality is decreased and urine sodium is decreased:
  • extrarenal loss of sodium (e.g. gastrointestinal tract, burns);
  • fluid retention associated with cardiac failure, hepatic failure or nephrotic syndrome;
  • psychogenic polydipsia;
3 Serum osmolality is normal:
  • usually spurious, e.g. in severe hyperlipidaemia when the amount of sodium in the aqueous phase of plasma is normal, but its concentration is expressed in terms of the volume of the aqueous and lipid phase.

Management

Salt depletion is corrected with NaCl, either orally (slow sodium tablets) or as intravenous normal saline (0.9%, 150 mmol/l each of Na^+ and Cl^-). Water excess in inappropriate ADH secretion and psychogenic polydysia is treated by water restriction (<600 ml/24 h).

Serum sodium increased (hypernatraemia)
Aetiology
Too much sodium or too little water.

Investigation
Check urine sodium (normal 10–20 mmol/l) and whether urine osmolality is low (<300 mosmol/l), or high (>800 mosmol/l).

If:

1 Urine osmolality decreased and urine sodium increased:
   • excess sodium load, either iatrogenic (including dialysis) or endocrine (e.g. Conn's, Cushing's);
   • previous renal loss of water and sodium (e.g. osmotic diuresis due to glucose);
2 Urine osmolality decreased and urine sodium decreased:
   • diabetes insipidus (p. 212);
3 Urine osmolality increased and urine sodium decreased:
   • previous and continuing extrarenal loss of sodium and water (e.g. from sweat, gastrointestinal tract);
4 Urine osmolality increased and urine sodium increased or normal:
   • previous and continuing extrarenal loss of water but not sodium (e.g. from lungs during febrile illness).

Management
Patients with hypernatraemia need water which can be given orally or as intravenous 5% dextrose. The underlying cause should be determined and treated.

SERUM POTASSIUM
Around 98% of potassium is intracellular (in contrast to sodium which is predominantly extracellular). Normal potassium intake = 60–200 mmol/day.

Serum potassium decreased (hypokalaemia)
Aetiology
   • Gastrointestinal losses: diarrhoea and/or vomiting (colonic tumours, particularly villous adenomata, may secrete large amounts of potassium), laxative abuse.
   • Renal loss:
      (a) diuretic therapy (thiazides, loop diuretics)
      (b) mineralocorticoid excess (renin secreted by the juxtaglomerular apparatus in the kidney converts angiotensinogen to angiotensin. Angiotensin stimulates aldosterone secretion from the adrenal cortex which causes urinary sodium retention and potassium loss). Causes include Conn's, Cushing's, corticosteroid therapy, ectopic adrenocorticotrophic hormone (ACTH;

tumours), Bartter's syndrome (renal potassium loss associated with juxta-glomerular cell hyperplasia and hyperreninaemia)

(c) osmotic diuresis (e.g. uncontrolled diabetes)

(d) renal tubular acidosis (renal tubular defect associated with potassium loss and an inability to acidify urine — causes hyperchloraemic, hypokalaemic acidosis (p. 289)).

• Shift to intracellular compartment (e.g. insulin therapy, familial periodic paralysis).

• Poor intake (including eating disorders, which may be associated with laxative or diuretic abuse).

Clinical features

Weakness and lethargy. The electrocardiogram (ECG) shows flat T and prominent U waves.

Management

Treat the underlying cause.

• Give oral potassium as potassium chloride.

• Where oral administration is not possible (e.g. diabetic ketoacidosis), potassium is given intravenously: 2 g (26 mmol) per litre of intravenous solution.

Serum potassium increased (hyperkalaemia)
Aetiology

• Potassium retention

(a) renal failure (prerenal, renal, postrenal)

(b) decreased mineralocorticoids: Addison's disease, spironolactone (aldosterone antagonist), angiotensin-converting enzyme inhibitors (e.g. captopril, enalapril)

(c) potassium-retaining diuretics (e.g. amiloride).

• Increased supply of potassium — potassium is predominantly intracellular, and released following cell destruction, e.g. haemolysis, trauma, cytotoxic therapy.

Clinical features

Severe hyperkalaemia (>6–7 mmol/l) may be associated with life-threatening ECG abnormalities.

Management

Stop oral or intravenous intake.

Ion exchange resins, e.g. calcium resonium 15 g 6-hourly orally (or rectally).

In emergency states, intravenous calcium (10 ml 10% calcium gluconate) antagonizes the cardiac effects of hyperkalaemia. Intravenous dextrose and insulin (e.g. 100 ml of 50% dextrose with 20 units of soluble insulin) moves potassium into the intracellular compartment. Dialysis may be required.

METABOLIC ACIDOSIS
Aetiology

- Exogenous acids (e.g. poisoning by salicylate, methanol, ethylene glycol).
- Accumulation of endogenous acids such as lactic acid (tissue hypoperfusion in cardiac arrest or shock) or acetoacetic acid in diabetic ketoacidosis.
- Loss of alkali (e.g. gastrointestinal loss in severe diarrhoea, biliary or enteric fistulae; or renal loss in proximal tubular acidosis).
- Failure of renal elimination of acid (renal failure and distal tubular acidosis).

Management

Treat the underlying cause.

The value of correcting acidosis in diabetic ketoacidosis or salicylate poisoning remains doubtful. In chronic renal failure acidosis is corrected by dialysing against a bicarbonate-based dialysis fluid (acetate which is converted to bicarbonate in liver and muscle can also be used).

Bicarbonate deficit can be calculated as the measured serum bicarbonate below normal standard bicarbonate $\times$30% body weight in kg. Bicarbonate can be replaced as 8.4% sodium bicarbonate solution (contains 1 mmol/ml). This should be rapid (give 50–100 ml) following sustained cardiac arrest as arrhythmias are difficult to revert in the presence of acidosis.

In *distal renal tubular acidosis (type 1)* there is a failure of hydrogen ion secretion in the distal tubule. Urine pH remains inappropriately high despite severe systemic acidosis. It may be inherited as an autosomal dominant or occur as a result of damage to the renal medulla from pyelonephritis, obstructive uropathy, medullary sponge kidney or ischaemia. In all, 70% of patients have nephrocalcinosis, and osteomalacia (or rickets in children) is common. Treatment is with oral bicarbonate, often with potassium supplements.

Proximal renal tubular acidosis (type 2) is less common. It is due to a defect of proximal tubular bicarbonate reabsorption.

METABOLIC ALKALOSIS
Aetiology

- Excess intake of alkali, e.g. milk-alkali syndrome, massive blood transfusion (citrate is metabolized to bicarbonate), overtreatment of metabolic acidosis.
- Loss of gastric acid, e.g. pyloric stenosis.
- Increased renal losses of acid with bicarbonate generation, as in hyperaldosteronism, elevated corticosteroids or severe hypokalaemia.

Management

Identify and treat the underlying cause.

HYPERCALCAEMIA
Aetiology
Hyperparathyroidism
- Primary (parathyroid adenoma or hyperplasia)
- Secondary (increased PTH secretion occurs in response to hypocalcaemia (e.g. in renal failure, malabsorption)—by definition the calcium is normal).
- Tertiary hyperparathyroidism: if secondary hyperparathyroidism gets 'out of control' an autonomous parathyroid adenoma develops, causing elevation of both PTH and serum calcium.

Malignancy
- Bone metastases (commonly breast, lung, prostate, kidney, thyroid).
- Multiple myeloma, leukaemia, Hodgkin's.
- Secretion of a PTH-like factor.

Sarcoid
Increased sensitivity to vitamin D — hypercalcaemia often precipitated by exposure to sunlight.

Drugs
- Excess vitamin D.
- Calcium-containing antacids (milk-alkali syndrome).
- Rarely thiazides.

Endocrine (rare)
Thyrotoxicosis, adrenal insufficiency.

HYPOCALCAEMIA
Aetiology
Hypoparathyroidism
- Idiopathic
- Post-thyroid or parathyroid surgery
- Pseudohypoparathyroidism (reduced sensitivity to PTH).

Inadequate dietary intake of vitamin D or calcium (rarely, vitamin D resistance)

Malabsorption

Renal disease

Acute pancreatitis

HYPOMAGNESAEMIA

Magnesium is the second most abundant intracellular cation. Normal requirement is 150 mg/day. Normal intake is 300–400 mg/day.

Aetiology

Occurs in starvation, enteral nutrition, prolonged diarrhoea, enteric fistulae and drugs (diuretics, aminoglycosides, amphotericin, carbenicillin). Usually associated with hypocalcaemia.

Reduced calcium and magnesium are often found in the seriously ill where nutrition has been inaccurately estimated.

Clinical features are paraesthesia, cramp, tetany, apathy.

HYPERPHOSPHATAEMIA

Aetiology

- Reduced loss:
  (a) renal failure
  (b) hypoparathyroidism

Increased load:
  (a) phosphate enemas or laxatives
  (b) excessive vitamin D intake.

HYPOPHOSPHATAEMIA

Aetiology

- Increased loss:
  (a) diuretic therapy
  (b) hypoparathyroidism
  (c) renal tubular defects (e.g. Fanconi's syndrome—glycosuria, aminoaciduria, phosphaturia, renal tubular acidosis).
- Decreased absorption:
  (a) malabsorption
  (b) phosphate-binding agents (e.g. antacids such as aluminium hydroxide, calcium carbonate)
  (c) vitamin D deficiency or resistance
  (d) malnutrition.
- Intracellular shift:
  (a) diabetes mellitus
  (b) 'refeeding syndrome' (after starvation or severe illness).

CHAPTER 16

Liver Disease

The commonest liver disease is acute viral hepatitis. Drug jaundice, gallstones, biliary tract obstruction and carcinomatous secondary deposits are fairly common.

Acute hepatitis

This refers to inflammation of the liver with little or no fibrosis and little or no nodular regeneration. There may be minor distortion of lobular architecture. If there is extensive fibrosis with nodular regeneration (and hence distortion of architecture) the condition is called cirrhosis. These diagnoses are made histologically and there may or may not be clinical evidence of previous hepatic disease.

Inflammation with necrosis of liver cells results from:

- *Infection*, most commonly acute infectious hepatitis A, but also with the viruses of hepatitis B, C and E, infectious mononucleosis, cytomegalovirus (CMV) and yellow fever, and associated with septicaemia and leptospirosis. Amoebic hepatitis is common on a worldwide basis, and usually presents as a hepatic abscess or amoeboma.
- *Chemical poisons* and *drugs* are less frequent causes of acute hepatitis. Toxic chemicals include carbon tetrachloride, vinyl chloride, and ethylene glycol and similar solvents (glue sniffing). Toxic drugs include alcohol (ethanol and methanol), halothane (after repeated exposures), periodic acid–Schiff, isoniazid and rifampicin, paracetamol, methotrexate, chlorpromazine and the monoamine oxidase inhibitors.
- *Pregnancy* (rare).

If the patient recovers this is usually complete but, rarely, progressive necrosis may affect almost the entire liver (fulminant hepatic failure or acute massive necrosis) causing hepatic coma (p. 299) and death.

VIRAL HEPATITIS

The clinical features of acute hepatitis A, B, C and E are similar, although they differ in severity, time course and progression to chronic liver disease.

Hepatitis A

Hepatitis A (infectious hepatitis) is a single-stranded RNA picornavirus of the enterovirus family which is excreted in the stool towards the end of the incubation period and disappears as the illness develops. Anti-hepatitis A virus immunoglobulin M (IgM) appears at the onset of the illness, and indicates recent infection. The disease is endemic but small epidemics may occur in schools or institutions. Spread is usually via the faecal–oral route by food products such as shellfish. The young (5–14 years) age group are chiefly involved.

Clinical presentation

After an incubation period of 2–6 weeks there is gradual onset of influenza-like illness with fever, malaise, anorexia, nausea, vomiting and upper abdominal discomfort associated with tender enlargement of the liver and, less commonly, the spleen. In smokers, there may be a distaste for cigarettes. After 3–4 days the urine becomes characteristically dark and the stools pale — evidence of cholestasis. Symptoms usually become less severe as jaundice appears, although pruritus may develop. Jaundice and symptoms tend to improve after 1–2 weeks and recovery is usually complete, although mild symptoms continue for 3–4 months in a few patients. Recurrent hepatitis A is extremely rare, and immunity probably lifelong.

Diagnosis

Diagnosis depends on detecting anti-hepatitis A virus IgM in serum.

Differential diagnosis

• Obstructive jaundice, either in the early cholestatic phase, or in the rare case where cholestatic jaundice persists after other clinical and biochemical evidence of liver cell damage has settled. It is dangerous to diagnose infective hepatitis in patients over 40 years old — a safeguard against misdiagnosing major bile duct obstruction.
• Drug jaundice (p. 303).
• Glandular fever.
• Yellow fever (travellers).
• Acute alcoholic hepatitis may present with enlargement and tenderness of the liver and, sometimes, obstructive jaundice. There are usually other signs of alcoholism.
• Wilson's disease must not be overlooked (pp. 147 and 303).

Management

If hospitalized, the patient should be isolated. Virus is present in stools for 1–2 weeks before the onset of jaundice, and for 1 week after. Symptomatic treatment only is required in the active disease state. No dietary restriction, other than alcohol, is necessary. Liver function tests usually return completely to normal in 1–3 months.

Recovery is the rule in virtually every case. Occasionally jaundice may be prolonged by intrahepatic cholestasis, and corticosteroids can be used to reduce the jaundice rapidly, particularly if associated with pruritus.

Fulminant hepatic failure is rare but has a mortality of about 50%. Management should be in a specialized centre where liver transplantation can be considered.

Prophylaxis

Active immunization with inactivated virus is recommended for travellers to endemic areas.

Passive immunization with pooled human immunoglobulin gives partial, short-lived immunity, but is effective immediately after the injection.

Hepatitis B

Hepatitis B is a double-stranded DNA hepadnavirus. It is spread by infected blood and serum and also occurs in saliva, semen and vaginal secretions. Transmission occurs through percutaneous exposure (contaminated needles), sexual contact and maternal–neonatal infection. It is most frequently seen in drug addicts and homosexuals. Haemodialysis patients are now regularly screened.

Clinical presentation

After a long incubation period of 6 weeks to 6 months, there is a gradual onset of lethargy, anorexia, abdominal discomfort, jaundice and hepatomegaly. It is often asymptomatic in infants. Occasionally a serum sickness-like illness occurs with polyarthritis, skin rashes and glomerulonephritis. Cholestatic hepatitis is very rare, about 1% develop fulminant hepatic failure.

Diagnosis

Hepatitis B virus has three different antigens: a surface antigen (HepB$_s$Ag), a core antigen (HepB$_c$Ag) and an internal component (HepB$_e$Ag). HepB$_s$Ag appears in the blood about 6 weeks after acute infection and has usually gone by 3 months. HepB$_e$Ag occurs at a similar time and denotes high infectivity. HepB$_c$Ag is usually found only in the liver. The development of antibodies to HepB$_s$Ag usually follows acute infection and indicates immunity. In about 5% antibodies do not appear and HepB$_s$Ag persists in the blood (carrier state).

Delta agent. The δ agent is a defective RNA virus which depends on the hepatitis B virus to replicate. It can cause recurrent hepatitis in HepB$_s$Ag-positive patients. Chronic infection is usually associated with progressive liver disease.

Management

Isolate if hospitalized. In the majority of cases spontaneous recovery occurs and treatment is supportive, as for hepatitis A. The carrier state is usually asymptomatic but is associated with chronic hepatitis and hepatocellular carcinoma. Some 30–40% of carriers respond to interferon-α (5 million units daily or 10 million units three times a week for 16 weeks) by losing HepB$_e$Ag and hepatitis B virus DNA from serum.

Immunization

Immunization using recombinant HepB$_s$Ag is advised for high-risk groups, including health workers who have contact with blood, patients with chronic renal failure, intravenous drug abusers, homosexual men and prostitutes. Three doses are given at 0, 1 and 6 months, and antibody status is checked 2–4 months thereafter. Booster is recommended every 5 years.

Hepatitis B immune globulin (HBIg) can be given with the vaccine to those accidentally infected.

Hepatitis C

Hepatitis C is a single-stranded RNA flavivirus, also known as parenterally transmitted non-A non-B virus. It predominantly affects intravenous drug abusers, and patients who have received multiple blood transfusions. Testing of blood products for hepatitis C has now virtually eradicated post-transfusion hepatitis.

Clinical features

Frequently asymptomatic — fewer than 25% of adults become jaundiced. Acute hepatitis following blood transfusion has been virtually eradicated by the introduction of testing of blood products for hepatitis C. The incubation period varies from 2 to 26 weeks.

Diagnosis

Antibody detection: first-generation enzyme-linked immunosorbent assays (ELISA) using recombinant antigen C100 were relatively non-specific. Newer assays using putative core antigens are more specific, although false-positives still occur. Mean time from infection to antibody detection is 12 weeks.

Hepatitis C virus RNA determination is essential for monitoring hepatitis C infection.

Management

Progression to chronic active hepatitis and cirrhosis is much commoner in hepatitis C than hepatitis B infection. Half of patients with chronic infection respond to interferon-α (3 million units three times a week for 6 months), with a sustained fall in transaminase levels, although 50% of these relapse on stopping treatment.

Hepatitis E

Hepatitis E virus is a newly identified RNA calicivirus, also known as enterically transmitted non-A non-B hepatitis. Transmission is faecal–oral. It is prevalent in the developing world, where it is the commonest cause of hepatitis in adults.

Clinical features

It is generally more severe than hepatitis A. The incubation period is 20–40 days. Progression to chronic liver disease does not occur.

AUTOIMMUNE HEPATITIS

Autoimmune hepatitis has recently been classified by the International Autoimmune Hepatitis Group (*Hepatology* 1993; **18**: 998–1005).

Type I autoimmune hepatitis is the commonest type, with a female:male ratio of 8:1. It is characterized by the presence of antinuclear antibody (50–70%), or antismooth muscle cell antibody (50–80%). Antimitochondrial antibodies are present in 20%. IgG concentrations and serum aminotransferases are elevated. Liver histology reveals plasma cell infiltrates, liver cell rosettes and piecemeal necrosis. An association with hepatitis C virus infection has been reported in some studies.

Type II autoimmune hepatitis typically affects girls aged 2–14 years, although 20–30% of cases occur in adults. Onset is often acute, with rapid progression to liver failure. It is characterized by the presence of anti-liver kidney microsome antibodies in the absence of antinuclear or antismooth muscle cell antibodies. It has been further classified according to the absence (IIa) or presence (IIb) of hepatitis C virus infection.

Management

Immunosuppressive therapy improves survival in the majority of cases. A total of 70% of patients respond to steroids, alone or in combination with azathioprine. In patients who fail to respond, 5-year survival rates following orthotopic liver transplantation exceed 90%.

ALCOHOLIC HEPATITIS

Moderate alcohol consumption is associated with a reduction in mortality compared with either abstinence or heavy drinking. Drinking in excess of 3 units of alcohol daily may increase mortality, but sensitivity to alcohol varies between individuals (8 g = 1 unit of ethanol is present in half a pint of beer, a glass of wine or a single measure of spirits). The clinical features of alcoholic liver disease vary from no clinical evidence at all, through nausea, episodes of right abdominal pain associated with tender hepatomegaly, fever and polymorphic leukocytosis, to cirrhosis with portal hypertension and fulminant hepatic failure. Marked jaundice is not always present.

The pathological spectrum includes fatty liver, alcoholic hepatitis, cirrhosis and hepatocellular carcinoma. Alcoholic hepatitis is characterized by liver cell damage, inflammatory cell infiltration and fibrosis. Injured hepatocytes are swollen, with pale granular cytoplasm ('ballooning degeneration'). In some cells Mallory's bodies are seen by haematoxylin and eosin stain as purple-red aggregates of material, predominantly around the nucleus. The γ-glutamyltransferase, which reflects levels of microsomal enzyme induction, and the mean corpuscular volume may be the best indices of persistent ethanol ingestion.

TRIALS

Doll et al. studied mortality prospectively in 12 321 male doctors with various drinking patterns. Moderate alcohol consumption (1 or 2 units daily) was associated with lower all-cause mortality than consumption of no or substantial amounts. Alcohol consumption reduced ischaemic heart disease, irrespective of amount. *Br Med J* 1994; **309**: 911–918.

Fuchs et al. followed 85 709 women aged 34–59 prospectively over a 12-year period. Light-to-moderate alcohol consumption (1.5–3.0 g daily) was associated with a reduced mortality rate, principally due to a decreased risk of death from cardiovascular disease. Heavier drinking was associated with an increased risk of death from other causes, particularly breast cancer and cirrhosis. *N Engl J Med* 1995; **332**: 1245–1250.

The only effective treatment is total abstinence from alcohol, if necessary with the help of a support group. Nutritional deficiencies are common. Vitamin B preparations and dietary supplementation are usually given.

ACUTE LIVER FAILURE

Fulminant hepatic failure refers to hepatic encephalopathy occurring within 8 weeks of the onset of symptoms of acute liver failure. Profound hypotension and multiple organ failure are common. Cerebral oedema and sepsis are the commonest causes of death.

Management

Management should be in a specialist unit and include:
- prophylactic antibiotics and antifungal treatment;
- inotropic support;
- early elective ventilation;
- intracranial pressure monitoring; and
- renal replacement therapy.

Prolonged administration of *N*-acetylcysteine may be of benefit in acute liver failure due to paracetamol overdose and other causes.

Chronic liver disease

Chronic hepatitis and cirrhosis are pathological diagnoses, and therefore imply liver biopsy in all suspected cases.

CHRONIC HEPATITIS

The International Association for the Study of the Liver (*Hepatology* 1994; **19**: 1513–1520) and the World Congress of Gastroenterology (*Am J Gastroenterol* 1994; **89**: S177–S181) have published guidelines for the revised classification of chronic hepatitis. It is proposed that the terms chronic persistent hepatitis, chronic lobular hepatitis and chronic active hepatitis should be replaced by a description of the aetiology (commonly hepatitis B, C or D; drug-induced; α_1-antitrypsin; Wilson's), the grade of necrosis and inflammation in portal or periportal and lobular regions, and the stage of fibrosis or cirrhosis.

Cirrhosis is a pathological diagnosis. It is characterized by widespread fibrosis with nodular regeneration. Its presence implies previous or continuing hepatic cell damage. Liver function tests are normal in inactive disease (p. 49).

Identified causes include viral hepatitis B and C, alcoholic hepatitis, haemochromatosis, hepatolenticular disease, α_1-antitrypsin deficiency, chronic severe heart failure and a few drugs (isoniazid, methyldopa).

Classification

Micronodular (portal cirrhosis) is characterized by regular thick fibrotic bands joining the portal tracts to hepatic veins, and with small regenerative nodules. The liver is initially large with a smooth edge but subsequently shrinks with progressive fibrosis. It is often alcoholic in origin.

Macronodular (post-necrotic cirrhosis) is less common and characterized by coarse irregular bands of fibrosis and loss of normal architecture and large regenerative nodules. It is believed usually to follow viral hepatitis with widespread necrosis. The liver is enlarged and very irregular due to large nodules.

Biliary cirrhosis is less common and is characterized by fibrosis around distended intrahepatic ducts. It may follow chronic cholangitis and biliary obstruction, or be idiopathic (primary).

PRIMARY BILIARY CIRRHOSIS

There is progressive damage to intrahepatic bile ducts. It chiefly (90%) affects women between 40 and 60 years of age, and presents with features of cholestasis, namely pruritus, jaundice with pale stools, dark urine and steatorrhoea, pigmentation and xanthelasma.

Osteodystrophy results from a combination of osteomalacia secondary to impaired vitamin D absorption and osteoporosis. The liver and spleen are usually palpable. Antimitochondrial antibodies are present in 95% of patients and this helps with the differential diagnosis from drug cholestasis, sclerosing cholangitis, carcinoma of the bile duct and biliary cirrhosis from chronic obstruction.

Histology shows progression from granulomatous changes around the bile ducts through bile duct proliferation to fibrosis and finally cirrhosis.

Management

The anion exchange resin cholestyramine which binds bile acids in the gut relieves pruritus.

Supplementary fat-soluble vitamins are given. The role of oestrogens in preventing osteoporosis in women with primary biliary cirrhosis is unclear. The bile acid ursodeoxycholic acid slows disease progression, leading to an improvement in both liver biochemistry and long-term survival. In patients with decompensated liver disease, liver transplantation should be considered. Five-year survival rates of over 70% post liver transplant have been reported.

Immunosuppressive agents are of little benefit. Prednisolone may promote further bone loss, and azathioprine is of doubtful value.

PRIMARY SCLEROSING CHOLANGITIS

This condition is diagnosed by endoscopic retrograde cholangiography. Inflammatory bowel disease coexists in 70% of cases. The radiological picture may be mimicked by bacterial and parasitic cholangitis, polycystic liver disease and cholangiocarcinoma, which is a recognized complication.

Management

Immunosuppression increases the risk of secondary bacterial cholangitis, although this may be required for coexistent inflammatory bowel disease. Endoscopic stenting of strictures carries the same risk. Assessment for liver transplantation is recommended if cirrhosis is present.

Other rare causes of cirrhosis include autoimmune hepatitis, haemochromatosis and Wilson's disease. Cardiac cirrhosis may occur in chronic cardiac failure. Centrilobular congestion leads to necrosis and fibrosis, but nodular regeneration is not marked.

NB   Schistosomiasis causes periportal fibrosis and is not a form of cirrhosis. Liver involvement is more common (50%) in *Schistosoma mansoni* (bowel) infections than in *S. haematobium* (bladder) due to the portal rather than the systemic drainage of the primary infected area in the former. The schistosomes cause a granulomatous fibrosis in the portal tracts and enlargement of the liver. In severe cases the liver shrinks and extensive fibrosis develops leading to portal hypertension. There is little or no hepatocellular failure since the disease is presinusoidal. Late spread may occur to the lungs (cor pulmonale) and to the spinal cord (paraplegia).

Clinical features of chronic liver disease relate mostly to the development of hepatocellular failure and complications of portal hypertension.

HEPATOCELLULAR FAILURE

Marked jaundice is uncommon. The oestrogen effects of gynaecomastia, spider naevi, liver palms and testicular atrophy may be present. In alcoholics, other features of alcoholism may be present (wasting, polyneuropathy, Korsakoff's psychosis, dementia, delirium tremens and Wernicke's encephalopathy). Pigmentation, fetor hepaticus, clubbing, white nails, cyanosis and peripheral oedema may occur.

Encephalopathy (hepatic coma or pre-coma) may be absent or may completely dominate the picture. Pre-coma is characterized by irritable confusion, drowsiness, flapping tremor, fetor and other signs of hepatocellular failure. Exaggerated reflexes and upgoing plantar responses may be present. Constructional apraxia may be demonstrated in inability to draw or copy a star. In the electro-encephalogram (EEG), δ waves (3–4 c/s) are characteristic. (They also occur in hypoglycaemia, uraemia, carbon dioxide retention and cerebral abscess.)

Hepatocellular failure may be precipitated acutely by:
- excess protein in the bowel, e.g. after gastrointestinal haemorrhage;
- acute alcoholic intoxication;
- intercurrent infection, particularly Gram-negative septicaemia;
- morphine and other alkaloids;
- minor or major surgical procedures including paracentesis; and
- electrolyte imbalance (potassium and/or sodium depletion), usually from the diuretics used to treat oedema and ascites.

Specific management

- *Identify any site of bleeding* by fibroscopy, and treat as appropriate: gastric or duodenal ulceration, see p. 314; variceal bleeding, see p. 301.
- *Maintenance of fluid and electrolyte balance.* Sodium restriction may be required despite hyponatraemia which may be dilutional. Hypokalaemia should be treated with standard potassium preparations. Diuretics (spironolactone followed if necessary by loop diuretics) may be given for ascites (p. 301). The blood glucose may be very low, and should be maintained with dextrose infusions (up to 300 g daily).
- *Infection.* Take blood cultures and send ascitic fluid for bacteriological examination, including tuberculosis. Treat infection as indicated, remembering that altered liver function may influence drug choice and dosage.
- *Lactulose* 50 ml tds produces osmotic diarrhoea, thereby removing protein and blood (if present) from the bowel, and prevents proliferation of ammonia-producing organisms.
- *Selective intestinal decontamination* by the administration of non-absorbable antibiotics (e.g. neomycin, nystatin and colistin) or norfloxacin may reduce the risk of spontaneous bacterial peritonitis.
- *Sedation* may be required. Short-acting benzodiazepines (e.g. oxazepam) are suitable.
- *Correct coagulation defects* with fresh frozen plasma or clotting factors.
- Give parenteral *B vitamins*.
- *Orthotopic liver transplantation* is becoming more widely available for all forms of liver failure. Auxiliary liver transplantation (either replacing part of the native liver with the equivalent section of donor liver or placing the donor liver adjacent to the native liver) has been used for the treatment of fulminant liver failure.

NB   A reduced level of consciousness in hepatocellular failure may be due to septicaemia, raised intracranial pressure from cerebral oedema, subdural haematoma, hypoglycaemia or epilepsy.

PORTAL HYPERTENSION

Cirrhosis accounts for 80% of the portal hypertension seen in the UK. The other post sinusoidal causes (which have poor hepatic function) are exceedingly rare and result from cardiac failure, constrictive pericarditis and hepatic vein thrombosis (Budd–Chiari syndrome; p. 302). Presinusoidal obstruction causes portal hypertension with normal hepatic function in schistosomiasis (granulomatous portal tract fibrosis), and in obstruction to the portal vein by tumours or following venous thrombosis with umbilical sepsis.

Collateral circulation may be evident in the oesophagus (varices), anus (anorectal varices rather than haemorrhoids) and at the umbilicus where a venous hum may be heard. Tests of liver cell function are usually slightly abnormal though not always so, and there may be hypersplenism.

Haematemesis is the commonest presenting symptom and may be precipitated by non-steroidal anti-inflammatory drugs, including aspirin. Bleeding is often from peptic ulceration or erosions in the alcoholic, and H_2 blockade or proton pump inhibitors are then useful.

Management of bleeding varices

The mortality is 30–50%, even in experienced hands. The initial aim is to replace blood and correct coagulation defects. Endoscopic techniques remain the mainstay of treatment. Therapeutic options are:
• Injection sclerotherapy controls bleeding in up to 95% of cases, although rebleeding is common, and sclerotherapy has no influence on the mortality rate at 6 weeks. Complications include oesophageal ulceration and stricture formation.
• Variceal banding ligation is as effective as sclerotherapy in controlling acute bleeding.
• Vasopressin reduces splanchnic blood flow and can be used prior to more definitive treatment. It causes coronary artery constriction and may precipitate myocardial ischaemia and infarction.
• Octreotide, a synthetic somatic analogue, also reduces collateral splanchnic blood flow, and when combined with sclerotherapy is more effective than sclerotherapy alone in controlling acute bleeding.
• A Sengstaken–Blakemore tube is now only used during transfer to a specialist centre, or when the above measures have failed.
• β-Blockers reduce portal pressure and are effective in preventing first bleed from varices, and as secondary prophylaxis after variceal bleeding.
• Surgical oesophageal transection or portosystemic shunting can be considered in patients with recurrent or intractable variceal bleeding.

Management of ascites

Ascites is due to a combination of factors, including portal hypertension, hypoalbuminaemia and secondary hyperaldosteronism. Management involves:
• sodium restriction;
• diuretics—aldosterone antagonists (e.g. spironolactone), alone or in combination with loop diuretics in patients with marked sodium retention;
• paracentesis is safe and effective, although expansion of plasma volume with albumin is required if large quantities of ascitic fluid are removed;

- peritoneovenous shunting or ultrafiltration and reinfusion of ascitic fluid are rarely employed in the setting of refractory ascites.

Spontaneous infection of ascites is common in cirrhotic patients. Most episodes respond to intravenous cephalosporins or oral quinolones (e.g. ciprofloxacin), but the overall prognosis is poor—30% die in hospital following an episode.

BUDD–CHIARI SYNDROME

This results from obstruction of the hepatic veins. Causes are:
- hepatic venous thrombosis, usually in association with a hypercoagulable state;
- occlusion of the hepatic veins by tumour, abscess or cyst; and
- webs of the suprahepatic segment of the inferior vena cava (IVC).

Patients present acutely with tender hepatomegaly (without hepatojugular reflux), resistant ascites and hepatic failure. Chronic onset is associated with weight loss, upper gut bleeding and spider naevi. All patients have abnormal liver function tests, but the pattern is variable and similar to other chronic liver diseases. Only half have the diagnostic liver scintiscan finding of maximum uptake in the caudate lobe (which drains directly into the IVC) with decreased uptake in the rest of the liver. Liver biopsy shows congestion around the hepatic venules. Laparotomy may produce abrupt deterioration. Treatment is surgical by side-to-side portocaval shunting or orthotopic liver transplantation. If there is a web, surgical correction may be attempted by transatrial membranectomy.

Rare cirrhoses

IDIOPATHIC HAEMOCHROMATOSIS (bronzed diabetes)

An autosomal recessive error of metabolism associated with human leukocyte antigen (HLA) A3 and HLA B14, resulting in excess iron absorption and deposition chiefly in the liver, pancreas and heart and synovial membranes, but also in endocrine glands. First-degree male relatives should be screened with serum iron and transferrin saturation. Females may present postmenopausally because continuous menstruation until then reduces the iron load.

Clinical presentation

It occurs almost entirely in men over the age of 30 years who present with:
- diabetes mellitus;
- skin pigmentation (due to melanin rather than iron);
- hepatomegaly (large, regular, firm); portal hypertension and hepatocellular failure are not common;
- progressive pyrophosphate polyarthropathy (40%) and chondrocalcinosis;
- arrhythmias (30%) and cardiac failure (15%);
- testicular atrophy, loss of body hair and loss of libido; and
- osteoarthritis of the first and second metacarpophalangeal joints.

Diagnosis

The serum iron is raised so that the serum iron-binding capacity is nearly saturated. The serum ferritin is raised. The patient is not anaemic or polycythaemic. The glucose tolerance test is usually abnormal.

Biopsy of most tissues (skin, marrow, testes) shows excess iron deposits but diagnosis is usually made on liver biopsy which shows iron staining of the liver with perilobular fibrosis.

Treatment

Deplete the body of the excess iron (up to 50 g) by weekly venesection of 500 ml (which contains 250 mg iron). This is continued until a normal serum iron is established and/or the patient becomes anaemic (in about 2 years). Maintenance venesection will be required (about 500 ml every 3 months depending on the serum iron).

Treat appropriately the diabetes, hypogonadism, heart failure and arrhythmias, hepatic cell failure and portal hypertension. High alcohol intake must be stopped. The arthropathy and testicular function do not improve but other features do.
NB   Primary hepatic carcinoma occurs in up to 20% of cases, whether treated or not. Alphafetoprotein is a suitable screen.

Overload of the tissues with iron can follow either repeated blood transfusions (about 100 units), as for instance in thalassaemia, or rarely after excessive iron ingestion. If the iron is in the reticuloendothelial cells only, the patients tend not to develop serious sequelae and the condition is called haemosiderosis.

HEPATOLENTICULAR DEGENERATION (Wilson's disease; p. 147)

An autosomal recessive disorder of copper metabolism. Symptoms appear during adolescence or early adult life.

Drug jaundice

Drugs are responsible for up to 10% of all patients admitted with jaundice.

Hypersensitivity reactions

These are the commonest cause of drug jaundice. They are dose-independent.

Cholestasis

Clinically and biochemically this is an obstructive jaundice. Histologically there are bile plugs in the canaliculi and there may be an inflammatory infiltrate of eosinophils in the portal tracts.

The classical example is chlorpromazine jaundice which occurs 3–6 weeks after starting the drug. The prognosis is excellent if the drug is discontinued (and never given again).

Other drugs producing cholestasis are other phenothiazines, carbimazole, erythromycin estolate (but not the stearate), sulphonylureas, sulphonamides, rifampicin and nitrofurantoin. Occasionally there may be a more generalized reaction with fever, rash, lymphadenopathy and eosinophilia.

Acute hepatitis syndrome

Occasionally with acute necrosis. This is much less common, but much more serious (mortality up to 20%). It occurs 2–3 weeks after starting the drug, and is caused by halothane (after multiple exposure), monoamine oxidase inhibitors, methyldopa (which more commonly gives haemolytic jaundice) and the antituberculous drugs, ethionamide and pyrazinamide (p. 348).

Direct hepatotoxicity

In some cases this is dose-dependent, though individual susceptibility is extremely variable.

The mechanisms are:

• cholestasis (without inflammatory infiltrate or necrosis). Chiefly due to C17-substituted testosterone derivatives, i.e. anabolic and androgenic steroids, including methyltestosterone and most contraceptive pills; and

• necrosis due to organic solvents, e.g. methotrexate, 6-mercaptopurine, azathioprine.

Haemolytic jaundice

This is a rare complication of therapy. It may occur with methyldopa (which more commonly gives a positive Coombs' reaction without jaundice), and the 8-amino-quinolines (e.g. primaquine) in patients with glucose-6-phosphate dehydrogenase deficiency.

CHAPTER 17

Gastroenterology

Symptoms arising in the gastrointestinal tract are extremely common, usually due to gastroenteritis or food poisoning. In clinics most are due to disturbances in motility. Over a third may have irritable bowel syndrome. Peptic ulcer, hiatus hernia, appendicitis, diverticulitis, haemorrhoids, ulcerative colitis and carcinoma of the colon are common. Carcinoma of the stomach and carcinoma of the oesophagus are less common.

GASTRIC AND DUODENAL ULCERATION

Peptic ulcer affects 1–2% of adults, and is a chronic disorder characterized by frequent recurrences.

Aetiology

The presence of *Helicobacter pylori* and the use of anti-inflammatory drugs, both steroidal and non-steroidal (including aspirin), are the commonest precipitating factors. Smoking increases the rate of ulcer recurrence, and slows ulcer healing. Rarely ulceration is associated with Zollinger–Ellison syndrome (p. 313), multiple endocrine neoplasia (MEN) syndrome (p. 219), hyperparathyroidism (p. 253) or stress (e.g. extensive burns)—Curling's ulcer.

Helicobacter pylori colonize the mucus layer overlying gastric epithelium. Infection is often asymptomatic, although a chronic superficial gastritis invariably affects the underlying mucosa. *H. pylori* infection is associated with peptic ulceration, and an increased incidence of gastric cancer. Production of urease and cytotoxins, and disruption of the gastric mucosal barrier, are thought to contribute to disease production.

There is an association between *H. pylori* infection and the development of B-cell gastric lymphomas of mucosa-associated lymphoid tissue (MALTomas). Tumour regression following eradication of *H. pylori* has been reported.

Clinical presentation

It is usually impossible, on the basis of history and examination alone, to differentiate between duodenal ulceration, benign ulceration of the stomach and carcinoma of the stomach, but carcinoma is much rarer.

Duodenal ulceration is the most common and classically presents with a history of periodic epigastric pain, often waking the patient at 1–3 a.m., relieved by food, milk or alkalis.

Gastric ulcer pain may be epigastric, or occur anywhere in the anterior upper abdomen. Anorexia, vomiting and weight loss are more frequent and severe in carcinomatous ulcers of the stomach than in benign peptic ulceration. Food occasionally precipitates pain immediately (as it may in reflux oesophagitis).

Examination

The patient characteristically puts the hand over the upper abdomen or may point to the epigastrium with a forefinger when asked where the pain is, and this is the point of maximum tenderness. The presence of an epigastric mass suggests a carcinoma. A gastric splash (or succussion) indicates pyloric obstruction due to benign duodenal stricture or to carcinoma of the pyloric antrum.

Complications

- Bleeding (p. 314).
- Perforation (usually duodenal ulceration).
- Pyloric stenosis. This presents with recurrent vomiting of food ingested up to 24 h previously with immediate relief. Visible gastric peristalsis may be seen. Conservative management with gastric aspiration and intravenous fluids may sometimes allow time for a benign active ulcer to heal and relieve the obstruction. Surgery is usually required either on the first or subsequent admission. These patients may vomit profusely and become dehydrated and alkalotic. Fluid and electrolyte replacement is obligatory and particularly so prior to surgery.

Investigation

Endoscopy with biopsy in experienced hands is important in establishing the diagnosis, and allows identification of *H. pylori* infection. Duodenal ulcers are virtually always benign.

Gastric carcinomas are commoner on the greater curve and in the antrum, but lesser curve ulcers may nevertheless be malignant. The size of the ulcer is no guide to whether a carcinoma is present. Carcinomas may have a rolled edge.

Biopsy can give histological confirmation. Repeat endoscopy after 4 weeks of treatment should show healing of a gastric ulcer. If this has not occurred the presence of a carcinoma becomes more likely.

Barium meal should be performed if endoscopy is not available, or dysphagia is present.

H. pylori is rich in the enzyme urease which hydrolyses urea to NH_4 and CO_2. This observation is utilized in the urea breath test which measures the amount of $^{14}CO_2$ released after a dose of ^{14}C-labelled urea.

Management

Antacids and diet often ameliorate symptoms, but do not hasten healing. The patient should stop smoking.

H₂-receptor antagonists reduce gastric acid output. Maintenance treatment prevents ulcer relapse. In patients with a history of bleeding duodenal ulcer, long-term treatment with H_2-antagonists appears safe and effective in preventing recurrent haemorrhage.

H+, K+-ATPase (proton pump) inhibitors cause a profound reduction in gastric acidity. Long-term treatment with omeprazole has been associated with the development of atrophic gastritis.

Misoprostol, a synthetic prostaglandin analogue, is effective in reducing gastrointestinal damage induced by non-steroidal anti-inflammatory drugs.

Treatment of *H. pylori* infection

The National Institutes of Health Consensus Development Panel on *Helicobacter pylori* in peptic ulcer disease (*JAMA* 1994; **272**: 65–69) suggested the following:

• patients with *H. pylori* infection and duodenal or gastric ulcer should be given treatment aimed at eradicating the bacteria

• the value of treatment in patients with *H. pylori* infection without peptic ulceration remains to be determined

• the relationship between *H. pylori* infection and gastric cancer requires further exploration

One of the most effective regimes for eradicating infection is triple therapy with a bismuth chelate (e.g. De-Nol), metronidazole and tetracycline. Failure may result from metronidazole resistance. Omeprazole in combination with amoxycillin eradicates infection in two-thirds of patients.

Indications for surgery

Duodenal ulcer

Acute indications include:

• perforation;

• pyloric obstruction; and

• persistent haemorrhage.

• *Failed medical management* is infrequent with the treatments available. Highly selective vagotomy reduces the incidence of side effects (diarrhoea, malabsorption and dumping), compared with truncal vagotomy with drainage (pyloroplasty or gastroenterostomy) or partial gastrectomy.

Gastric ulcer
* Acute indication: persistent haemorrhage.
* Non-acute indications:
  (a) carcinoma;
  (b) failed medical treatment, either if there is a possibility of carcinoma or for persistent symptoms.

Gastric carcinoma

Gastric carcinoma is the eighth leading cause of cancer mortality worldwide. It affects mainly the pylorus and antrum. Symptoms are those of a gastric ulcer in the early stages but pyloric obstruction or dysphagia may occur. Occasionally the patient may complain of no more than weight loss.

The prognosis is poor, with 5-year survival rates of 10%. Curative resection with removal of the primary tumour and regional lymph nodes is the most effective treatment, but only 40% of patients are potential candidates. Fluorouracil is the most commonly used chemotherapy for advanced disease.

Hiatus hernia and gastro-oesophageal reflux

Aetiology
Weakness of the diaphragmatic sphincter allows the lower oesophagus and cardia of the stomach to rise into the thorax. Gastro-oesophageal reflux may occur in the presence or absence of a hiatus hernia, and is aggravated by smoking or alcohol.

Symptoms
Retrosternal burning pain, usually episodic, with acid regurgitation into throat and flatulence which may give relief; worse on lying flat or bending. It is relieved by milk and antacids. Bleeding may give positive occult blood tests and anaemia. Peptic oesophagitis may lead to ulceration and/or stricture.

Investigations
If persistent and symptoms severe or if associated with dysphagia (to exclude benign or malignant stricture) or weight loss (to exclude oesophageal or gastric carcinoma), barium swallow will reveal the hernia and the presence of gastric acid reflux.

Management
* Weight reduction and stop smoking. Avoid clothes which constrict and

increase intra-abdominal pressure, and avoid foods which induce symptoms if recognized. Sleep propped up (raise head of the bed).
• Antacids for symptoms. Metoclopramide increases oesophageal sphincter contraction, and increases gastric emptying. It is a dopamine antagonist and may induce acute dystonic reactions which respond to procyclidine. Cisapride increases gastric motility, probably by release of acetylcholine. A course of an H_2-receptor antagonist or a proton pump inhibitor usually relieves symptoms if severe.
• Surgery for hiatus hernia is very rarely indicated in the absence of stricture formation as it is a major procedure and the results are uncertain.

In *Barrett's oesophagus* reflux is associated with columnar metaplasia of the normal stratified squamous epithelium of the lower oesophagus. It predisposes to carcinoma of the oesophagus and gastric cardia.

Inflammatory bowel disease (ulcerative colitis and Crohn's disease)

Aetiology

The aetiology of ulcerative colitis and Crohn's disease remains unknown. A genetic predisposition is suggested by the increased incidence in first-degree relatives, higher prevalence in monozygotic versus dizygotic twins and migrant studies. The incidence is highest in whites, and lowest in Asians. Antineutrophil cytoplasm antibodies (p. 182) are found in 50–70% of patients with ulcerative colitis, and 20–40% of patients with Crohn's disease. Their significance is unclear.

Clinical features

Ulcerative colitis usually presents in the 20–40-year age group, but may occur at any age. First presentation over 65 years is uncommon but carries a greater mortality. At presentation 30% have disease confined to the rectum, and 20% have extensive disease. Intermittent diarrhoea with mucus and blood in the stool, associated with fever and remissions to near normal, are the most frequent symptoms.

Three patterns may be distinguished:

1 The disease may occasionally present as a single short mild episode of diarrhoea which appears to settle rapidly but may relapse at any time.

2 Usually the history is of months or years of general ill health, with continuous or intermittent diarrhoea. In these cases the disease is usually restricted to the rectum and descending colon, and then usually termed proctocolitis. General symptoms may be mild or severe. Secondary complications are frequent.

3 Approximately one-fifth present with a severe acute episode of bloody diarrhoea with constitutional symptoms of fever and toxaemia and abdominal discomfort from toxic megacolon which may proceed to perforation.

Crohn's disease usually starts in the teens and early 20s. There is a second peak of colonic Crohn's disease in the elderly. The terminal ileum is most frequently diseased but any part of the alimentary tract may be involved. The colon is involved in 10–20% of cases. It usually presents (80–90%) as intermittent abdominal pain with diarrhoea and abdominal distension in a young thin person. Less commonly it presents as an 'acute abdomen' with signs of acute appendicitis with or without a palpable mass. A mass in the right iliac fossa from terminal ileitis must be differentiated from a caecal carcinoma and an appendix abscess. Amoebic abscess and ileocaecal tuberculosis are less common causes.

The granulomatous inflammatory process affects short lengths of the intestine, leaving normal bowel between — skip lesions. The wall is thickened and the lumen narrowed. Mucosal ulceration and regional lymphadenopathy are present. The characteristic microscopic features are of submucosal inflammation, less marked than in ulcerative colitis. There are numerous fissures down to the submucosa with or without chronic granulation tissue, consisting of non-caseating granulomata not unlike those found in sarcoid.

Diagnosis

This is suggested by the clinical picture and may be confirmed, except in the very ill, by sigmoidoscopy with biopsy and barium examination.

ULCERATIVE COLITIS
Sigmoidoscopy

The rectal mucosa is virtually always abnormal in *ulcerative colitis*; it is a distal disease with a variable extension proximally up the large bowel. Abnormal appearances, in order of severity, are:
- granular mucosa with loss of normal vascular pattern;
- presence of pus and blood; and
- visible ulceration with contact bleeding at the rim of the sigmoidoscope.

Radiology

Barium enema shows loss of normal haustral pattern with shortening of the large intestine. The bowel takes on the appearance of a smooth tube (hosepipe appearance). Undermined ulcers and pseudopolypi may be seen. Stricture formation or carcinoma produces fixed areas of narrowing.

Plain abdominal film will show acute dilatation when present, and bowel gas may outline mucosal ulceration. Barium enema examination in such circumstances may produce perforation.

The *differential diagnosis* of *ulcerative colitis* includes:
- carcinoma of the colon, which may present with bloody diarrhoea;
- infective enteritis. The acute case may resemble *Campylobacter* enteritis or bacillary dysentery, and the chronic case amoebic colitis (these should be excluded by stool examination);
- antibiotic-associated pseudomembranous colitis. On sigmoidoscopy, characteristically there are patchy yellowish areas of necrotic mucosa. Histology shows mucosal destruction with characteristic exudation of fibrin and inflammatory cells in the cross-sectional shape of a mushroom. *Clostridium difficile* and its toxin may be found in the stool, and the condition responds to oral vancomycin;

- very rarely, acute ischaemic colitis may occur and affect the rectosigmoid junction (but not the rectum); and
- irritable bowel syndrome.

CROHN'S DISEASE

Crohn's disease of the large bowel may resemble ulcerative colitis. The diagnosis of Crohn's disease is favoured by little blood loss, a normal rectal mucosa on sigmoidoscopy, the presence of perianal sepsis and the radiological differences.

Radiology

Barium enema. The terminal ileum is most commonly involved and may produce incompetence of the ileocaecal valve. Mucosal ulceration may be deep and 'spikes' of barium may enter deep into the bowel wall (rose thorn). Lesions may be multiple with normal bowel between (skip lesions). Coarse cobblestone appearance of the mucosa appears early. Later in the disease fibrosis produces narrowing of the intestine (string sign) with some proximal dilatation.

Small-bowel enema. There may be mucosal ulceration, luminal narrowing or pooling of barium in irregular clumps at the site of an inflammatory mass.

Indium-labelled white cell scanning is helpful in localizing active inflammatory bowel disease.

Histology

In *ulcerative colitis* histology shows superficial inflammation with chronic inflammatory cells infiltrating the lamina propria with crypt abscesses, with little involvement of the muscularis mucosa and with reduction of goblet cells.

In *Crohn's disease* the characteristic microscopic features are of submucosal inflammation, less marked than in ulcerative colitis. There are numerous fissures down to the submucosa with or without chronic granulation tissue consisting of non-caseating granulomata not unlike those found in sarcoid.

Complications

Fever, anaemia and weight loss. Hypoalbuminaemia results from loss of protein, and in small-bowel disease malabsorption. Clubbing is fairly common. Occasionally uveitis (5%), arthritis (5%) and skin rashes (erythema nodosum and pyoderma gangrenosum) occur. Fistulae, perianal sepsis and intestinal sepsis may complicate Crohn's disease. Renal stones occur in 5–10%.

The benefit of colonoscopy surveillance for colorectal carcinoma in ulcerative colitis remains unclear. The risk is greater if the entire colon is involved, if the history is prolonged (10% after 10 years), if the first attack was severe and if the first attack occurred at a young age. Medical treatment appears to lessen the risk of carcinoma. In Crohn's disease there is an increased risk of both colorectal and small-bowel cancer.

Management

- Attention to nutritional deficiencies (p. 260) and electrolyte imbalance is essential.
- *Aminosalicylates* are of value in inducing and maintaining remission in colitis. Their value in small-bowel Crohn's is less clear. Sulphasalazine is a combination of 5-aminosalicylic acid (5-ASA) and sulphapyridine, which acts as a carrier to deliver 5-ASA to its site of action in the colon. Mesalazine is 5-ASA by itself, and olsalazine is two linked molecules of 5-ASA which separate in the lower bowel. These newer aminosalicylates lack sulphonamide-related side effects, and may be of more benefit in treating Crohn's disease.
- *Corticosteroids* are of benefit in moderate to severe active ulcerative colitis and Crohn's disease. Side effects limit their long-term use. Enemas or suppositories are used for localized rectal disease.
- *Azathioprine* and *6-mercaptopurine* are of value as a steroid-sparing agent in both ulcerative colitis and Crohn's disease.
- *Methotrexate* has also been used for its steroid-sparing effect. Long-term benefits are unclear.
- *Cyclosporin A* has successfully healed refractory fistulas in Crohn's disease. Variable responses of active colitis to cyclosporin A have been reported.
- *Antibiotics: metronidazole* has been used in Crohn's, particularly for perianal disease. *Ciprofloxacin* may also be of value.
- *Elemental diets* may be of benefit in Crohn's disease.
- Smoking aggravates Crohn's disease, but can improve the clinical course of ulcerative colitis. *Nicotine* may be of value in maintaining remission in ulcerative colitis.

Surgery

In *ulcerative colitis*, surgery is indicated if there is:
- severe haemorrhage;
- perforation;
- acute toxaemia with dilatation of the colon which fails to respond within 24–48 h to high-dose steroids;
- prophylactic colectomy should be performed if regular colonoscopy shows high-grade dysplasia or carcinoma.

'Continent' ileostomy and ileoanal anastomosis are becoming the operations of choice.

In Crohn's disease surgery is used for relief of acute emergencies (obstruction), abscesses and fistulae. Surgery eventually becomes necessary in about 30% of cases. Resection of diseased intestine and bypass operations may become necessary for severe chronic ill health, but these are not curative. Fistula formation may result and recurrence is the rule. Intestinal obstruction is best managed conservatively in the first instance with gastric aspiration and intravenous feeding to allow time for the acute inflammation to resolve.

Endocrine tumours of the gut

All are very rare.

APUDOMAS

Amine precursor uptake and decarboxylation (APUD) cells: these are the hormone-secreting cells found chiefly along the length of the gastrointestinal tract. They have molecular and functional similarities with each other and may form various kinds of functioning tumour. They secrete a number of hormones including gastrin, cholecystokinin, secretin, glucagon and vasoactive intestinal peptide (VIP).

ZOLLINGER–ELLISON SYNDROME

This rare disorder is characterized by multiple recurrent duodenal and jejunal ulceration associated with a very high plasma gastrin level (>300 mg/l with the patient off H_2-receptor blockade), gross gastric acid hypersecretion and the presence of a gastrin-secreting adenoma (which may be malignant), usually in the pancreas but sometimes in the stomach wall.

Diarrhoea sometimes with steatorrhoea may be a feature (lipase is inactivated by the low pH). The volume of gastric secretion is enormous (7–10 l/24 h) and acid secretion persistently raised (and raised little further by pentagastrin). Normal fasting gastrin is <100 pg/ml. In Zollinger–Ellison syndrome there is a rise in serum gastrin level >200 pg/ml after infusion of secretin 2 units/kg.

The presence of an adenoma may be associated with adenomata of other endocrine glands, i.e. adrenals, parathyroids and anterior pituitary (p. 219).

Treatment is by removal of the tumour, which is usually benign. If it cannot be found, give either omeprazole or H_2-blockade long term.

OTHER ENDOCRINE TUMOURS OF THE GUT

These are very rare indeed but are sometimes discussed in examinations.

Insulinoma

A tumour of the pancreatic islet β cells which produces episodic hypoglycaemic attacks which may present as epilepsy or abnormal behaviour. Fasting produces prolonged hypoglycaemia with high insulin levels in the serum. In all, 10% are malignant and 5% are multiple.

Glucagonoma

A tumour of the α cells which produces a syndrome of mild diabetes with diarrhoea, weight loss, anaemia, glossitis and a migratory necrolytic rash.

Vipoma (WDHA syndrome)

A variant of the Zollinger–Ellison syndrome with severe watery diarrhoea, hypokalaemia with or without achlorhydria caused by a pancreatic tumour producing a VIP. Abdominal pain and flushing are typical features. Vipomectomy may be curative.

•   *Benign tumours* account for 40% of cases.
•   *Malignant tumours* account for 60% of cases. Two-thirds have metastasized at diagnosis.

Gastrointestinal haemorrhage

UPPER GUT
Aetiology

Acute
•   Duodenal ulcer: 35%
•   Gastric ulcer: 20%
•   Gastric erosions: 20%
•   Mallory–Weiss (mucosal tears) and oesophagitis: 10%
•   Oesophageal varices: 5%*
•   Others: 10%

*Up to 50% in France and parts of USA.

Half the patients are over 60 years old. Bleeding from gastric ulcers is rare under the age of 50 years, as is bleeding from duodenal ulcers in females. Melaena as a presenting symptom suggests less severe bleeding than haematemesis.

Clinical presentation
Haematemesis is a reliable indication of bleeding above the duodenojejunal flexure, and bright red rectal bleeding of the lower colon or rectum. The colour of altered blood passed per rectum is related to transit time more than to the site of bleeding.

Faintness, weakness, sweating, palpitation and nausea often precede the evidence of bleeding. The patient is pale and sweating, and has tachycardia and hypotension.

Chronic
Bleeding from hiatus hernia and gastric carcinoma is usually insidious (but not always).

Initial treatment
•   Take blood for grouping and cross-matching, liver function tests including the prothrombin time and full blood count with platelets.
•   Treat shock if present with transfusion of blood, and monitor by pulse and blood pressure recording. Conventionally give blood when the pulse is over 100 beats/min or the systolic arterial blood pressure under 100mmHg and the haemoglobin under 10g/dl if the trends are adverse. If bleeding is continuous or severe a central venous pressure monitor should be inserted as a guide to further

transfusion and rebleeding. A central venous pressure of $+5$ to $+10$ cm of saline should be maintained. Oxygen should be given.

• Sedate the patient if anxious. Diazepam probably causes less hypotension than morphine or diamorphine.

• When bleeding has stopped (steady pulse, blood pressure and central venous pressure), assess progress with repeat haemoglobin.

Variceal bleeding—see p. 301.

Investigation (for site and cause of bleeding)

Within 24 h, as soon as the patient's condition allows, upper gastro-intestinal endoscopy should be performed and this shows the site of bleeding in up to 90% of cases. Local diathermy or injection of a sclerosant may arrest bleeding. Selective angiography may show the site of active bleeding if not previously determined, particularly when angiodysplasia must be excluded. If bleeding is sufficiently fast (2 ml/min) a labelled red blood corpuscle isotope scan or selective angiography may help to locate bleeding, e.g. from a Meckel's diverticulum.

If bleeding continues or recurs, surgery may be necessary (see below). If bleeding has stopped the patient should be given oral iron and a normal diet. H_2 blockade is usually given and may reduce blood loss. Patients should be advised not to smoke.

Indications for surgery (in haemorrhage from peptic ulcer)

Although there are no absolute indications, surgery is indicated if bleeding does not stop spontaneously or the patient rebleeds in hospital (the central venous pressure may be the first indication of this, but slower continuous bleeds are indicated by a persistently low haemoglobin). The overall mortality is worse in older patients (10% in the over-60s) than in the young (2% in the under-60s). Bleeds from gastric ulcers (mortality up to 20% in the over-60s) carry twice the mortality of bleeds from duodenal ulcers. Also the operative risk for gastric ulcer surgery is less than for duodenal ulcers.

Hence the tendency is to operate early in older patients, particularly if bleeding from a gastric ulcer. Supplies of compatible blood may be a controlling factor.

LOWER GUT

Acute loss may occur from haemorrhoids, fissures, ulcerative colitis and Crohn's disease, ischaemic colitis, colonic and caecal carcinoma and diverticular disease. Chronic and occult bleeding usually presents with lethargy and iron-deficiency anaemia and is confirmed by positive faecal occult blood tests. Any of the causes of upper or lower gut bleeding given above may be responsible. Other very rare causes include polyps, and vascular abnormalities, such as arteriovenous malformations, angiodysplasia of the ascending colon, Peutz–Jeghers syndrome (small intestinal polyposis and blotchy pigmentation around the mouth) and Rendu–Osler–Weber (hereditary (autosomal dominant) haemorrhagic telangiectasia in which thin-walled dilated blood vessels rupture causing GI bleeding, epistaxis, haemoptysis or haematuria) syndromes. Meckel's diverticulum, polyps and endometriosis may also present with bleeding.

Steatorrhoea and malabsorption

Malabsorption signifies impaired ability to absorb one or more of the normally absorbed dietary constituents, including protein, carbohydrates, fats, minerals and vitamins.

Steatorrhoea signifies malabsorption of fat, and is defined as a faecal fat excretion of more than 18 mmol/day (6 g/day) on a normal fat intake (50–100 g). Apart from the occasions when the cause of steatorrhoea is obvious (such as obstructive jaundice), the diagnostic problem revolves around the differentiation between enteropathy (commonly gluten-induced) and other causes of steatorrhoea.

Diarrhoea is not necessarily a presenting symptom and malabsorption may present with one or more of its complications (e.g. anaemia, weight loss, osteomalacia).

GLUTEN-SENSITIVE ENTEROPATHY (coeliac disease)
Aetiology

There is mucosal sensitivity to wheat gluten (in particular α-gliadin, a polypeptide in gluten) and to barley and rye, and occasionally oats (though not rice or maize). IgA α-gliadin antibodies are present in 80–90% of patients with coeliac disease. It is associated with human leukocyte antigen (HLA) B8, A1, DR3, DR7, DQW2 and antibodies to reticulin may be present. There is an increased incidence in near relatives and there is a high incidence of gut lymphoma and carcinoma.
NB   Virtually all patients with dermatitis herpetiformis have gluten-sensitive enteropathy.

Clinical presentation

There is usually a history of intermittent or chronic increased bowel frequency, classically with pale, bulky, offensive frothy greasy stools which flush only with difficulty. There may be a history of intermittent abdominal colic, flatus and abdominal distension. Depending on the severity and duration of the disease, there may be weakness and weight loss. If the malabsorption started in childhood, the patient may be short compared with unaffected siblings or parents. Children may present with irritability, failure to gain weight or failure to thrive.

The malabsorption involves not only fat and the fat-soluble vitamins but also minerals and water-soluble vitamins (Table 17.1).

Examination

In addition to the features mentioned above there may be:
- evidence of weight loss;
- pigmented, scaly and bruised skin; and

VITAMIN AND MINERAL DEFICIENCIES

Vitamin B_{12}	To produce megaloblastic anaemia (p. 420)
Iron (rare)	To produce iron-deficiency anaemia (p. 419)
Vitamin D and calcium	Resulting in osteomalacia with bone tenderness and muscle weakness. Tetany may occur. Children may develop rickets
Vitamin B group	Glossitis and angular stomatitis
Vitamin K	Deficient prothrombin formation to produce bruising and epistaxis
Associated impairment of amino-acid absorption	May produce hypoproteinaemia and oedema
Potassium	May produce weakness

Table 17.1 Vitamin and mineral deficiency following malabsorption.

- distended abdomen with increased bowel sounds.

NB The anaemia has many causes including anorexia, blood loss, mucosal damage, folate deficiency, and bacterial overgrowth.

Clubbing may occur. Signs of subacute combined degeneration of the cord are very rare.

OTHER CAUSES OF MALABSORPTION

Bile salt deficiency

Patients present with obstructive jaundice usually secondary to carcinoma of the head of the pancreas or to gall stones (which may sometimes be seen on plain abdominal X-ray) or, rarely, in primary biliary cirrhosis or bile duct stricture.

Pancreatic enzyme deficiency

Usually due to chronic pancreatitis or carcinoma affecting the pancreatic ducts (also rarely, fibrocystic disease, pancreatic calculi and benign pancreatic cystadenoma). The differentiation of these two diseases may be very difficult at presentation. Tests for malabsorption, glucose tolerance, serum bilirubin and barium meal are of little help. Tests of pancreatic secretion (secretin–pancreozymin–cholecystokinin stimulation) are said to give low volumes in carcinoma and low enzyme levels in chronic pancreatitis. Indirect tests of exocrine pancreatic function include the N-benzoyl-L-tyrosyl-p-aminobenzoic acid (BT-PABA) test (measure urinary excretion of para-amino benzoic acid specifically split from BTP-PABA by pancreatic chymotrypsin) and the pancreolauryl test (measure urinary excretion of fluorescein specifically split from fluorescein dilaurate by pancreatic esterase in the presence of bile salts). Calcification of the pancreas on straight abdominal X-ray favours chronic pancreatitis. Similarly, duodenal fibroscopy with endoscopic retrograde cholangiopancreatography (ERCP) may help to distinguish between carcinoma of the pancreas and chronic pancreatitis. Carcinoembryonic antigen (CEA) studies are useful only for assessing completeness of resection of a CEA-producing tumour. Symptoms of pancreatic malabsorption are improved by a low-fat diet (40 g/day), replacing minerals and vitamins, and giving pancreatic supplements (e.g. Nutrizym, Creon, Pancrex V Forte), preferably with H_2 blockade. Avoid alcohol.

Other intestinal disease

- *Post surgical.* Incomplete food mixing may follow gastrectomy or gastroen-terostomy and there may be a diminished area for absorption following small bowel resection.
- *Abnormal intestinal organisms.*

Bacterial overgrowth can be distinguished from ileal disease using the early (40 min) peak in breath hydrogen after lactulose (10 g) or glucose (50 g).

The normal bacterial count in jejunal juice is $<10^3-10^5$ organisms/ml. The organisms (*Escherichia coli* and *Bacteroides*) break down dietary tryptophan to produce indoxylsulphate (indican) which is excreted in the urine. Overgrowth can be detected by urinary indican excretion of more than 80 mg/24 h.

An aetiological role of the cultured organisms in malabsorption is difficult to prove but the steatorrhoea may respond to antibiotic therapy (e.g. tetracycline or erythromycin). There may be a close association between bacterial overgrowth and stasis from blind loops, diverticula and strictures. It may occur after gastrectomy due to reduced acid and pepsin, and in diabetic autonomic nephropathy.

In the radioactive bile acid breath test ^{14}C glycine-labelled bile salt is given orally, and anaerobic bacteria in the intestine deconjugate the bile acid. The released ^{14}C amino acid is transported to the liver and metabolized to $^{14}CO_2$ which can be detected in the breath.

- *Crohn's disease* (p. 311).

Rare causes

The following are very uncommon but well-recognized:
- *Zollinger–Ellison syndrome* (p. 313).
- *Disaccharidase deficiency.* Malabsorption of lactose, maltose and sucrose may occur in isolation due to primary enzyme deficiency, or as part of a general malabsorption picture in any disease which damages the intestinal brush border. The most important is isolated lactase deficiency which presents, usually in children, with milk intolerance and malabsorption. Patients have abdominal pain, diarrhoea, distension and borborygmi (i.e. symptoms of bacterial fermentation of unabsorbed sugars) after 50 g lactose by mouth and the blood glucose rises by <1.1 mmol/l over the following 2 h. The diagnosis is confirmed by the absence of lactase activity in the jejunal mucosa on biopsy. Management consists of withdrawal of milk and milk products from the diet.
- *Other intrinsic disease* of the intestinal wall due to tuberculosis, Hodgkin's disease, lymphosarcoma, diffuse systemic sclerosis, amyloidosis and Whipple's disease (intestinal lipodystrophy), associated with the organism *Trophenyma whippoli*.

• *Tropical sprue* is a disorder which produces steatorrhoea and occurs almost exclusively in Europeans in or from the tropics, especially in India and the Far East. The aetiology is unknown. The most common associated deficiency is folic acid. The disease frequently remits spontaneously on return from the tropics. In some cases which do not remit, a course of parenteral folic acid, metronidazole or oral tetracycline may be curative.

Very rarely, malabsorption is associated with diabetes, cardiac failure and giardiasis.

Investigation of malabsorption

In a patient with a characteristic history, the investigation with the greatest likelihood of achieving a diagnosis is jejunal biopsy.

However, tests of absorption may quantitate the degree of malabsorption and help with the differential diagnosis between pancreatic and intestinal steatorrhoea.

Using the hydrogen breath test, after an oral dose of lactose (2 g/kg up to 50 g, in 250 ml water), normal subjects show no rise in breath hydrogen over the following 3 h because they absorb the disaccharide completely. If, because it is not absorbed higher up the gut, the disaccharide reaches the colon, the anaerobic bacteria there ferment it so that hydrogen can be detected in the breath at about 90 min. The hydrogen breath test can also be used to assess small-bowel transit time using lactulose.

NB   Intestinal malabsorption tends to give a total malabsorption. Pancreatic malabsorption (p. 317) is much less common and tends to affect the absorption only of fat and proteins and to leave the absorption of sugars, minerals and water-soluble vitamins relatively unaffected.

Blood tests

• Anaemia is common and may be iron-deficient, megaloblastic or both (dimorphic).
• Serum and red cell folate, iron and transferrin may be low.
• Serum albumin may be reduced and the prothrombin time prolonged.
• Serum calcium, phosphate and magnesium may be low and the serum alkaline phosphatase increased (osteomalacia pattern).

Tests of absorption

Faecal fat excretion. The diagnosis of steatorrhoea is made by measuring faecal fat excretion over 3–5 days on a normal diet (50–100 g of fat in 24 h). The upper limit of normal is 6 g/24 h (18 mmol/24 h).

Butter fat absorption test. This is a screening test that has replaced faecal fat collection. Change in plasma turbidity is measured following a standard fatty meal.

D-*xylose excretion.* More than 20% (5 g) of an oral load of 25 g is normally excreted in the urine in the 5 h after ingestion. Less than 4 g is excreted in intestinal malabsorption and also if there is renal dysfunction (and if the urine collection is incomplete). The 2-h blood xylose level is normally 2.1–3.8 mmol/l. The test is normal in pancreatic steatorrhoea but points to upper small-bowel disease if abnormal.
NB   Xylose was originally used because it was thought not to be metabolized (it is a little). It is absorbed mainly in the jejunum.

Glucose tolerance test. In intestinal malabsorption, the curve is usually flat. In chronic pancreatitis and pancreatic carcinoma the curve may be diabetic. In postgastrectomy dumping, there may be a lag curve.

Other disaccharide (sucrose or lactose) absorption tests. The blood glucose should normally rise more than 20 mg/dl after a 50 g oral dose. Those with disaccharidase deficiency have a smaller rise and tend to develop abdominal colic and diarrhoea during the test.

Schilling test. Megaloblastic anaemia may be caused by vitamin B_{12} deficiency in malabsorption syndromes if the terminal ileum is involved (e.g. Crohn's disease). In this case the absorption of radiocobalt-labelled B_{12} is not improved by the addition of intrinsic factor (unlike pernicious anaemia).

Radiology
A small intestinal barium meal with a flocculable contrast medium may show flocculation and segmentation of barium — evidence of excess mucus secretion. Of more significance are widening of the small intestinal calibre and increased distance between adjacent loops of bowel, indicating thickening of the intestinal wall. All these changes are non-specific and the main purpose of the barium meal is to detect diverticula, fistulae or Crohn's disease.

The bones may show evidence of osteomalacia and/or osteoporosis, and even of hyperparathyroidism (secondary or tertiary) if very severe and prolonged.

Jejunal biopsy
In gluten-induced enteropathy, dissecting microscopic examination usually reveals flattening of the mucosa, with partial or total villous atrophy.

Management of gluten-induced enteropathy
Gluten-free diet. In adults the response may take several months. Repeat biopsy is performed and the diagnosis is confirmed by a return to normal appearances.
NB   There may be a predisposition to malignancy — lymphomas and gut carcinoma (particularly oesophagus) — in gluten-induced enteropathy and there is some evidence that gluten-free diets may reduce the incidence of these. Hence the diet is continued for life.
Replace vitamins and minerals as indicated, and, if necessary, parenterally.

Diverticular disease

Diverticula occur anywhere in the alimentary tract but chiefly in the colon — diverticulosis. They are due to a weakening of the colonic wall and increased intra-colonic pressure. They affect chiefly the descending and sigmoid colon. It is a disorder of mid and late age (5% of the population over 50 years in the UK), more common in women than men and is usually discovered incidentally during barium enema performed to exclude colonic carcinoma.

Clinical features

Inflamed diverticula produce diverticulitis with:
- pain, discomfort and tenderness in the left iliac fossa (there may be a mass from pericolic abscess)—'appendicitis of the left side';
- change in bowel habit with constipation and/or diarrhoea sometimes alternating (NB exclude carcinoma);
- rectal bleeding, which may be acute and sometimes massive and the first symptom;
- subacute obstruction;
- frequency of micturition and cystitis, due to vesicocolic fistula; and
- perforation with peritonitis or fistulae.

Management

Acute diverticulitis may be extremely painful and require rest in bed, analgesia, local warmth and antibiotics (ampicillin or metronidazole or co-trimoxazole). Occasionally surgery is required, particularly colostomy and resection for obstruction.

Dietary fibre

Diverticulosis is rare in communities which take a fibre-rich diet, where there is also far less carcinoma of the colon and appendicitis. A diet high in dietary fibre results in bulkier stools and rapid intestinal transit times. The soft stool prevents straining which may help to prevent diverticulosis. In the established disease added dietary fibre (2 teaspoonsful to 2 tablespoonsful daily) reduces symptoms in most patients. Fibre-rich diets also decrease serum cholesterol and increase faecal excretion of bile salts and their relative absence from western diets has been suggested as a possible contributory factor in coronary artery atheroma and gallstones.

Irritable bowel syndrome

Clinical presentation

One of the commonest bowel disorders, affecting about 20% of adults in the industrialized world, more often female than male. It presents with colicky abdominal pain eased by bowel movement, often frequent and loose at the onset of pain, altered bowel habit, bloating and a sense of incomplete evacuation. Examination is normal though there may be tenderness in the left iliac fossa. There may be symptoms unrelated to the gastrointestinal tract, including lethargy, urinary symptoms and dyspareunia. About 50% of patients have symptoms of anxiety and/or depression.

The cause of the disturbed gastrointestinal function is unknown, but increased sensitivity to distension of the bowel and abnormalities of motility are found in some patients.

Investigation

Diagnosis is usually made on history and examination, but exclusion of more serious disease is necessary, particularly in patients over 45.

If the history is typical, the examination and sigmoidoscopy normal, and blood count, erythrocyte sedimentation rate, C-reactive protein and serum proteins normal and at least three faecal occult blood examinations negative, serious alternative diagnoses are effectively excluded. If there are changes in bowel habit, barium enema can exclude carcinoma and demonstrate diverticula.

Treatment

There is no uniformly successful treatment. Antispasmodics may be tried, e.g. hyoscine (Buscopan) 10–20 mg tds before meals. If a cause of anxiety can be identified and treated, symptoms may be markedly reduced. Occasionally specific foods may produce symptoms of irritable colon and these should be excluded from the diet. Bran makes symptoms worse in 50% of patients, but fibre is indicated when there is associated constipation.

Ischaemic colitis

Clinical features

This is a disorder of middle and old age which often presents as an acute abdomen with the sudden onset of pain followed by bloody diarrhoea, sometimes copious.

Diagnosis

If subacute, it must be distinguished from the bleeding of diverticular disease and of ulcerative colitis. Any part of the colon can be affected though, because it has the most precarious blood supply, the splenic flexure is usually involved. If the colon looks normal on sigmoidoscopy, ulcerative colitis is virtually excluded, though large-bowel Crohn's disease or diverticular disease is not. Barium enema shows mucosal oedema with characteristic 'thumb-printing', as if a thumb had been pressed along the outside of the affected colon.

Prognosis

In mild cases there may be complete recovery but colonic strictures can develop later. In colonic gangrene, surgical resection is necessary. The differential diagnosis includes *Campylobacter* enteritis, and diverticular disease, in which bleeding can be torrential. Pseudomembranous colitis does not usually cause bloody diarrhoea.

Pancreas

CARCINOMA

A total of 75% of tumours occur in the head. It is commoner in men and in cigarette smokers.

Clinical presentation

Patients present with one or more of the following features.
- Anorexia and weight loss.
- Indigestion or epigastric pain often indistinguishable from duodenal or gastric ulceration. Back pain suggests pancreatic disease (and posterior ulcers).
- Obstructive jaundice. Intermittent jaundice suggests a gallstone in the bile duct (rarely, carcinoma of the ampulla of Vater).
- About 20% of patients have diabetes, usually of short duration, and some present with it. In the elderly, sudden onset or worsening of diabetes may indicate malignancy.

Investigation

Ultrasound or computed tomographic (CT) scan may show the tumour.

ERCP may confirm the diagnosis and allows palliative stenting of the obstructed common bile duct to relieve pruritus and jaundice.

Management

Ampullary carcinoma presents early with obstructive jaundice and can be resected.

Carcinoma of the head and body of the pancreas is usually fatal within 1 year.

Islet cell tumours

See Zollinger–Ellison syndrome and insulinoma (p. 228).

ACUTE PANCREATITIS

Aetiology

About 90% are associated with gall bladder disease (especially gallstones) and alcoholism. It is uncommon after cholecystectomy.

Clinical presentation

There may be a previous history of cholecystitis as biliary colic associated with gallstones. Pancreatitis occurs occasionally in association with mumps, drugs (e.g. thiazides) or severe hypertriglyceridaemia.

Abdominal pain, often very severe, occurs suddenly, usually in the epigastrium or across the upper abdomen with radiation to the back or shoulder. It spreads to involve the entire abdomen, which is tender with guarding and rebound tenderness. Hypotension with sweating and cyanosis occurs in severe attacks. There may be bruising around the umbilicus or in the flanks.

Differential diagnosis

It presents initially as an 'acute abdomen' and resembles:

- cholecystitis;
- acute myocardial infarction, dissecting aortic aneurysm, mesenteric vascular occlusion; and
- intestinal perforation, particularly duodenal ulcer (though shock is not often a feature of a perforated duodenal ulcer).

Investigation

The serum amylase is very high (over 1000 units/ml) within 24 h of onset. The level falls rapidly. Posterior duodenal ulcers can also cause very high amylase levels but not usually above 1000 units. Peritoneal fluid also has high amylase levels.

Straight abdominal X-ray may show gallstones, pancreatic calcification (indicating previous inflammation) and a distended loop of jejunum or transverse colon if they are close to the inflamed pancreas. Check serum calcium (which may fall due to the formation of calcium soaps). There is usually a leukocytosis.

Management

- If the diagnosis is definite, conservative management is preferred by most clinicians.
- Relieve pain with pentazocine or pethidine.
- Gastric aspiration and intravenous rehydration.
- Maintain the circulating volume.
- Monitor the blood glucose.
- If shock is present, give plasma expanders (e.g. dextran, plasma) whilst monitoring the central venous pressure, and give oxygen.

Other measures are of less certain value:

- Propantheline 15–30 mg 6-hourly to block the vagus and relax the sphincter of Oddi.
- H_2 blockade.
- Antibiotics to prevent infection.
- Calcium if the serum level falls.
- In very severe cases, peritoneal lavage and parenteral nutrition may be tried.

Prognosis

Complete recovery occurs in over 95% of patients and recurrence is uncommon. Pancreatic abscess or pseudocyst may complicate acute pancreatitis. Patients should be investigated to exclude gallstones (<5%). Alcohol should be avoided if it is a possible cause.

CHRONIC PANCREATITIS
Clinical presentation
- Recurrent though mild attacks resembling acute pancreatitis.
- Malabsorption and steatorrhoea from pancreatic insufficiency (p. 317).
- Diabetes mellitus when the islet cells are involved.
- Obstructive jaundice, which may be intermittent.
- In association with cystic fibrosis and haemochromatosis.

Investigation
Straight abdominal X-ray for pancreatic calcification and gallstones. There is a reduction in bicarbonate output in the duodenal juice in a response to secretin pancreozymin (secretin cholecystokinin) stimulation in most cases. CT scan may show dilated ducts. ERCP shows duct anatomy (ectasia or stricture) and calculi. The serum amylase is valueless in chronic pancreatitis, though it is sometimes slightly raised, and isotope scanning of the pancreas is of little value. Investigate for malabsorption (p. 316), pancreatic exocrine function (p. 317), diabetes mellitus (p. 221) and obstructive jaundice (p. 49) if relevant.

Treatment
- There is no specific therapy for chronic pancreatitis.
- Treat pancreatic malabsorption with low-fat diet (45 g/day), fat-soluble vita-mins, calcium and pancreatic enzymes (e.g. Pancrex V, Creon) plus H_2 blockade.
- Treat diabetes mellitus (p. 221).
- Remove gallstones if present.
- Treat recurrent attacks and consider sphincterotomy or pancreatectomy.
- Alcohol is forbidden.
- Chronic severe pain is common and may lead to opiate addiction.

Gall bladder

ACUTE CHOLECYSTITIS
Clinical features
The story is of fever, occasionally with rigors, abdominal pain, usually right sub-costal with acute pain on palpation over the gall bladder region. The disease is more common in obese females over 50, but may occur in young adults. Gall-stones are present in over 90% of cases. Occasionally, acute cholecystitis may be difficult to distinguish from a high appendix and right basal pneumonia and even perforated peptic ulcer, pancreatitis and myocardial infarction.

Management
The acute inflammation usually settles with bed rest, analgesia (pethidine) and antibiotics. Penicillin and co-trimoxazole are both secreted in the bile but a third of biliary coliforms are now ampicillin-resistant. Cefotaxime is probably the antibi-otic of choice. The gall bladder is removed 2–3 months later, after the inflamma-

tion has settled, although some surgeons elect to operate within 48 h because this is technically easier.

Rarely, an empyema develops or the gall bladder perforates.

CHRONIC CHOLECYSTITIS
Clinical presentation

Recurrent episodes of cholecystitis are usually associated with gallstones. The attacks are often less severe than classical acute cholecystitis, and may resemble peptic ulceration and peptic oesophagitis. Myocardial ischaemia may be confused if the site of the pain is high.

GALLSTONES

Twice as common in women as men. There is an increased incidence in women taking oral contraceptives. The incidence rises with age. Stones occur in 10% of women over 40, classically in the fair, fat, fertile, female of 40–50 on a low-fibre diet. They are usually cholesterol or mixed. Rarely they are pigment stones associated with haemolytic anaemia.

Clinical features

Most stones produce no symptoms, but they may cause:
- flatulence upwards;
- biliary colic;
- acute cholecystitis;
- chronic cholecystitis; and
- obstructive jaundice, which may be intermittent, giving attacks of fever, jaundice and upper abdominal pain—Charcot's triad. Gall bladder empyema from bile duct obstruction is uncommon

Gallstones are associated with acute and chronic pancreatitis and their presence indicates a higher risk of gall bladder carcinoma, although this is still extremely rare.

Investigation

Straight abdominal X-ray and ultrasonography with acoustic shadow will reveal many stones. Cholecystogram will confirm and reveal the rest but contrast medium will not concentrate in the gall bladder if the bilirubin is above 35 μmol/l and intravenous cholangiography then becomes necessary, though it only shows stones in the biliary tree.

Although surgeons may explore the bile duct at surgery, stones are sometimes missed and may later produce symptoms. Operative cholangiography and/or fibreoptic examination of the bile duct make this less likely.

Management

If causing symptoms, the gall bladder and stones should be removed. It is at this stage that pigment stones are detected and indicate investigation for haemolysis.

In elderly patients or if surgery is contraindicated, sphincterotomy via ERCP may release the stones if they are in the common bile duct. Ursodeoxycholic acid may dissolve radiolucent stones if the stones are under 2 cm in diameter, and if the gall bladder is functioning. The stones may recur after treatment. Rowachol (a monoterpene mixture including menthol) is an adjuvant to bile acid therapy.

Respiratory Disease

The commonest respiratory diseases are infections of the upper respiratory tract, e.g. the common cold. The commonest diseases of the lower respiratory tract are bronchitis (acute and chronic), asthma and carcinoma of the bronchus.

Chronic bronchitis and emphysema

Definitions

Daily cough with sputum for at least 3 months a year for at least 2 consecutive years. This defines the hypersecretory form of chronic bronchitis. Airflow obstruction in small airways >2 mm in diameter is more dangerous and is not necessarily associated with hypersecretion. It is a clinical definition and radiological, pathological and biochemical features are judged by this standard. The definition is chiefly of use epidemiologically: patients whose respiratory disease does not satisfy this definition may nevertheless have bronchitis. It causes about 30 000 deaths per annum in the UK.

Emphysema is a histological diagnosis and is therefore usually made with precision only at postmortem. It is defined as enlargement of the air spaces distal to the terminal (smallest) bronchioles with destructive changes in the alveolar wall. In centrilobular emphysema, damage is limited to the central part of the lobule around the respiratory bronchiole, whereas in panacinar emphysema, there is destruction and distension of the whole lobule. If the air spaces are >1 cm in diameter, they are called bullae.

Aetiological factors

- *Tobacco smoking.* The increased mortality risk from bronchitis has an approximately straight-line relationship with numbers of cigarettes smoked per day (increased risk = $1/2 \times$ cigarettes smoked per day)
- *Atmospheric pollution*
- There is a relationship to lower social class, industrial environment and to being British, although mortality from chronic bronchitis has fallen progressively in the last 10 years. This is probably due to the considerable drop in cigarette tar and nicotine content. Other factors include control of air pollution and an improment in living standards and working conditions
- α_1-*Antitrypsin deficiency* is a recessive disorder which accounts for about 5% of all patients with emphysema (and about 20% of neonatal cholestasis). Five per cent of homozygotes tend to develop emphysema by the age of 40 years and heterozygotes are at risk. The emphysema is predominantly of the lower zones and is much worse in smokers.

Clinical presentation

Initially, the patient has a productive morning cough and an increased frequency of lower respiratory tract infections producing purulent sputum. The organisms responsible are usually *Haemophilus influenzae*, *Streptococcus pneumoniae* and the respiratory viruses. Over the years there is slowly progressive dyspnoea with wheezing, exacerbated in the acute infective episodes. There is clinical emphysema with hyperinflation of the lungs. Respiratory failure (p. 336) or chronic right heart failure (cor pulmonale) are long-term complications.

Investigation

Chest X-ray. This may be normal. Abnormalities correlate with the presence of emphysema and are due to:
- overinflation with a low, flat, poorly moving diaphragm and a large retrosternal window on lateral X-ray;
- vascular changes with loss of peripheral vascular markings but enlarged hilar vessels—the heart is narrow until cor pulmonale develops; and
- bullae if present.

The chest X-ray is an important investigation because it excludes other disease (carcinoma, tuberculosis, pneumonia, pneumothorax).

Ventilatory function tests. Spirometry shows a greater reduction in forced expiratory volume in 1 s (FEV_1) than in vital capacity (VC—and their ratio, the FEV%, is thus also reduced).

The peak expiratory flow rate (PEFR) is reduced. This airways obstruction is usually only partially reversible.

Arterial blood gas estimations. These may be normal. In later stages the Po_2 falls and the Pco_2 rises, particularly with exacerbations.

Electrocardiogram (ECG). This records the presence and progression of cor pulmonale (right atrial and ventricular hypertrophy).

Sputum for bacterial culture and sensitivity. This is useful in acute infective episodes when infections other than *Haemophilus influenzae* or *Streptococcus pneumoniae* may be present.

Haemoglobin estimation may show secondary polycythaemia.

Management

- Stop smoking and control excess weight.
- Treat acute bacterial exacerbations with antibiotics — oral amoxycillin or a macrolide (erythromycin or clarithromycin).
- Bacterial sensitivities are useful if clinical improvement has not occurred.
- *Bronchodilators:* the β_2-agonists, e.g. salbutamol (Ventolin), terbutaline (Bricanyl) or the anticholinergic ipratropium (Atrovent) are suitable and are given by metered aerosol or nebulizer.
- Oral theophylline preparations may help.
- Treat right heart failure with diuretics.
- Secondary polycythaemia is sometimes managed by venesection at 3–6-month intervals if the haematocrit is over 0.52 down to 0.48. Supplementary iron should be given.
- Physiotherapy—with emphasis on coughing and relaxation.
- Home oxygen (controlled concentrations and no smoking) is useful for hypoxic cor pulmonale and may reduce pulmonary hypertention. The UK Department of Health suggest the following criteria: $Pao_2 < 7.3\,kPa$; $Paco_2 > 6\,kPa$; $FEV_1 < 1.5$ litres and FVC < 2 litres.
- Mucolytic agents are probably useless.

NB   Steroids are not usually indicated either orally or by aerosol. In severe cases steroids may be given a short trial while ventilatory function is monitored. At least 25% improvement in FEV_1 or PEFR should be achieved. If not, steroids are not given long term.

Bronchiectasis

Bronchiectasis means dilation of the airways. It only becomes of clinical significance when infection and/or haemoptysis occurs within these dilated airways. Severe forms are now rare, especially in the young.

Aetiology

- Following acute childhood respiratory infection, particularly measles and whooping cough and pneumonia.
- Cystic fibrosis.
- Bronchial obstruction predisposes to bronchiectasis (e.g. peanuts).

- Tuberculosis has become less common as a cause.
- Congenital (rare): the immotile cilia syndrome, e.g. Kartagener's syndrome.

Clinical features

- Chronic cough, often postural.
- Sputum, often copious, especially with acute infections. Halitosis.
- Febrile episodes.
- Haemoptysis: may be the only symptom ('dry bronchiectasis') and is occasionally severe.
- Dyspnoea, coarse basal crepitations and wheeze.
- Cyanosis and clubbing.
- Loss of weight and cor pulmonale in advanced cases.

Management

Stop smoking.

The object is to get rid of chronic sepsis. Twice-daily postural drainage will help empty dilated airways and decrease the frequency of further infections. Bronchodilators will often help improve clearance of sputum. Antibiotics, as for chronic bronchitis, are given for acute infections and exacerbations. Treatment is unnecessary in the absence of symptoms.

Surgery is virtually never indicated unless there is uncontrolled bleeding because the disease is seldom limited to one or two lung segments. Patients with severe disease may develop respiratory failure.

Cystic fibrosis

Autosomal recessive disorder affecting 1/3000 live births which occurs equally in males and females and usually presents in early childhood. It is caused by mutations of the cystic fibrosis transmembrane conductance regulator (CFTR) gene located on chromosome 7. CFTR functions as a cyclic adenosine monophosphate (cAMP)-regulated chloride channel on the apical surface of airway and other epithelial cells. Abnormally thick secretions are produced by glandular tissue. It predominantly affects the pancreas and respiratory tract, leading to pancreatic insufficiency and lung damage from recurrent chest infections. Secondary bronchiectasis or lung abscess may result. Recurrent small haemoptyses and finger clubbing are common, and pneumothorax occurs. Persistent productive cough is associated initially with *Staphylococcus aureus*, *Haemophilus influenzae* and Gram-negative bacilli. Later *Pseudomonas aeruginosa* predominates and is associated with a poor prognosis.

Other manifestations are meconium ileus (15% of newborns), diabetes mellitus (20%), biliary obstruction (15%) and azoospermia (over 90% of males).

Most males are sterile and women subfertile. A high sodium concentration in the sweat (above 70 mmol/l) is characteristic.

> ### TRIAL
>
> **Fuchs *et al.*** compared inhaled rhDNase with placebo in patients with cystic fibrosis. Over a 24-week period rhDNase improved pulmonary function and reduced the frequency of respiratory exacerbations requiring intravenous antibiotics. *N Engl J Med* 1994; **331**: 637–642.

Management
Pancreatic enzymes and fat-soluble vitamins
Clearance of pulmonary secretions and treatment of infections
- Chest physiotherapy with postural drainage.
- Bronchodilators.
- Inhaled recombinant human deoxyribonuclease 1 (rhDNase) reduces the viscoelasticity of sputum by digesting viscous extracellular DNA in mucus (it is expensive).
- Antibiotics—exacerbations are usually treated with two parenteral antibiotics (to reduce antibiotic resistance). Choice is guided by sensitivity of isolated organisms but usually includes an aminoglycoside with an antipseudomonal penicillin (e.g. ticarcillin), cephalosporin or quinolone. The benefits of maintenance antibiotic therapy have to be weighed against the risks of antibiotic resistance. Inhaled aminoglycosides may allow delivery of high concentrations to the lungs with less risk of toxicity.

Respiratory failure with or without cor pulmonale usually occurs in early adult life, when lung or heart–lung transplantation should be considered.

The social and emotional problems can be enormous and, for this reason, as well as the complexity of clinical management, the condition should be supervised from specialist centres.

Asthma

Asthma affects 5–7% of the population of Europe and North America. It is characterized by recurrent shortness of breath, wheeze or cough caused by reversible narrowing of the airway lumen. The principal cause of increased airways resistance is contraction of smooth-muscle cells as a result of hypersensitivity to many different stimuli such as cold air, smoke, exercise and emotion, as well as antigens. Thickening of the airways by oedema and cellular infiltrates, as well as blockage of airways by mucus and secretions, also contributes. Wheeze is not an essential feature.

Asthma is sometimes classified into extrinsic and intrinsic, although treatment is the same.

Clinical features

Acute attacks

These may be fairly abrupt in onset and brief in duration (hours), or longer (a week or two), remittent and less severe. Longer severe attacks are called status asthmaticus (see p. 334). In an attack the patient feels tightness in the chest and both inspiratory and expiratory effort difficult. There may be a cough which is initially dry but later becomes productive, particularly if there is infection. The patient usually sits up with an overinflated chest, an audible expiratory wheeze and a fixed shoulder girdle using the accessory muscles of respiration. The respiratory rate may be little altered but the pulse is invariably rapid. Acute attacks are precipitated by specific allergens (e.g. pollens or house dust mite), exertion, excitement, cold air, a respiratory infection or β-blockers.

Recurrent asthma

Mild asthmatics (particularly with extrinsic asthma) usually have normal respiratory function between attacks, but those with long-standing severe asthma tend to develop emphysema and some degree of dyspnoea and persistent airways obstruction between acute attacks.

Investigation

Investigation includes chest X-ray (for regional collapse, pneumonia, pneumothorax) and measurement of ventilatory function (FEV_1 or PEFR, preferably at several times in a day on several days at home) and the response to bronchodilators. Variability through the day, especially with a 'morning dip' in PEFR, is characteristic. Skin hypersensitivity tests performed by pricking standard allergens into the skin can help the patient recognize and avoid environmental precipitants. Bronchial reactivity may be more precise but should be tested only in carefully controlled conditions. Adrenaline (0.5 ml of 1 : 1000) must be available in case of acute anaphylactic reactions (see *Acute anaphylaxis*, p. 337).

Management

The patient should be asked about precipitant factors, including the relationship of attacks to upper respiratory tract infection, season (grass pollen and fungal spores), cold, exercise, food, house dust (contains the mite *Dermatophagoides*), smoke, emotion and drugs (e.g. aspirin, β-blockers). New patients, and those being further investigated, should be given a peak flow meter to document waking and end-of-day values at home. Increasing morning dips provide an early warning of deterioration.

Most patients and almost all extrinsic asthmatics respond to simple therapy and may be controlled by:

* removing known allergies, e.g. feather pillows and cats;
* β₂-agonists, e.g. salbutamol as required by inhaler;
* disodium cromoglycate (Intal), 2–4 Spincaps daily or aerosol for children;
* inhaled steroids;

- oral steroids may be required for exacerbations; and
- hyposensitization is of value in only a small number of patients who demonstrate specific allergies.

NB When metered aerosols are used, always check inhaler technique. A number of simpler inhalers are now available (spacers, discs, rotahalers, breath-actuated aerosols). A β_2-agonist delivered by nebulizer at home has helped many patients with severe recurrent asthma. In some patients the PEFR tends to fall for a few days before an acute attack and prophylactic therapy with steroids may then abate it. Such patients may be given a peak flow meter and prednisolone to use at home.

SEVERE ASTHMA

Status asthmaticus is defined as an asthma attack of over 24 h duration. This is not a clinically useful definition since, of those who die in an acute asthma attack, half are dead within 24 h. Moreover, death is frequently sudden and sometimes unexpected as the patient may not appear severely ill. It is this lack of recognition of severity plus inadequate early treatment which is so dangerous. Most patients have some degree of respiratory failure at presentation.

Clinical presentation

Dyspnoea. Inability to speak or difficulty in maintaining speech is one criterion of

---

British Thoracic Society Guidelines (*British Medical Journal* 1993; **306**: 776–782) described a stepwise approach to the management of asthma:

Step 1   As required use of inhaled bronchodilators (β-agonists)
Step 2   As required inhaled bronchodilators with regular inhaled anti-inflammatory agents (steroids, cromoglycate or nemocromil sodium)
Step 3   As required inhaled bronchodilators with high-dose inhaled steroids
Step 4   Regular bronchodilators and high-dose inhaled steroids
Step 5   Addition of regular steroid tablets

TRIAL

The **National Heart, Lung, and Blood Institute's Asthma Clinical Research Network** compared regular with as-needed use of a β-agonist (albuterol) in mild asthma. Regular use provided neither beneficial nor deleterious effects, and as-needed use was recommended. *N Engl J Med* 1996; **335**: 841–847.

severity. It also implies inability to drink and therefore dehydration. Hypoxaemia is usually then present, and wheeze frequently absent due to poor ventilation. Confusion and drowsiness are evidence of a perilous situation whatever the cause (abnormal blood gases, sedation or fatigue).

Cyanosis is also ominous and tends to occur at a lower Po_2 than in the chronic bronchitic (because the bronchitic tends to have polycythaemia).

Absence of wheeze may denote very severe airways obstruction. A severe attack may be suggested by tachycardia, a peak flow rate <50% of predicted values, a heart rate >110 beats/min, pulsus paradoxus >10 mmHg and arterial hypotension.

NB   The clinical signs of drowsiness, cyanosis, bradycardia or hypotension are those of a very severe attack and vigorous treatment is essential before they are apparent.

Investigation

A chest X-ray is mandatory to exclude a pneumothorax. Blood gases provide the most useful guide to the severity of the attack and to the success of treatment. PEFRs can usually not be obtained, though one should always try, and are less than a quarter of the predicted values.

Management

All asthma attacks which do not respond to treatment with standard bronchodilators (β_2-agonist drugs such as salbutamol and theophylline preparations) within a few hours should be regarded as severe. They usually merit admission to hospital. Sedation may depress respiration further and is contraindicated.

• *Continuous oxygen* should invariably be given in high concentration, e.g. by nasal cannula. It is not necessary to give controlled (28%) oxygen unless there is evidence of some chronic respiratory failure.

• *Bronchodilators*: β_2-agonists (e.g. salbutamol, terbutaline) by nebulizer or intravenous infusion.

• If life-threatening features are present aminophylline bolus followed by ipratropium bromide by nebulizer.

NB   Too rapid infusion may cause circulatory collapse. This can be dangerous in patients already on oral preparations, including theophylline-containing cough mixtures, because of toxicity: check blood theophylline levels first. Children are particularly at risk.

• *Corticosteroids.* Hydrocortisone is given early and in large doses intravenously, e.g. 4 mg/kg immediately and 3 mg/kg 6-hourly if the patient cannot swallow. The patient is transferred to oral prednisolone (e.g. 40–60 mg daily) when he or she can swallow and this is subsequently withdrawn gradually.

• *Intravenous fluids* are required both to make up the initial dehydration and for as long as oral fluids are not taken. Monitor urine output.

• *Bacterial infection* is a rare trigger but *antibiotics* are given if it is present or strongly suspected. The usual organisms are *Strepcococcus pneumoniae* or *Haemophilus influenzae* (p. 338).

- *Mechanical ventilation* may be necessary. Persistent or increasing elevation of arterial $P\text{CO}_2$, especially with accompanying exhaustion, indicates the need for artifical ventilation.

NB   Check the chest X-ray for pneumothorax.

Respiratory failure

Respiratory failure can be defined as a reduction in arterial $P\text{O}_2$ below 8 kPa with or without an increase in arterial $P\text{CO}_2$ above 6.0 kPa.

NB   The mean $P\text{O}_2$ is about 13 kPa. Normally values of $P\text{O}_2$ are about 1.3 kPa (10 mmHg), lower in the elderly.

The $P\text{O}_2$ may fall while the $P\text{CO}_2$ remains normal. This may occur with alveolar parenchymal lung disease: infiltrations, fibrosing alveolitis and 'pure' emphysema. Much more commonly, both arterial gas levels are abnormal. This occurs with ventilatory failure.

Acute
- Patients with normal lungs, with upper airways obstruction (e.g. croup and acute anaphylaxis) or mechanical failure (e.g. flail chest, drug overdosage) or sleep apnoea.
- Patients with abnormal lungs (e.g. asthma, chronic bronchitis).

Chronic
Usually in patients with abnormal lungs, especially chronic bronchitis. These patients are particularly likely to develop acute failure if infection occurs.

In restrictive disorders, lung expansion is limited by:
- lung disease such as fibrosis collapse, oedema, consolidation;
- pleural disease such as fibrosis, effusion or mesothelioma;
- chest-wall disease such as costospinal rigidity and deformity, or abdominal splinting by obesity, ascites or pregnancy; and
- neuromuscular disease such as muscular dystrophy, myasthenia or phrenic nerve paralysis.

Sleep apnoea syndrome is defined as absence of airflow in periods of at least 10 s occurring not less than 30 times per night's sleep.

ACUTE ON CHRONIC RESPIRATORY FAILURE
Usually chronic bronchitis.

Clinical presentation
- Peripheral vasodilatation with headache, engorged veins in the fundi, warm hands and a bounding pulse, all due to carbon dioxide retention.
- Varying degrees of agitated confusion, drowsiness and coma.
- Increasing cyanosis.

- Signs of right heart failure.
- Flapping tremor of the outstretched hands and papilloedema are late signs.

NB   Unfortunately the physical signs are a poor guide to the presence of respiratory failure and to its degree. It is therefore necessary to measure blood gases in all patients in whom the diagnosis is suspected.

Management

This consists of the measures used for chronic bronchitis as given above, with the addition of controlled oxygen therapy. The danger to life in this situation is hypoxia but paradoxically, relief of hypoxia may make the situation worse because of the patient's reliance on hypoxic drive. Oxygen is given at 24% or 28% by Ventimask (or other controlled technique) if the arterial Po_2 is low. Oxygen is not required unless the Po_2 is <6.7 kPa (50 mmHg). It is given continuously until the acute situation (including infection and heart failure) has recovered. The Pco_2 is monitored either by the mixed venous rebreathing method or from the arterial blood. Intravenous aminophylline (10 ml) very slowly and doxapram infusion may be valuable. For chronic failure ($Po_2 < 7.3$ kPa; $Pco_2 > 6$ kPa; $FEV_1 < 1.5$ litres; FVC < 2 litres), controlled oxygen can be given continuously at home, usually from an oxygen concentrator for not less than 15 h in 24, over several months with improvement in symptoms and an increase in life expectancy.

NB   Sedatives are absolutely contraindicated.

Indications for mechanical ventilation

If the Pco_2 falls or rises only slightly (e.g. by 1.3 kPa (10 mmHg)), conservative therapy should be continued and reassessed periodically. If the Pco_2 rises, this indicates that the patient's ventilation is inadequate and is the prime indication for mechanical positive-pressure ventilation. Patients should be ventilated before they become exhausted. The final decision to ventilate a patient is determined mainly on the basis of respiratory function before the acute illness: if very poor, it may not be possible to wean the patient off.

Acute anaphylaxis

This rare condition occurs in previously healthy people following drug therapy, e.g. penicillin, or insect stings. Patients with known previous hypersensitivity or allergy should not be given immune serum, live vaccine or known allergens.

Clinical features range from mild with flushing of the face, pruritus and blotchy wheals, to severe with asthma, which may proceed to respiratory obstruction from oedema of the larynx and to hypotension.

Immediate treatment is with adrenaline 0.5–1.0 ml of 1 : 1000 solution (1 mg/ml) given intramuscularly or subcutaneously and repeated every 15 min until improvement is observed to reverse the type 1 acute reaction. Hydrocortisone takes 20–30 min to act and is not the immediate therapy of choice. It is given (after the first injection of adrenaline), in a dose of 200 mg intravenously, with chlorpheniramine 10 mg slowly intravenously or intramuscularly.

Hereditary angioedema due to C_1 esterase deficiency is a rare autosomal dominant condition and gives erythema but not wheals, patchy oedema and colicky abdominal pain. It responds to danazol prophylaxis and fresh frozen plasma to correct the deficiency during attacks.

Pneumonia

Community-acquired pneumonia affects approximately 12 per 1000 adults per year. One in 1000 require hospitalization, and mortality in these patients is around 10%.

Clinical presentation

Symptoms of cough, sputum, pleurisy and dyspnoea are less common in the elderly.

Clinical findings include fever (80%), tachypnoea (>20 breaths/min), crackles (80%) and signs of consolidation (30%).

The commonest organism in UK studies is *Streptococcus pneumoniae* (60–75%), followed by *Mycoplasma pneumoniae* (5–18%). *Haemophilus influenzae*, *Legionella* species, *Chlamydia psittaci* and *Staphylococcus aureus* account for most of the remainder. Gram-negative bacilli, *Coxiella burnetii* and anaerobes were rare.

Viruses (including influenza) account for up to 15%.

Investigations

Investigations are performed to establish the diagnosis and assess severity:
- *Chest X-ray* shows infiltrates. Computed tomographic (CT) scanning is more sensitive and may be useful in detecting interstitial disease, cavitation or empyema.
- *Blood gases* to assess severity and guide oxygen treatment.
- *Blood count*—white cell count $\geq 15 \times 10^9$/l suggests bacterial infection; white cell count $>20 \times 10^9$/l or $\leq 4 \times 10^9$/l indicates poor prognosis. Haemoglobin for haemolysis.
- *Urea, electrolytes and liver function tests* for underlying or associated renal or hepatic disease.
- *Gram staining and culture of sputum*—but cough is unproductive in one-third of patients, and negative results are common, particularly if antibiotics have been given.
- *Blood culture.*
- *Pleural fluid*, if present, should be aspirated for culture.
- *Acute-phase serum* is usually taken for later analysis.

Management

- Oxygen—to maintain Pao_2 above 8 kPa.
- Antibiotics—the organism is usually unknown initially. Treatment should cover

British Thoracic Society guidelines report an increased risk of death associated with the following features:

Clinical
Respiratory rate ≥30 breaths/min
Diastolic blood pressure <60 mmHg
Age ≥60 years
Atrial fibrillation
Underlying disease, confusion, multilobar involvement

Laboratory
Urea ≥7 mmol/l
Albumin ≤35 mmol/l
Pao_2 ≤8 kPa
White blood cells ≤4000 × 10^9/l or ≥20 × 10^9/l
Bacteraemia

Streptococcus pneumoniae. In uncomplicated pneumonia treatment is usually started with oral amoxyclinin or a macrolide (erythromycin or clarithromycin). In severe pneumonia intravenous therapy is given, often using a combination of a macrolide and a second- or third-generation cephalosporin (cefuroxime or cefotaxime).
- *Intravenous fluids* may be required.
- *Analgesia* for pleuritic pain.

Pneumococcal pneumonia is the commonest bacterial pneumonia. *S. pneumoniae* is a Gram-positive diplococcus. It affects all ages, but is commoner in the elderly, after splenectomy, in the immunosuppressed, alcoholics, patients with chronic heart failure, and those with pre-existing lung disease. It typically presents acutely with fever, pleuritic pain and rust-coloured sputum. It causes both lobar and bronchopneumonia. Treatment is with penicillin, or erythromycin in the penicillin-sensitive. A polysaccharide pneumococcal vaccine is available for those at high risk. It should be given at least 2 weeks before splenectomy and before chemotherapy.

Staphylococcal pneumonia produces widespread infection with abscess formation. It may complicate influenzal pneumonia, and this makes it relatively common during epidemics of influenza. It also occurs in patients with underlying disease, which prevents a normal response to infection, e.g. chronic leukaemia, Hodgkin's disease, cystic fibrosis. Flucloxacillin and fusidic acid are the drugs of choice. Lung abscess, empyema and subsequent bronchiectasis are relatively common complications.

Legionnaire's disease was first described in a group of American army veterans (legionnaires). The causative Gram-negative bacillus flourishes in the cooling waters of air conditioners and may colonize hot-water tanks kept at <60°C. It begins as an influenza-like illness with fever, malaise and myalgia, and proceeds with cough (little sputum), dyspnoea and sometimes severe anorexia, marked confusion and coma. Diarrhoea and vomiting are common and renal failure may develop. Examination shows consolidation which usually affects both lung bases. X-ray changes may persist for more than 2 months after the acute illness.

Erythromycin or ciprofloxacin are the antibiotics of choice, but the mortality remains high (20%).

NB   Legionnaire's disease (and *Mycoplasma pneumoniae* or psittacosis) should be suspected in all patients who develop atypical pneumonia which does not respond to standard antibiotics.

Mycoplasma pneumonia is caused by *M. pneumoniae*, the only mycoplasma definitely pathogenic to humans. The clinical picture resembles bacterial pneumonia, although cough and sputum are absent in one-third of cases.

Respiratory symptoms and signs and X-ray changes (patchy consolidation with small effusions) are usually preceded by several days of flu-like symptoms. Polyarthritis occurs and may persist for months. Malaise and fatigue may persist long after the acute illness is over. The diagnosis is confirmed by a positive *Mycoplasma*-specific IgM titre. Erythromycin or tetracycline are the antibiotics of choice.

Psittacosis is a pneumonia due to *Chlamydia psittaci*. It is transmitted in the excrement of infected birds (the bird need not be ill). Headache, fever and dry cough may be accompanied by a rash and splenomegaly. Hepatitis, encephalitis, renal failure and haemolysis also occur. Treatment is with tetracycline or erythromycin.

Viral pneumonia The commonest virus causing pneumonia in children in the UK and USA is the respiratory syncytial virus (RSV) — so called as it is a respiratory virus which produces syncytium formation when grown in tissue culture. Infection may be indistinguishable from acute bacterial bronchitis or bronchiolitis in children and infants. The presence of a skin rash supports the likelihood of RSV infection.

Acute viral pneumonia in adults is less common, but occurs during epidemics of influenza. Fever, headache and myalgia are followed after a few days by dry cough and chest pain. Treatment is largely symptomatic (paracetamol, rest, fluids). Influenza vaccines are available for those at high risk. The most common cause of pneumonia during influenza epidemics results from secondary bacterial infection, the most serious being staphylococcal pneumonia. The viruses of measles, chickenpox and herpes zoster may directly affect the lung. The diagnosis is confirmed by a rise in specific antibody titre.

Aspiration pneumonia. There are two main varieties, differentiated from each other by the type of fluid aspirated and the circumstances in which it occurs.

Aspiration of gastric contents may produce a severe chemical pneumonitis with considerable pulmonary oedema and bronchospasm (Mendelson's syndrome). The acute respiratory distress and shock can be very rapidly fatal and very difficult to treat. It tends to occur in states of reduced consciousness such as general anaesthesia, drunks and when gastric lavage (for drug overdose) has been performed inexpertly.

Aspiration of bacteria from the oropharynx may follow dental anaesthesia and can occur in bulbar palsies. The bacteria, apart from *Bacteroides*, are nearly all penicillin-sensitive and amoxycillin (or ampicillin) with metronidazole are the antibiotics of choice until sensitivities of isolated organisms are known. Recurrent episodes occur in some oesophageal disorders, including hiatus hernia, stricture, achalasia of the cardia, and in patients with diverticula or pharyngeal pouch.

Recurrent bacterial pneumonia. In the absence of chronic bronchitis, recurrent pneumonia arouses suspicion of:
*   bronchial carcinoma preventing drainage of infected areas of lung;
*   bronchiectasis;
*   cystic fibrosis;
*   achalasia of the cardia, 25% of which present as chest disease, pharyngeal pouch and neuromuscular disease of the oesophagus, e.g. bulbar palsy; and
*   hypogammaglobulinaemia and myeloma.

Opportunistic infection of the lungs occurs in patients immunosuppressed as a result of treatment, e.g. for myeloproliferative disorders or acquired immunodeficiency syndrome (AIDS; p. 451).

LUNG ABSCESS
Aetiology
*   Aspiration (see above).
*   Bronchial obstruction, usually by carcinoma or a foreign body (especially peanuts and teeth).
*   Pneumonia partially resolved or treated, particularly when caused by the *Staphylococcus*, *Klebsiella* or *Pneumococcus* organisms.

Clinical features
There is a swinging fever and the patient is very ill. The sputum is foul and purulent and there is a high polymorph cell count. Clubbing may develop.

Investigation
Sputum is sent for Gram stain and culture, and blood for culture. Chest X-ray shows round lesions which usually have a fluid level, and serial X-rays monitor progress. It may be necessary to proceed to bronchoscopy to exclude obstruction and to obtain a biopsy and sputum trap specimen.

Treatment

Antibiotic therapy is given according to sensitivities and continued until healing is complete. Repeated postural drainage is started. In resistant cases, repeated aspiration, antibiotic instillation and even surgical excision may be required.

Carcinoma of the bronchus

Incidence

This causes about 40 000 deaths per year in the UK, half of them under 65 years of age. About 30% are squamous cell (epidermoid) and 25% oat cell (anaplastic small cell). They are 2–3 times commoner in men than women. Fifteen per cent are undifferentiated large cell tumours and about 30% are adenocarcinoma. Alveolar cell carcinoma is very rare.

Aetiological factors

Cigarette smoking. The increased mortality risk of carcinoma of the bronchus (squamous and oat cell) has an approximately straight-line relationship with numbers of cigarettes smoked per day (increased risk of death = cigarettes smoked per day, numerically). Stopping smoking decreases the risk by one-half in 5 years, and to only twice that of lifelong non-smokers in 15 years. Other atmospheric pollution (coal smoke and diesel fumes) may prove to be aetiologically relevant, but quantitatively small compared with cigarettes.

Exposure to chromium, arsenic, radioactive materials or asbestos (which in addition produces interstitial fibrosis and mesotheliomata) is associated with a higher incidence of bronchial carcinoma.

Clinical presentation

The patient is usually a cigarette smoker. Cough or the accentuation of an existing cough is the commonest early symptom, and haemoptysis the next. Dyspnoea, central chest ache or pleuritic pain, or slowly resolving chest infection are common early manifestations. The patient may present with metastatic deposits involving brain, bone, liver, skin, kidney, adrenal glands or other site, or symptoms from local extension (superior vena cava obstruction, Horner's syndrome, Pancoast syndrome, hoarseness, cervical lymph glands, dysphagia, cardiac arrhythmia or pleural effusion). Occasionally patients are identified following a routine chest X-ray.

The presence of systemic and non-specific symptoms (anorexia, weight loss and fatigue) usually, but not always, implies late and possibly inoperable disease.

Blood and marrow

Anaemia (often normochromic or normocytic). Polycythaemia is uncommon.
Marrow infiltration is common in small cell carcinoma.

Neuromuscular

Dementia or focal neurological deficit (due to cerebral secondaries or rarely cortical atrophy), cerebellar syndrome, mixed sensorimotor peripheral neuropathy, proximal myopathy, polymyositis (p. 167) and the myasthenic syndrome (p. 168).

Skin, connective tissue, bone

Clubbing, hypertrophic pulmonary osteoarthropathy, dermatomyositis and acanthosis nigricans.

Endocrine

Syndromes due to ectopic hormone production, the pituitary-like ones (adrenocorticotrophic hormone (ACTH), antidiuretic hormone (ADH), prolactin) usually from oat cell tumours, and parathyroid hormone from squamous cell tumours. Hypercalcaemia is usually due to bone secondaries.

Cardiovascular

Atrial fibrillation (local extension) and migratory thrombophlebitis. Pericarditis.

Diagnosis

Chest X-ray:
- the tumour may be visible often as a unilaterally enlarged hilum or peripheral circular opacity occasionally cavitated;
- collapse/consolidation due to bronchial obstruction by the tumour;
- effusion, raised hemidiaphragm of phrenic paralysis, and bone erosion suggest local extension.

CT scan shows the tumour position better and demonstrates bronchial narrowing and mediastinal involvement. Exfoliative cytology may be diagnostic.

Fibreoptic bronchoscopy with biopsy is performed if possible to establish histological diagnosis and assess operability. The site of the tumour is a guide to operability (not less than 2 cm from the carina).

Treatment

Surgery offers the only 'cure': 15–20% of all cases are resectable and only 30% of these survive 5 years. Surgery is contraindicated by metastasis (present in 60% at the time of presentation—in bone and liver), local spread and inadequate respiratory function.

Radiotherapy is valuable for relief of distressing symptoms (major airway narrowing, haemoptysis, mediastinal compression, Pancoast syndrome and relief of pain produced by bony secondaries). Small cancer carcinoma may respond to chemotherapy, often using a combination of cyclophosphamide, etoposide, doxorubicin and cisplatin (an alkylating agent) (pp. 431–432).

Bronchial adenoma

This rare tumour is usually benign but locally invasive. Ninety per cent are histologically 'carcinoid' tumours but only a few cases present with the carcinoid syndrome. They usually present with cough and haemoptysis. The tumour may either occur anywhere within the thoracic cavity and appear as a well-circumscribed peripheral mass on chest X-ray, or more often, in the major bronchi and appear as a pedunculated intrabronchial mass seen bronchoscopically. The tumours are removed in view of the risk of neoplastic change.

Sarcoidosis

This is a disease of unknown aetiology. It appears to be a systemic granulomatous reaction to various stimuli which may involve any tissue. It most commonly affects the lungs, mediastinal lymph nodes and skin.

Clinical presentation

Pulmonary sarcoid (90%)

Most commonly it presents as a subacute syndrome in young people (20–40 years, and in females five times more commonly than males) with fever, malaise and lassitude, erythema nodosum (sarcoid is the most common cause in the UK), polyarthralgia, usually of the ankles and knees, and mediastinal hilar lymphadenopathy. Dyspnoea is not usually a feature of this acute form, which is self-limiting (2 months–2 years).

Less commonly and more seriously it presents as a chronic insidious disease with respiratory symptoms of cough and progressive dyspnoea with malaise and fever leading to progressive pulmonary fibrosis.

Non-pulmonary sarcoid

Apart from erythema nodosum, this is relatively uncommon.
• Skin (70%). Erythema nodosum (not sarcoid tissue) in the acute syndrome; infiltration of scars: lupus pernio.
• Hypercalcaemia occurs in about 10% of patients with sarcoidosis and may be the presenting abnormality (p. 290). Hypercalciuria is even more common. This is probably due to an excessive sensitivity to vitamin D and responds to steroids.
• Eyes (15%). Uveitis and keratoconjunctivitis sicca. Blindness may result.
• Parotitis (5%).
• Hepatosplenomegaly (12%).
• Generalized lymphadenopathy (30%).
• Bone and joints, producing cystic lesions most commonly in the phalanges (4%).
• Nervous system, causing isolated cranial nerve lesions and peripheral neuropathy (3%).

- Endocrine, producing diabetes insipidus from pituitary involvement (very rare).
- Renal damage from hypercalcaemia or an associated interstitial nephritis or glomerulonephritis.

Investigation

Chest X-ray shows symmetrical lobulated bilateral hilar gland enlargement (inter-bronchial rather than tracheobronchial; 80%) or, less commonly (40%), parenchymal mottling or diffuse fibrosis. CT scan will help distinguish gland enlargement from prominent pulmonary artery shadows.

'Blind' transbronchial lung biopsy at bronchoscopy often shows non-caseating epithelioid granulomata.

The Mantoux test is usually negative (70%): a positive test is not uncommon but a strongly positive test is very unusual.

Kveim test (intradermal inoculation with 0.1 ml splenic homogenate from a previous case of sarcoid). The skin becomes indurated and biopsy of the papule at 4–6 weeks shows characteristic sarcoid granulomata. False-negative reactions occur in up to 25%, depending partly on the quality of the antigen. It is rarely performed now.

Hypercalcaemia (10%) returns to normal with steroids.

Polyclonal increase in γ-globulins is non-specific but common.

Management

The differential diagnosis of bilateral hilar lymph node enlargement is from Hodgkin's disease (and other reticuloses), and any deviation of the patient's syndrome from the usual pattern makes a definite diagnosis by biopsy imperative. Treatment, other than simple analgesics and non-steroidal anti-inflammatory agents, is usually unnecessary.

Indications for corticosteroids in sarcoidosis (e.g. prednisolone 20 mg daily reducing after 1 month to the minimum dose necessary to suppress activity for 1 year) include:
- Progressive lung disease, to try to prevent fibrosis. The indication is progressive pulmonary shadowing or increasing breathlessness. The effect of therapy is monitored by symptoms, chest X-rays and lung function tests, including carbon monoxide transfer factor, $T_{L}CO$.
- Hypercalcaemia.
- When vital organs are threatened, e.g. eyes, nervous system, kidneys and heart.

Prognosis (of pulmonary sarcoid)

The chest X-ray remains abnormal in about half of all cases (Table 18.1). Clinical disability due to the disease is much less common and is related to:
- age—the younger, the better;
- presence of erythema nodosum where over 95% recover by 1 year;

PROGNOSIS OF PULMONARY SARCOID			
Chest X-ray appearance	Recovery stage	X-ray (%)	Clinical (%)
Bilateral hilar lymphadenopathy alone	I	75	90
Bilateral hilar lymphadenopathy with fine pulmonary reticular–nodular shadowing	II	50	60
Coarse reticular–nodular shadowing or fibrosis	III	30	30

Table 18.1 Prognosis of pulmonary sarcoid.

• extent of extrapulmonary involvement. Bone or chronic skin lesions indicate chronicity and the more widespread it is, the worse the prognosis; and
• extent of intrathoracic involvement.
NB   In systemic sarcoidosis, the activity and clinical course of the disease in any one tissue (e.g. skin, eyes) is a guide to the activity in any tissue less easily observed (e.g. lungs).

Tuberculosis

Infection with the acid alcohol-fast bacillus (AAFB) of *Mycobacterium tuberculosis* affects predominantly the lungs, lymph nodes and gut. Some features of the disease vary with the patient's sensitivity to tuberculin.

PRIMARY TUBERCULOSIS

This is the syndrome produced by infection with *M. tuberculosis* in non-sensitive patients, i.e. in those who have not previously been infected. There is a mild inflammatory response at the site of infection (subpleural in the mid-zones of the lungs, in the pharynx or in the terminal ileum), followed by spread to the regional lymph nodes (hilar, cervical and mesenteric respectively)—the primary complex. One to two weeks following infection, with the onset of tuberculin sensitivity, the tissue reaction changes at both the focus and in the nodes, to the charateristic caseating granuloma. The combination of a focus with regional lymph node involvement is called the *primary complex*. Patients are usually symptomless. The complex heals with fibrosis and, frequently, calcifies without therapy. The enlarged lymph node may be obvious in the neck or cause obstruction to a bronchus with consequent collapse-consolidation. Blood dissemination of the organisms occurs rarely from the primary complex to cause widespread miliary disease, especially in infants.

POST-PRIMARY TUBERCULOSIS

This is the syndrome produced by infection with *M. tuberulosis* in the previously infected and therefore tuberculin-sensitive patient. Reactivation (or reinfection) is followed by an immediate brisk granulomatous response which tends to localize the disease and regional lymph node involvement is uncommon. As with primary tuberculosis, the lesion may:

- heal with fibrosis (and calcification);
- rupture into a bronchus giving tuberculous bronchopneumonia;
- spread via the blood to produce miliary tuberculosis of liver, spleen, lungs, choroid, bone and/or meninges.

Presenting features

Symptoms occur relatively late and therefore in established disease. The earliest are non-specific, such as malaise, fatigue, anorexia and weight loss. Of more specific symptoms, the most common is cough, often with mucoid sputum. Other symptoms include repeated small haemoptysis, pleural pain, slight fever or occasionally exertional dyspnoea. Frequently the diagnosis is made presymptomatically on routine chest radiography. Signs also occur late in the disease and are not very specific, e.g. crepitations (usually apical) and, later, signs of consolidation, pleural effusion or cavitation.

Diagnosis

Clinical suspicion should be particularly high in high-risk groups:

- the hostel-dwelling 'down-and-out', and the alcoholic;
- Pakistani and Indian immigrant (lymph node tuberculosis is common in Indian and Pakistani patients);
- diabetics;
- patients with AIDS;
- patients on immunosuppressive therapy (steroids or cytotoxic drugs); and
- occupations at risk—doctors and nurses.

Ideally the diagnosis is made by repeated examination for AAFB in sputum and bronchial washing on direct smear or culture. Six to 12 specimens (or more) may be required. Sometimes the diagnosis can only be made radiologically and activity is suggested by:

- changing 'soft' shadows;
- progression of apical lesions;
- cavitation; and
- strongly positive Heaf test.

It may be necessary to treat on clinical grounds alone and response to specific therapy in 2 weeks is taken as proof of diagnosis.

NB   AAFB on smear may not be pathogenic mycobacteria, particularly in urine specimens.

Management

Isolate patients who are sputum-positive for the first week of treatment (this is standard practice in the UK but the Madras trials suggest that this may not be necessary). Tuberculosis is notifiable in the UK.

Investigate family and social contacts for infection (or via the local community physician) by chest X-ray and tuberculin sensitivity (Mantoux or Heaf) immediately and 6 weeks later. Then:

- if both tests are negative, give bacillus Calmette-Guérin (BCG), check for conversion and follow up for 2 years;
- if the initial test is negative and the 6-week test positive this indicates recent infection. These patients are treated with two antituberculous drugs (ethambutol and isoniazid) for 12–18 months unless primary resistance is discovered in the contact;
- if the initial tuberculin test is positive, give isoniazid for 1 year to children under 7 years not previously inoculated with BCG, and follow up all other patients for 2 years and then annually for 3 years.

Start therapy if AAFB are detected in sputum. If the clinical suspicion of tuberculosis is high but the sputum smear is negative, collect sputa for culture and start therapy with three of the first-line drugs (see also p. 460):

- Rifampicin 450–600 mg daily
- Isoniazid 300 mg (with pyridoxine 10 mg) daily
- Ethambutol 15 mg/kg daily
- Streptomycin 1 g by intramuscular injection daily
- Pyrazinamide 1.5–2.0 g daily.

Therapy should be started with a warning about possible adverse effects and early clinic review. Continue triple therapy until sensitivities are reported (6–8 weeks). If the organism is sensitive to all three drugs, stop ethambutol and continue rifampicin and isoniazid for 6 months with 3-monthly follow-up, radiographic and clinical. The patient's sputum is tested regularly to detect relapse (failure to take drugs is the most common reason).

For tuberculous meningitis see p. 156.

Common drug complications

- Rifampicin: abnormal liver function tests. Colours the urine pink
- Isoniazid: peripheral neuropathy and encephalopathy — these are extremely rare, occur in slow acetylators and respond to pyridoxine, often given prophylactically
- Ethambutol: optic neuritis with colour vision and acuity reduced
- Streptomycin: vertigo and nerve deafness. In the elderly and in the presence of raised blood urea, the dose is reduced to 0.75 g or 0.5 g daily to maintain blood levels of 1–2 μg/ml.

Second-line drug complications

- Ethionamide: nausea and vomiting; hepatotoxic

- Pyrazinamide: hepatotoxic (rare but severe)
- Cycloserine: neurotoxicity with confusion and depression
- Para-aminosalicylic acid: nausea, vomiting and skin rash.

NB   Twice-weekly treatment with streptomycin and high-dose isoniazid or rifampicin with isoniazid has been shown to be effective. Other combinations of two, three and four antituberculous drugs given for shorter periods are under trial.

Corticosteroids

Steroids are indicated for severely ill tuberculous patients at the onset of chemotherapy; for tuberculous meningitis, and in miliary tuberculosis to try and prevent fibrosis. The value of steroids other than when life is immediately threatened remains unproven and they probably do not affect long-term morbidity.

Occupational lung diseases

There are four main groups: dust diseases, asthma, extrinsic allergic alveolitis and irritant gases.

DUST DISEASES

These include the pneumoconioses, asthma, allergic alveolitis and the effects of irritant gases.

- coal pneumoconiosis;
- silicosis in rock drilling and crushing—also occurs in coal miners;
- asbestosis in insulation workers; this can produce fibrosis, carcinoma and pleural mesothelioma; and
- benign (no fibrosis).

These are radiographic diagnoses made in the light of the patient's known occupational hazards; the shadows are due to the metals themselves, e.g. siderosis (iron) and stannosis (tin). All are rare.

Clinical features

In the early stages there are no symptoms but X-ray changes occur; later there is dyspnoea on exertion, cough, sputum and attacks of bronchitis. In coal miners, progressive massive fibrosis may occur and Caplan's syndrome (rheumatoid arthritis and pulmonary nodules) occurs in association with rhematoid arthritis. The patients may eventually develop cor pulmonale.

ASTHMA

Occupational asthma can occur in response to precipitants of animal, vegetable, bacteriological or chemical origin. Some of the commoner occupations are: animal laboratory workers (urinary proteins), grain and flour workers (mites and flour), sawmill operatives and carpenters (hardwoods), those who manufacture biological detergents (inhalation of *Bacillus subtilis* proteolytic enzymes), in the electronics industry (colophony in solder flux), paint sprayers and polyurethane workers (isocyanates), and workers with epoxy resins or platinum salts, and in the pharmaceutical industry. All these are recognized for compensation under industrial injuries legislation in the UK.

EXTRINSIC ALLERGIC ALVEOLITIS

Inhalation of organic dusts may give a diffuse allergic (type III precipitin-mediated) reaction in the alveoli and bronchioles.

Aetiology

Exposure to mouldy hay (*Micropolyspora faeni*) causes farmer's lung, to mouldy sugar cane causes bagassosis, to mushroom dust causes mushroom picker's lung, to bird droppings (containing avian serum proteins) causes bird fancier's lung, to contaminated malting barley (*Aspergillus clavatus*) causes malt worker's lung and to pituitary snuff (containing foreign serum protein) causes pituitary snuff-taker's lung. Precipitating antibodies against the offending antigen can be found in the patient's blood.

Clinical features

Acute (i.e. 4–6 h after exposure). Dyspnoea, dry cough, malaise, fever and limb pains occur, and examination shows fine inspiratory crepitations with little wheeze. The symptoms subside in 2–3 days.

Chronic. After repeated acute attacks fibrosis occurs with persistent inspiratory crepitations, respiratory failure and cor pulmonale.

Investigation

Chest X-ray shows a diffuse haze initially and later micronodular shadowing develops, progressing to honeycombing. Ventilatory function tests initially show a reversible restrictive defect with low T_{LCO} during the acute attacks. This becomes permanent as the chronic disorder develops. There is little or no obstruction. The P_{O_2} falls and P_{CO_2} is normal or reduced by the hyperventilation. There is no eosinophilia.

Treatment

Separate the patient and the allergen. Masks are of little use and positive-pressure helmets should be worn. High-dose steroids are tried in serious cases and should be continued only if there has been a measured response in lung function.

Irritant gases. Cause pulmonary oedema.

Pulmonary embolism

Emboli usually arise in the veins of the pelvis or legs, and rarely from the right atrium.

They occur more frequently:
- following surgery (classically, though not always about 10 days);
- following myocardial infarction;
- following a stroke;
- in disseminated malignancy;
- in prolonged bed rest associated with illness;
- following trauma, especially to the pelvis and legs (including caesarean section);
- in antiphospholipid syndrome;
- in hypercoagulable states — antithrombin III, protein C and S deficiencies. In factor V Leiden a single point mutation in the factor V gene causes resistance to activated protein C.

The risk may increase if other factors are present:
- advancing age;
- obesity;
- pregnancy and postpartum;
- treatment with oestrogens (oral contraceptive or hormone replacement therapy);
- previous venous thrombosis.

About 50% of those who die from pulmonary embolism have had premonitory signs and symptoms of small emboli (unexplained breathless attacks) or venous thrombosis in the previous weeks. A deep vein thrombosis should be regarded as potential pulmonary embolus and must be suspected, diagnosed and treated early.

Clinical features

The clinical features of deep venous thrombosis are:
- erythema and warmth of the affected leg (30%);
- swelling and tenderness (75%); and
- the thrombosed vein may be palpable.

Homan's sign is neither specific nor sensitive.

Thromboses which extend above the knee are more likely to produce clinically recognizable pulmonary emboli.

NB   Diagnosis is confirmed by Doppler ultrasound with vein compression or venography. Swelling of the calf also occurs in rupture of a Baker's cyst behind the knee. An effusion of the knee makes this more likely. The cyst can often be shown on ultrasound.

Clinical presentation (of pulmonary embolus)

This depends upon the size of the embolus. Multiple small acute emboli may

remain undetected until up to 50% of the vascular bed is involved and present with effort dyspnoea:
- *Small.* Transient faints and dyspnoea, with slight pyrexia.
- *Medium.* Usually results in infarction and produces, in addition, haemoptysis, pleurisy and occasionally a pleural effusion.
- *Large.* (Affecting over 60% of the pulmonary bed.) Acute cor pulmonale with sudden dyspnoea and shock. There is a small-volume rapid pulse, with hypotension, cyanosis, peripheral vasoconstriction and a raised jugular venous pressure. There may be a gallop rhythm.

Investigation

Chest X-ray to demonstrate:
- pulmonary oligaemia of the affected segment (usually present but difficult to diagnose except in retrospect);
- the corresponding pulmonary artery is sometimes dilated at the hilum;
- small areas of horizontal linear collapse, usually at the bases, with a raised diaphragm;
- a small pleural effusion.

With larger emboli, the heart enlarges acutely and the superior vena cava distends.

Electrocardiogram changes usually occur only with larger emboli but are then common. The characteristic changes are as follows (see also p. 90):
- tachycardia;
- right ventricular 'strain' pattern (inverted T waves in leads V1–4);
- acute, often transient, right bundle branch block pattern;
- S_1, Q_3, T_3 pattern; and
- transient arrhythmias, e.g. atrial fibrillation.

Arterial blood gases. With larger emboli, a fall in Pao_2 and $Paco_2$ is common.

Lung perfusion scan is a useful non-traumatic investigation in doubtful cases and may show underperfusion of one or more parts of the lung which are radiologically normal (and ventilated normally on ventilation scan).

Combined ventilation and perfusion scans may be helpful in pre-existent lung disease in which ventilation and perfusion defects are usually matched. A normal scan virtually excludes pulmonary embolism.

Pulmonary angiography is the most precise for cases presenting difficulty in diagnosis.

Treatment

Prophylaxis pre- and postoperatively, especially lower abdomen and lower limb, and in patients confined to bed or with predisposing disorders (e.g. cardiac failure).

Low-molecular-weight heparins are prepared by depolymerization of standard (unfractionated) heparin. They have a longer duration of action than standard

TRIALS

Imperiale and Speroff performed a meta-analysis of methods to prevent venous thromboembolism following total hip replacement. Low-molecular-weight heparin was more effective than low-dose heparin. *JAMA* 1994; **271**: 1780–1785.

Lensing et al. performed a meta-analysis of trials comparing the efficacy and safety of low-molecular-weight heparin versus standard heparin in the initial treatment of deep venous thrombosis. Low-molecular-weight heparins were more effective and safer than standard heparin. *Arch Intern Med* 1995; **155**: 601–607.

heparin, and given as a once-daily subcutaneous dose produce a more predictable anticoagulant response. They are safe and effective as low-dose prophylaxis, and can be used in weight-adjusted doses for treatment of deep vein thrombosis without laboratory monitoring.

For established deep vein thrombosis or pulmonary embolism, patients are usually treated with heparin initially, followed by warfarin for a minimum of 3 months.

In massive pulmonary embolism, cardiac massage and correction of acidosis with urgent intravenous heparin may improve survival. With large emboli, oxygen in high concentration and thrombolytic therapy with urokinase or streptokinase may be valuable. The operative removal of large emboli with bypass surgery may be life-saving.

Placement of a vena caval filter should be considered when anticoagulation is hazardous or in patients who develop emboli despite adequate anticoagulation.

Pneumothorax

Aetiology

Spontaneous

This is the most common type and usually occurs in normal thin young men following rupture of a small subpleural bulla. The history is of the sudden onset of one-sided pleuritic pain and/or dyspnoea. Dyspnoea rapidly increases in tension pneumothorax and the patient becomes cyanosed. The classical signs are of diminished movement on the affected side with deviation of the trachea to the other side. There is hyperresonance to percussion and reduced pulmonary sounds (breath sounds, tactile fremitus and vocal resonance). All pneumothoraces are best diagnosed by seeing a lung edge on X-ray which is clearest on an expiratory film. Conditions predisposing to pneumothorax include:

- emphysematous bullae;

- tuberculosis—often with a small effusion; and
- bronchial asthma.

Other rare causes include staphylococcal pneumonia, carcinoma, occupational lung disease and connective tissue disorders, e.g. Marfan's and Ehlers–Danlos syndrome

Management (of spontaneous pneumothorax)

Often no therapy is required if the pneumothorax is small. Spontaneous recovery occurs in 3–4 weeks. Indications for aspiration of air are:

- tension pneumothorax (an acute emergency)
- severe dyspnoea
- collapse of more than 50% of the total lung field on chest X-ray.

Aspirate using a 16-gauge cannula and three-way tap. If this fails, insert an intercostal tube with a valve or water seal. When the lung is re-expanded, X-ray the chest. If the lung remains expanded for 24h the tube may be removed and if not, suction should be applied to the tube.

Rarely, a continuing air leak persists from the lung into the pleural space (bronchopleural fistula). Pleurodesis with defibrinated blood, camphor in oil or surgical pleurectomy may be required.

Hyperventilation syndrome

Breathlessness in the absence of abnormal clinical signs and increased by emotion (e.g. clinical examination and ward rounds) should never be described as psychogenic until the following diagnoses have been excluded:

- early pulmonary congestion of left ventricular failure;
- silent multiple pulmonary emboli (lung scan may be diagnostic);
- lymphangitis carcinomatosa;
- interstitial fibrotic pulmonary infiltrations;
- metabolic acidosis (e.g. uraemia, diabetic ketosis); and
- respiratory muscle weakness.

The chest X-ray may appear normal in all of these at the time of presentation.

The hyperventilation syndrome may be the presenting symptom of psychiatric disease and the patient should be asked about symptoms of anxiety, depression and enquiries made about personality previously. The breathlessness is usually episodic and not directly related in degree to exertion (often even occurring at rest). It is frequently described as an inability to take a deep breath or shortage of oxygen. There are associated symptoms of hypocapnia (tingling in the fingers, dizziness, headache, heaviness in the chest, cramp). Tetany may occur with carpopedal spasm. Spirometry usually gives a disorganized trace but the FEV_1 and FVC are normal when obtained.

Fibrosing alveolitis (diffuse interstitial pulmonary fibrosis)

Clinical features

The disease begins in middle age and presents with progressive dyspnoea and dry cough, usually without wheeze or sputum. The typical signs are clubbing, cyanosis and crepitations in the mid and lower lung fields. Polyarthritis is common. There is an association with the collagen diseases, particularly rheumatoid arthritis. The disease usually progresses slowly, but occasionally is very rapid (Hamman–Rich syndrome).

Investigation

The arterial Po_2 is reduced and hyperventilation may cause a reduction in Pco_2. Spirometry (p. 62) demonstrates a restrictive pattern, i.e. a grossly reduced FVC with rapid initial exhalation of this small volume, thus giving a normal or high FEV_1/FVC. The transfer factor is reduced.

Chest X-ray shows diffuse bilateral basal nodular–reticular shadowing which extends upwards as the disease progresses. The differential diagnosis of the chest X-ray includes other causes of diffuse pulmonary fibrosis and infiltration: occupational dust lung diseases, sarcoidosis, scleroderma, lymphangitis carcinomatosa, collagen diseases, miliary tuberculosis, radiation pneumonitis, drugs (busulphan and other cytotoxic drugs, nitrofurantoin, paraquat), histoplasmosis, coccidioidomycosis and histiocytosis X. Clinically the problem is less difficult. Lung biopsy, either open by thoracotomy or transbronchial via a bronchoscope, may be diagnostic. Bronchoalveolar lavage shows lymphocytes in sarcoidosis and neutrophils in fibrosing alveolitis.

Management

The disease is progressive and, though steroids are usually given, sometimes in combination with azathioprine or cyclophosphamide, response is variable. The patient eventually dies with severe hypoxia. Lung transplantation should be considered.

Adult respiratory distress syndrome

Adult respiratory distress syndrome (ARDS) refers to acute progressive respiratory failure starting hours to days after a number of pulmonary or systemic insults. These include sepsis, trauma (lung contusion or non-thoracic), aspiration (gastric contents, toxins, smoke), shock from any cause, disseminated intravascular coagulation, and air and fat emboli. It can occur in association with pneumonia, and may be drug-induced (heroin, barbiturates). The pulmonary oedema is due to capillary leakage rather than the elevated left atrial pressure of heart failure.

It is characterized by:
- arterial hypoxia;
- reduced thoracic compliance;

- normal pulmonary capillary wedge pressure; and
- diffuse infiltrates on chest X-ray.

Treatment should be aimed at the underlying condition, although in many cases the lung injury has already occurred. Ventilation with positive end-expiratory pressure is usually necessary. Neither steroids nor surfactant have been shown to be of benefit in sepsis-associated ARDS. Mortality is high (50–70%) and associated with sepsis, organ failure and age.

Cardiovascular Disease

Ischaemic heart disease

This presents as a cardiac chest pain or myocardial infarction. Less commonly, it presents as an arrhythmia or conduction defect, or heart failure.

Myocardial ischaemia is normally due to atherosclerosis but cardiac pain is also produced by:

- aortic valve disease (p. 381);
- paroxysmal tachycardias; and
- severe anaemia, cardiomyopathy, coronary artery embolism and vasculitis are all rare causes.

CORONARY ATHEROSCLEROSIS

Examination of atherosclerotic plaques suggests an interaction between blood constituents and cellular elements of the arterial wall. Alteration of normal endothelial cell function may allow accumulation of macrophages, which form foam cells and provoke proliferation of smooth-muscle cells and connective tissue. Cholesterol crystals and other lipids accumulate at the base of plaques, which is covered by a fibrous cap. Plaque rupture leads to thrombosis.

Factors associated with coronary atherosclerosis:

- Sex: men more than women, particularly before the menopause
- Age: steady increase with age
- Smoking is a powerful risk factor for coronary heart disease. Cessation is associated with significant reduction in risk, which decreases by half after 1 year, and approaching that of never-smokers after several years.
- Hypertension: risk of coronary heart disease rises progressively with increasing blood pressure. Although most antihypertensive trials have shown a lower than expected reduction in risk, this may reflect the short duration of the trials.
- Obesity: central adiposity is a better marker for coronary heart disease risk than the overall level of obesity.
- Hyperlipidaemia: coronary heart disease is associated with raised total cholesterol and low ratio of total cholesterol to high-density lipoprotein (HDL) cholesterol. Hypertriglyceridaemia appears to be associated more with risk of myocardial infarction than coronary atherosclerosis, possibly because it affects coagulation.
- Diabetes mellitus: hyperlipidaemia in diabetics is a powerful risk factor.
- Alcohol: the association between coronary heart disease and alcohol is J-shaped—the lowest risk is associated with moderate alcohol intake.

Diagnosis

The diagnosis of angina is clinical, based on the characteristic history:
- site—central chest;
- character—usually tight, heavy, crushing;
- radiation—to arms, epigastrium, jaw or back;
- precipitation—by effort or emotion, particularly after meals or in the cold;
- relief—within minutes by rest or sublingual or buccal glyceryl trinitrate.

There are no specific physical signs. A non-cardiac cause is favoured by continuation for several days, precipitation by changes in posture or deep breathing, the ability to continue normal activities, and lack of relief by rest. The commoner alternatives in the differential diagnosis are oesophageal pain and musculoskeletal pain.

Unstable angina refers to:
- angina of effort of recent onset with no previous history;
- increased frequency and/or severity of pre-existing angina; and
- angina at rest.

Investigation

Electrocardiogram

The electrocardiogram (ECG) is usually normal between attacks, but may show evidence of old myocardial infarction, T-wave flattening or inversion, bundle branch block or signs of left ventricular hypertrophy. ST segment depression is usually seen during attacks, and may be provoked by exercise testing. A negative exercise test indicates a very good prognosis. Coronary arteriography has a small morbidity and mortality (<0.1%) which varies from centre to centre. It may supply unequivocal evidence of arterial narrowing, and define its site to guide revascularization procedures. Radionuclide studies can give additional information (p. 96).

Management

Risk factors should be identified and advice given about stopping smoking, losing weight and taking regular exercise. Treat hypertension (p. 373) and specific hyper-lipidaemic syndromes (p. 231). Anaemia should be investigated and treated.

Sublingual glyceryl trinitrate remains the mainstay of treatment. The major side effect is headache. It should be taken for pain, and prophylactically before known precipitating events. Treatment with oral nitrates, β-blockers and calcium

TRIALS

The **RITA (Randomized Intervention Treatment of Angina) study** compared the long-term results of PTCA and CABG. Interim results after a mean follow-up of 2.5 years showed that both procedures were effective in relieving symptoms, although antianginal therapy was prescribed more widely following PTCA. Over 2 years, 38% of the PTCA group and 11% of the CABG group experienced a major cardiac event. *Lancet* 1993; **341**: 573–580.

EAST (Emory Angioplasty versus Surgery Trial) compared PTCA and CABG in 392 patients followed over 3 years. CABG achieved a more complete revascularization and was associated with a rein-tervention rate of 13% at 3 years, compared with 54% in patients undergoing PTCA. *N Engl J Med* 1994; **331**: 1044–1050.

The **CABRI (Coronary Angioplasty versus Bypass Revasculariza-tion Investigation) trial** compared PTCA and CABG in 1054 patients with symptomatic multivessel disease. Both treatments were effective in relieving angina at equivalent risk of myocardial infarc-tion or death. However, patients undergoing PTCA were more likely to require intervention and to have clinically significant angina at 1 year. *Lancet* 1995; **346**: 1179–1184.

The **BARI (Bypass Angioplasty Revascularization Investigation)**. Investigators compared angioplasty with coronary artery bypass surgery as initial treatment in 1829 patients with multivessel disease. Initial treatment by angioplasty did not compromise 5-year survival, although subsequent revascularization was required more often than in patients treated by surgery in the first instance. In diabetics 5-year survival was better in patients treated initially by surgery. *N Engl J Med* 1996; **335**: 217–225.

antagonists provides effective control of symptoms, although there is no evidence that they reduce the risk of myocardial infarction or death. Nicorandil, a potassium channel activator, can be useful. Low-dose aspirin (75 mg/day) reduces the risk of acute coronary events and myocardial infarction in patients with stable angina.

Medical management versus revascularization

Coronary angiography should be considered if non-invasive testing reveals:
* ST- or T-wave changes at low levels of exercise (exercise testing, p. 92)
* blood pressure fall during exercise
* significant left ventricular dysfunction (echocardiography, p. 93)
* multiple or large transient perfusion defects (radionuclide studies, p. 96).

Surgery improves prognosis in patients with left main stem, three-vessel disease and probably two-vessel disease. About 20% of coronary artery bypass grafts (CABG) occlude during the first year. Comparisons between CABG and percutaenous transluminal coronary angioplasty (PTCA) are currently in progress.

Patients with unstable angina should be admitted to hospital, and precipitating factors (anaemia, arrhythmia, fever) identified and treated. Anti-ischaemic drug therapy is escalated (nitrates and β-blockers with addition of calcium antagonist if symptoms persist) and heparin and aspirin given. The role of coronary arteriography and revascularization, and the timing of such therapy, are at present unclear.

Myocardial infarction

The World Health Organization (WHO) diagnosis of myocardial infarction depends on the presence of at least two of the following:
* typical chest pain for more than 20 min;
* ECG changes with development of Q waves, bundle branch block or ST segment elevation or depression of at least 0.1 mV for 24 h; and
* increased cardiac enzymes (creatine kinase, aspartate transaminase or lactate dehydrogenase).

Aetiology

The commonest cause is thrombosis in association with an atheromatous plaque which has cracked or ruptured. Necrosis of muscle supplied by the vessel is followed by scarring. Major risk factors are:
* smoking;
* hypercholesterolaemia;
* diabetes; and
* hypertension.

Rare causes (consider in young patients without risk factors) are:
* coronary artery embolism — from thrombus in left atrium or ventricle, or mitral or aortic valve lesions;

- congenital abnormalities such as anomalous origin of coronary artery from pulmonary artery;
- coronary artery vasculitis—consider Kawasaki disease in children; and
- dissecting aneurysm with coronary artery occlusion.

The size and location of the infarct depend on which artery is involved (Fig. 19.1), and the presence of any collateral supply. Occlusion of:
- left anterior descending affects the anterior wall of the left ventricle, and sometimes the septum;
- right coronary artery involves the inferior part of the left ventricle, as well as part of the septum and right ventricle;
- left circumflex involves the lateral or posterior walls of the left ventricle.

The infarct may extend from endocardium to epicardium (transmural), or involve only the subendocardial region.

Symptoms

Ask about:
- Pain—onset, duration (over 20 min), character (often tight or compressing), site and radiation (usually chest going to arms or neck). Associated sweating, breathlessness, nausea and vomiting are common. There may be a previous history of angina or myocardial infarction.

NB   Intensity is no guide to the extent of the infarct, especially in the elderly and diabetics where pain may be absent.
- Past history of hypertension, stroke, intermittent claudication, diabetes mellitus, hyperlipidaemia.
- Family history of cardiovascular disease, hyperlipidaemia.
- Smoking.

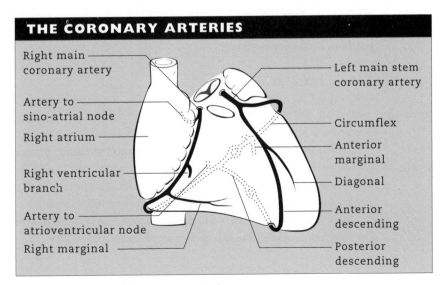

Fig. 19.1 Anatomy of the coronary arteries.

Examination

Once any distress has been alleviated by pain control there may be no signs. Examine:

- For evidence of associated diseases
  (a) xanthelasmata and xanthoma of hyperlipidaemia
  (b) evidence of diabetes, thyroid disease, diabetes mellitus, gout, cigarette smoking (smell and finger staining).
- Pulse for small volume (low cardiac output), arrhythmia.
- Blood pressure (hypotension usually indicates low cardiac output, hypertension may not be long standing).
- Jugular venous pressure (JVP) is usually normal or only slightly elevated.
- Listen to heart for
  (a) fourth heart sound (common); third heart sound if there is heart failure
  (b) pericardial friction rub
  (c) mitral regurgitation (papillary muscle dysfunction or ventricular dilatation)
  (d) ventricular septal defect (VSD; rare).
- Listen to lungs for basal crackles of heart failure.
- Fever is usual within the first few days.

Investigations

ECG

Serial ECGs typically show ST segment elevation and T-wave inversion in anterior or inferior leads, with the development of Q waves indicating full-thickness myocardial necrosis (Figs 7.9 and 7.10). Subendocardial myocardial infarction leads to ST segment and T-wave changes, but not Q waves. A normal ECG does not exclude myocardial infarction. Posterior infarction is rare and does not produce Q waves, but gives a tall R wave in V1.

Right ventricular infarction is usually associated with inferior infarction, and produces ST elevation which can be detected if right ventricular leads (V3R and V4R) are recorded by placing chest electrodes on the right side of the chest in positions equivalent to V3 and V4.

Cardiac enzymes

Creatine kinase (CK) is the marker of choice. Increase starts at 3–6 h, peaks within 24 h, and often returns to normal by 48 h. Subsequent rises imply reinfarction.

CK is formed by dimerization of two polypeptide chains, denoted B and M, giving rise to three different isoenzymes. The predominant isoenzyme in skeletal muscle is MM, whereas in brain it is BB. Cardiac muscle contains both MM and MB, and the MB isoenzyme is used in diagnosis of myocardial infarction.

Aspartate transaminase (AST) is found in cardiac and skeletal muscle, brain, liver and kidney. Peaks 24–48 h after myocardial infarction may return to normal by 72 h.

Lactate dehydrogenase (LDH) peaks at 3–4 days and may remain elevated for 2–3 weeks. It is also released from damaged skeletal muscle, liver and red cells (haemolysis).

Management

The early mortality (within 4 weeks) is 30–40%, chiefly within the first 2 h and usually from ventricular fibrillation.

Any patient suspected of having a myocardial infarction requires:
- pain relief—usually in the form of opiates;
- aspirin 300 mg to chew;
- specialist coronary care where facilities for defibrillation, resuscitation and administration of thrombolytic therapy are available.

Thrombolysis

Several studies (p. 366) in the late 1980s showed that intravenous streptokinase reduced mortality in patients reaching hospital with myocardial infarction from just over 10% to around 8%. ISIS-2 (p. 367) showed that aspirin gives additional benefit, and subsequent trials showed that other agents anisolyated plasminogen streptokinase activator complex (APSAC) and alteplase had similar effects.

Streptokinase 1.5 MU is given by intravenous infusion over 1 h. It is cheaper than alternatives, but can cause allergic reactions. It stimulates antibody formation, limiting its potential for repeated use.

APSAC shares these disadvantages, but can be given as a bolus injection. Alteplase (recombinant tissue plasminogen activator; rtPA) is not antigenic but is very expensive.

Contraindications to thrombolysis are any recent bleeding, severe hypertension (blood pressure >200/120 mmHg), active peptic ulceration, recent stroke (within last 2 months), proliferative diabetic retinopathy, severe liver or renal disease, pregnancy/lactation, bacterial endocarditis, acute pancreatitis.

β-Blockade

Intravenous β-blockade in the early stages of myocardial infarction may confer some benefit (see ISIS-1) (p. 366), but is contraindicated if there is bradycardia, hypotension, heart failure, asthma, sick-sinus syndrome or heart block (second degree, third degree or bifascicular). Long-term β-blockade beginning a few days postinfarction is routine in the absence of contraindications.

Angiotensin-converting enzyme inhibitors

Angiotensin-converting enzyme (ACE) inhibitors are beneficial in patients with heart failure following myocardial infarction, even if they are asymptomatic (ejection fraction ≤40%).

Calcium channel blockers, antiarrythmic agents, magnesium and nitrates

These should not be given routinely as they confer no benefit or are possibly harmful.

Anticoagulation

Anticoagulation should be considered to prevent deep venous thrombosis in patients slow to mobilize, or in the presence of atrial fibrillation or left ventricular aneurysm.

Complications

Shock (10% of hospital admissions)

The patient is hypotensive, pale, cold, sweaty, and cyanosed. A Swan–Ganz (left pulmonary artery flotation; p. 96) catheter will distinguish pump failure (pulmonary artery wedge pressure high) from hypovolaemia (wedge pressure low). Arrhythmias are common. Treatment is with:

- oxygen
- diuretics if pulmonary oedema and high pulmonary artery wedge pressure
- vasodilators — ACE inhibitors (arterial and venous) or nitrates (venous) if blood pressure allows
- inotropes—dopamine and dobutamine increase cardiac contractility by stimulating β_1-receptors in cardiac muscle. Low doses of dopamine ($<5\,\mu g/kg$ per min) induce vasodilatation and increase renal perfusion, whereas higher doses cause vasoconstriction and may exacerbate heart failure.

The overall mortality exceeds 70%. A pulmonary artery flotation catheter can also be used to monitor the response to treatment.

Arrhythmias

Sinus tachycardia. Usually requires no treatment. May be a sign of heart failure.

Supraventricular extrasystoles. Common, but rarely require treatment.

Supraventricular tachycardia. First try unilateral carotid sinus massage or Valsalva manoeuvre.

Adenosine (3 mg by rapid injection into central or large peripheral vein) usually causes rapid reversion to sinus rhythm. Its short half-life (10 s) means that side effects (facial flushing, bronchospasm, bradycardia) are usually short-lived.

Verapamil may be preferable in asthmatics, but should be avoided if hypotension or heart failure are present. Verapamil is contraindicated in patients taking β-blockers.

Disopyramide and amiodarone may be useful in resistant supraventricular tachycardia.

Cardioversion under short-acting general anaesthesia is used when rapid results are required and other procedures have failed.

Atrial flutter and fibrillation. Oral digoxin usually slows the ventricular rate. Amiodarone can also be used. Consider direct current (DC) cardioversion.

NB Supraventricular arrhythmias may be caused by digoxin toxicity (serum levels helpful), particularly if there is hypokalaemia. In this situation, stop digoxin and consider β-blockade. Avoid DC shock, which may produce resistant ventricular fibrillation.

Sinus or nodal bradycardia. May be due to sedation, particularly with opiates. If the rate is <50 beats/min, and the patient is hypotensive, give atropine 0.6 mg intravenously and repeat twice if necessary. If unsuccessful, consider cardiac pacing.

Heart block. All degrees of heart block are more serious if they complicate anterior rather than inferior infarcts.
* first-degree: requires no therapy
* second-degree: monitor and consider atropine. Many physicians would consider cardiac pacing for Mobitz type 2 with anterior infarcts
* third-degree (complete heart block): atropine and isoprenaline may be helpful while awaiting cardiac pacing.

NB Complete heart block is commoner in inferior myocardial infarctions because the atrioventricular nodal artery is a branch of the right coronary artery; complete heart block complicating anterior infarction is ominous since it implies a large muscle infarction.

Ventricular tachycardia. Try lignocaine 100 mg intravenously as a bolus over a few minutes. If successful, continue as an infusion of 2–4 mg/min. If this fails, mexiletine (100–250 mg intravenously over 10 min), or amiodarone (5 mg/kg into central vein over at least 20 min) can be used, but proceed to DC cardioversion without delay if no success.

NB Lignocaine does not reduce mortality when used prophylactically following myocardial infarction.

Ventricular fibrillation. This is frequently within 6 h of myocardial infarction. A precordial thump should be followed by DC cardioversion (200 J, then further 200 J, followed by 360 J if unsuccessful). If ventricular fibrillation persists, perform external cardiac massage with artificial ventilation if not already started; give adrenaline 1 mg intravenously and repeat DC cardioversion.

Electromechanical dissociation (complexes on ECG with no pulse). Consider and, if indicated, treat hypovolaemia, pneumothorax, cardiac tamponade, pulmonary embolism, electrolyte imbalance, hypothermia. External cardiac massage and artificial ventilation. Give adrenaline 1 mg intravenously and consider calcium chloride (10 ml of 10% intravenously).

TRIALS

GISSI-1 (Gruppo Italiano per lo Studio della Sopravvvenza nell'- Infarto Miocardio) studied the use of conventional treatment (including heparin, nitrates, calcium antagonists, antiplatelet drugs, β-blockers) with or without streptokinase in 11712 patients admitted within 12 h of chest pain suggestive of myocardial infarction. Streptokinase reduced both in-hospital and 1-year mortality, and was of most benefit if administered within 3 h. *Lancet* 1986; **i**: 397–401; *Lancet* 1987; **ii**: 871–874.

GISSI-2 compared streptokinase with alteplase, either with or without heparin, in up to 20891 patients within 6 h of myocardial infarction. Concomitant aspirin and atenolol was recommended. Streptokinase and alteplase had similar beneficial effects, but the addition of heparin had no apparent benefit. *Lancet* 1990; **336**: 65–71; *Lancet* 1990; **336**: 71–75.

GISSI-3 studied the effects of lisinopril and/or transdermal glyceryl trinitrate on 19394 patients admitted within 24 h of myocardial infarction. Lisinopril, but not nitrates, reduced early (6 weeks) development of heart failure and mortality. *Lancet* 1994; **343**: 1115–1122.

The **GUSTO (Global Utilization of Streptokinase and t-PA for Occluded Coronary Arteries)** investigators compared alteplase with heparin and/or streptokinase with heparin in 41021 patients within 6 h of myocardial infarction. Aspirin and atenolol were also given unless contraindicated. The results showed a small benefit in survival of alteplase over streptokinase. *N Engl J Med* 1993; **329**: 673–682.

MITI (Myocardial Infarction Triage and Intervention Investigators) found no benefit in terms of either mortality or the use of resources in a comparison of primary coronary angioplasty with thrombolytic therapy in patients with acute myocardial infarction. *N Engl J Med* 1996; **335**: 1253–1260.

The **ISIS-1 (First International Study of Infarct Survival) Collaborative Group** studied the effect of atenolol (5–10 mg iv followed by 100 mg daily for 6 days) in 16027 patients within 12 h of myocardial infarction. The results showed a short-term survival benefit of atenolol which was lost or reversed after the first year. *Lancet* 1986; **ii**: 57–66.

continued

ISIS-2 compared the use of streptokinase, or aspirin, or aspirin and streptokinase, or placebo in 41 299 patients within 24 h of myocardial infarction. Mortality at 5 weeks was reduced by all treatments, although aspirin and streptokinase was the most effective procedure. *Lancet* 1988; **ii**: 349–360.

ISIS-3 studied the effects of streptokinase, or alteplase, or APSAC in 41 299 patients within 24 h of myocardial infarction. Patients also received aspirin, alone or in combination with heparin. There was no significant difference in survival up to 6 months between patients treated with streptokinase, alteplase or APSAC. Fewer reinfarctions and more strokes were observed following alteplase compared with streptokinase. *Lancet* 1992; **339**: 753–770.

ISIS-4 studied the effect of oral captopril for 1 month, oral mononitrate for 1 month, and intravenous magnesium sulphate for 24 h in 58 050 patients presenting within 24 h of suspected myocardial infarction in a randomized factorial trial. There was a significant 7% reduction in 5-week mortality in patients treated with captopril compared with placebo. Intravenous magnesium was ineffective, and although mononitrate was safe it conferred no clear survival benefit. *Lancet* 1995; **345**: 669–685.

SAVE (Survival and Ventricular Enlargement) Trial compared the effect of captopril or placebo in 2231 patients up to 16 days post myocardial infarction with an asymptomatic ejection fraction ≤40%. Captopril was associated with a reduction of overall and cardiovascular mortality, and also reduced the risk of requiring treatment or hospitalization for heart failure. *N Engl J Med* 1992; **327**: 685–691.

In a **follow-up study of the SAVE trial patients** a substantial risk of stroke was observed during the 5 years after myocardial infarction (estimated 5-year rate of stroke 8.1%). Decreased ejection fraction and older age were independent risk factors. Anticoagulant therapy appeared to have a protective effect. *N Engl J Med* 1997; **336**: 251–257.

S4 (Scandinavian Simvastatin Survival Study) compared the effect of simvastatin or placebo in 4444 patients with established coronary heart disease (angina or post myocardial infarction) and cholesterol 5.5–8.0 mmol/l. Simvastatin reduced mortality and morbidity. *Lancet* 1994; **344**: 1383–1389.

continued

> **TRIALS** (continued)
>
> **West of Scotland Coronary Prevention Group** showed that treatment with pravastatin significantly reduced the risk of myocardial infarction and death from cardiovascular disease in middle-aged men with moderate hypercholesterolaemia and no history of myocardial infarction. *N Engl J Med* 1995; **333**: 1301–1307.
>
> The **CARE (Cholesterol and Recurrent Events)** investigators showed that cholesterol-lowering therapy may be of benefit in patients with coronary heart disease and normal cholesterol levels. *N Engl J Med* 1996; **335**: 1001–1009.

Late complications

Ventricular aneurysm occurs in 10–20%. Serious complications are heart failure, angina, arrhythmias, and emboli from thrombi within the aneurysm. There may be cardiac enlargement and abnormal cardiac pulsation (e.g. an impulse at the left sternal border). Its presence is suggested by ST segment elevation persisting in convalescence. The aneurysm may be demonstrated by echocardiography, radionuclide studies or left ventriculography. Surgical removal is indicated for heart failure or arrhythmias. Anticoagulants reduce the risk of emboli.

Papillary muscle dysfunction or rupture may cause heart failure. There is a pan-systolic or late sysytolic mitral regurgitant murmur. Echocardiography confirms the diagnosis. Surgery may be indicated.

Ruptured ventricular septum is rare. Urgent surgical repair may be required for severe heart failure.

Myocardial rupture leads to death from tamponade (unless immediate surgery is available). Dressler's (post myocardial infarction) syndrome occurs weeks or months after myocardial infarction or cardiac surgery. It is characterized by fever, pleurisy and pericarditis, and the presence of antibodies to heart muscle.

Rehabilitation

Many patients find a formal coronary rehabilitation programme valuable. It may be preceded by an exercise stress test to assess suitability. Dietary and health education is given. An optimistic attitude to the future, together with an active involvement in self-rehabilitation, should be encouraged. The importance of stopping smoking must be stressed, and strategies to help smokers, including repeated supportive advice and nicotine replacement therapy, used if needed.

The uncomplicated case may be discharged without excess risk at 7–10 days. Patients should be encouraged to increase activity gradually over 1–2 months, when return to work can be considered. Patients should not drive for at least 1 month after the event.

Long-term pharmacological treatments

The benefits of aspirin persist for at least 4 years.

β-Blockers, if tolerated, reduce mortality (mostly sudden death) and morbidity (non-fatal infarction for at least 2–3 years).

Diet and lipid-lowering drugs reduce mortality in patients with high cholesterol (see Trials above).

Heart failure

Heart failure has a prevalence in the UK, Scandinavia and the USA of about 1% overall, and 10% in the elderly. Annual mortality in severe cases exceeds 50%.

New York Heart Association classification
- Class I: no limitation of normal physical activity
- Class II: symptoms on moderate or severe exertion
- Class III: symptoms on mild exertion
- Class IV: inability to perform any physical activity without discomfort, which may be present at rest.

Pathophysiology

Cardiac size increases as a result of dilatation or muscle fibre hypertrophy.

In response to increased volume load, ventricular volume increases (the heart dilates). This is initially beneficial as the strength of contraction increases as the cardiac muscle is stretched (Starling's law). However, contraction declines as stretch becomes extreme.

Cardiac output is diminished by definition, resulting in reduced perfusion to vital organs.

Sympathetic nervous activity and plasma noradrenaline levels increase, leading to increased heart rate, myocardial contractility and arterial and venous tone.

Renal blood flow is reduced, leading to activation of the renin–angiotensin system (p. 373). *Angiotensin II* causes vasoconstriction and, by stimulating aldosterone, sodium and water retention. These mechanisms increase both preload and afterload.

Preload is the extent to which cardiac muscle is stretched prior to contraction; it is reflected by the ventricular volume at the end of diastole — the *end-diastolic volume*.

Afterload is the load the ventricle contracts against during systole, which is produced by the aortic valve and the arterial tree.

Heart failure is therefore associated with vasoconstriction through angiotensin II and sympathetic nervous activity, and salt and water retention. These mechanisms initially increase cardiac output (Starling's law) and blood pressure, but do so at the expense of reduced peripheral blood flow and circulatory congestion.

Aetiology

It is important to identify the underlying cause:
- ischaemic heart disease with left ventricular dysfunction (the commonest cause);
- hypertension;
- cardiomyopathy;
- valvular heart disease;
- congenital heart disease (atrial septal defect, ventricular septal defect);
- pericardial disease; and
- in high-output heart failure excessive cardiac workload may result from anaemia, Paget's disease and, thyrotoxicosis.

There may also be precipitating factors:
- anaemia;
- fluid retention (non-steroidal drugs, renal disease);
- infection (especially of the lungs with reduced Po_2; endocarditis);
- pulmonary emboli; and
- drugs with negative inotropism (β-blockers, most anti-arrhythmic drugs except digoxin).

Clinical features

In *left heart failure* left ventricular end-diastolic pressure (LVEDP) is increased. Pulmonary congestion causes dyspnoea, orthopnoea and paroxysmal nocturnal dyspnoea, and leads to acute pulmonary oedema. Fatigue results from reduced muscle blood flow. Signs are tachycardia, third heart sound, crackles at the lung bases and pulmonary effusions.

Right heart failure is usually due to pulmonary congestion of left heart failure. It also complicates lung disease (cor pulmonale), pulmonary hypertension, right ventricular infarction, or pulmonary or tricuspid valve disease. Signs are raised JVP, hepatomegaly (cardiac cirrhosis may occur if chronic), oedema and ascites.

Investigation

All patients require:
- Full blood count (FBC) to exclude anaemia.
- Urea and electrolytes to look for evidence of impaired renal function as a cause of fluid retention or a consequence of reduced renal perfusion.
- Chest X-ray for evidence of cardiomegaly, venous hypertension or pulmonary oedema
- ECG for evidence of myocardial ischaemia or infarction, left ventricular hypertrophy, arrhythmia.
- Echocardiography to exclude valvular or pericardial disease and assess left ventricular function.

Further investigations, including cardiac radionuclide studies, exercise testing and coronary angiography, may be indicated.

TRIALS

ACE inhibitors

The **Cooperative North Scandinavian Enalapril Survival Study (CONSENSUS)** compared the effect of enalapril (2.5–20 mg bd) or placebo (in addition to conventional treatment including digoxin, diuretics, vasodilators), on mortality, morbidity (NYHA class), and heart size in 253 patients with NYHA class IV heart failure. Enalapril reduced mortality, improved NYHA class and decreased heart size. *N Engl J Med* 1987; **316**: 1429–1435.

The **SLOVD (Studies of Left Ventricular Dysfunction)** trials studied the effects of enalapril in patients with symptomatic or asymptomatic left ventricular failure.

SOLVD Treatment compared enalapril (2.5 or 5 mg bd titrating up 10 mg bd) with placebo in the treatment of 2569 patients with symptomatic heart failure (ejection fraction ≤35%). Mortality and hospitalization rate were both reduced by enalapril. *N Engl J Med* 1991; **325**: 293–302.

SOLVD Prevention compared enalapril (2.5–10 mg bd) with placebo in 4228 patients with asymptomatic heart failure (ejection fraction ≤35%). Enalapril reduced the incidence of heart failure and related hospitalization and mortality, but did not affect overall mortality. *N Engl J Med* 1992; **327**: 685–691.

The **Acute Infarction Ramipril Efficacy (AIRE) and AIRE Extension (AIREX)** studies assessed the long-term (mean follow up 59 months) effect of ramipril compared with placebo in 603 patients with heart failure after myocardial infarction. Treatment with ramipril resulted in a large and sustained reduction in mortality (relative risk reduction 36%). *Lancet* 1997; **349**: 1493–1497.

Other vasodilators

The **Vasodilator–Heart Failure Trial (VHeFT II)** compared enalapril (5 mg bd increasing to 10 mg bd) with hydralazine and isosorbide dinitrate in 804 men. Enalapril improved prognosis, despite evidence that hydralazine and isosorbide had superior haemodynamic effects. *N Engl J Med* 1991; **325**: 303–310.

continued

TRIALS (continued)

Digoxin

The **Randomized Assessment of the Effect of Digoxin on Inhibitors of the Angiotensin Converting Enzyme (RADIANCE)** studied 178 patients with stable NYHA class II or III heart failure who were in sinus rhythm whilst taking digoxin, diuretics and an ACE inhibitor. Patients were randomized to continue digoxin or switch to placebo for 12 weeks. Patients withdrawn from digoxin suffered a significant reduction in functional capacity and quality of life. *N Engl J Med* 1993; **329**: 1–7.

Echocardiography (p. 93)

In dilated cardiomyopathy both end-diastolic and end-systolic dimensions are increased, and shortening fraction reduced.

Hypertrophic cardiomyopathy is suggested by thickening of the left and/or right ventricle or interventricular septum in the absence of aortic stenosis or hypertension. There is typically anterior motion of the mitral valve during systole, and mid systolic closure of the aortic valve. Doppler can be used to detect a pressure gradient across the left ventricular outflow tract.

Thickening of stenotic valves, often with calcification, gives rise to intense echoes with limited movement of the valve leaflets. Doppler can be used to assess pressure gradients across stenosed valves, and is extremely sensitive in detecting valve regurgitation.

Pericardial effusion appears as an echo-free space around the heart. If tamponade develops ventricular wall movement is reduced.

Radionuclide studies

Ejection fraction is reduced and there may be dilatation of the heart. A fall in ejection fraction on exercise is a poor prognostic sign.

Regional abnormalities of the ventricular muscle usually indicate myocardial ischaemia or infarction. Regional paradoxical movement suggests an aneurysm.

Treatment

- *Diuretics* form an essential part of therapy. Frusemide 40 mg daily or bumetanide 1 mg daily are usually effective. Higher doses may be required and synergism between thiazide and loop diuretics can be exploited. Careful monitoring of fluid status and renal function is required.
- *ACE inhibitors* have beneficial effects on all classes of heart failure (see Trials above). They should be considered in all patients, even if asymptomatic. Use may be limited by side effects which include hypotension, renal impairment, hyperkalaemia and cough.

- *Hydralazine* and *isosorbide* improve symptoms, exercise tolerance and possibly survival, but the survival benefit of ACE inhibitors appears superior.
- *Digoxin* is indicated for control of concomitant atrial fibrillation. Recent studies have also shown a benefit in patients with heart failure in sinus rhythm (see Trials, p. 371).

Hypertension

Aetiology

In over 90% of cases no specific cause is found and the hypertension is known as essential. The aetiology is probably multifactorial. Predisposing factors include:
- increasing age;
- obesity; and
- excessive alcohol intake.
  Hypertension may be secondary to:
- renal disease;
- endocrine disease — Cushing's syndrome, Conn's syndrome, phaeochromocytoma, arcomegaly;
- contraceptive pill;
- eclampsia; and
- coarctation of the aorta.

Genetic factors

Blood pressure levels show strong familial aggregation which cannot be accounted for by shared environment alone. However, the genetic and environmental factors contributing to hypertension are likely to be extremely diverse, confounding the search for responsible genes. Attention has principally been directed towards the identification of candidate genes. These include genes involved in the renin–angiotensin system, together with a number of important vasoconstrictor and vasodilator substances which have recently been identified.

Renin–angiotensin–aldosterone system

A number of factors, including hypotension, hypovolaemia and hyponatraemia, stimulate renin release from the juxtaglomerular apparatus. Renin converts angiotensinogen to angiotensin I, which is then converted by ACE to angiotensin II. Angiotensin II causes arteriolar vasoconstriction, activation of the sympathetic nervous system, and antidiuretic hormone (ADH) and aldosterone secretion. In the kidney angiotensin II causes a relatively greater increase in efferent (post glomerular) compared to afferent (preglomerular) arteriolar constriction, thereby maintaining glomerular filtration in the face of reduced renal perfusion.

Endothelins are a family of structurally related 21-amino-acid peptides and the most potent vasoconstrictors. At least three different isoforms exist. Endothelin-1 (ET-1) is the predominant peptide generated by vascular endothelial cells. It is generated from proendothelin-1 by the action of endothelin-converting enzyme, a metalloprotease. Two distinct endothelin receptors have been identified. ET_A receptors are highly expressed is smooth-muscle cells where they preferentially bind ET-1 and mediate vasoconstriction. ET_B receptors have equal affinity for all three endothelins. They are present on the luminal surface of vascular endothelial cells, where they promote release of endothelium-derived vasodilators, and to a lesser extent smooth-muscle cells, where they mediate vasoconstriction.

ET-1 has been implicated in the pathophysiology of a number of conditions involving vasoconstriction, including heart failure, pulmonary hypertension, sub-arachnoid haemorrhage, Raynaud's disease and Printzmetal angina.

Nitric oxide (NO, originally named endothelial-derived relaxing factor) is produced by oxidation of the guanidine-nitrogen terminal of L-arginine, forming NO and citrulline. Production of NO is regulated via activity of NO synthase, a predominantly cytosolic calcium-calmodulin-requiring enzyme which is similar in structure to cytochrome P450 enzymes. Two distinct types of the enzyme have been identified, designated constitutive and inducible.

Constitutive NO synthase is a calcium-calmodulin-requiring enzyme that is responsible for the transient release of small (picomolar) quantities of NO from vascular endothelium, platelets, mast cells, adrenal medulla and some neurons.

Enzyme activity is increased by:
- inflammatory mediators such as thrombin, histamine, bradykinin, serotonin and leukotriene C_4, which raise intracellular calcium;
- mechanical forces such as shear stress;
- acetylcholine.

Inducible NO synthase is not dependent on calcium-calmodulin and causes a sustained release of larger (nanomolar) amounts of NO from activated macrophages, neutrophils, vascular endothelium and microglial cells. It is induced by bacterial endotoxin, interleukin-1 (IL-1), tumour necrosis factor and interferon-γ.

Pharmacology of nitric oxide

NO mediates the action of some commonly used vasodilators. Glyceryl trinitrate and organic nitrate esters react with thiols such as cysteine and glutathione to yield unstable intermediates which release NO. Sodium nitroprusside spontaneously releases NO.

Analogues of L-arginine such as L-NG-monomethyl arginine (L-NMMA) and L-nitroarginine methyl ester (L-NAME) act as inhibitors of NO production. Although yet to enter clinical practice, such agents offer the possibility of novel therapies for conditions such as septic shock.

Prostacyclin is produced by endothelial cells, platelets and monocytes via a phospholipase A_2 (PLA_2)-dependent pathway, and causes smooth-muscle cell relaxation, and also inhibition of platelet aggregation, via intracellular increases in cyclic 3′,5′-adenosine monophosphate (cAMP). Prostacyclin is synthesized in response to the same inflammatory mediators which raise cytoplasmic free calcium as NO. IL-1 and tumour necrosis factor increase the activity of the enzymes mediating prostacyclin generation.

Atrial natriuretic factor is synthesized in atrial granules and released predominantly in response to atrial wall distension.

Vascular and renal effects include:

- vasodilatation and decreased blood pressure;
- increased renal blood flow and glomerular filtration rate (GFR); and
- inhibition of sodium and water reabsorption in proximal and distal renal tubules (natriuresis and diuresis).

The serum level is often elevated in oedematous conditions, but there may be tubular resistance to the hormone's actions.

Pathophysiology

In its early stages hypertension is thought to be characterized by increased cardiac output with normal peripheral resistance. As hypertension progresses peripheral resistance increases and cardiac output returns to normal.

Left ventricular hypertrophy (LVH) may be present even in mild hypertension, and is associated with increased risk of cardiac dysfunction, atherosclerosis, arrhythmias and sudden death.

Diagnosis

- ECG: S wave in V1 and R wave in V5 or V6 $\geq$ 35 mm. May be associated with ST segment depression or T-wave inversion ('strain pattern').
- Echo: much more sensitive than ECG. The left ventricular mass index (LVMI) is calculated from left ventricular wall thickness and left ventricular internal diameters in systole and diastole.
- LVH present if LVMI $>$ 110 g/m^2 in women or $>$ 131 g/m^2 in men.

There is good evidence that treatment of hypertension results in regression of LVH.

Symptoms

There are usually no symptoms of hypertension.

Ask about headaches or visual disturbance (in severe or accelerated hypertension), chest pain and intermittent claudication, family history and any medication.

Examination

Measure the blood pressure at rest. If high (systolic $>$ 160 mmHg, diastolic $>$ 90 mmHg), check in both arms, and unless very severe recheck on at least three separate occasions before considering treatment. A large cuff should be used in the 10% of the population with arm circumference over 33 cm. Phase V diastolic (disappearance) should be recorded together with the patient's posture and the arm used.

Mild or moderate hypertension usually gives no other abnormalities on examination. In long-standing or severe hypertension look for evidence of LVH with an aortic ejection murmur and loud aortic second sound. The optic fundi may show evidence of retinopathy with arterial narrowing and arteriovenous narrowing (indicating atherosclerosis), haemorrhages and exudates. Papilloedema indicates the presence of malignant hypertension.

It is essential to think of less common causes:

• Observe the face for evidence of Cushing's syndrome—usually due to steroid administration.

• Examine for aortic coarctation—feel both radials and measure blood pressure in both arms. Look for radial-femoral delay, weak femoral pulses, bruits of the coarctation and scapular anastomoses which may produce visible pulsations.

• Listen for an epigastric or paraumbilical bruit of renal artery stenosis.

• Feel for polycystic kidneys.

• Think of chronic renal disease, phaeochromocytoma (rare) and primary hyperaldosteronism (very rare).

Investigation

Routine investigation of hypertension is aimed at detecting treatable disease (usually renal), and assessing cardiac and renal function.

All patients require

• ECG to assess left ventricular size, and if abnormal a chest X-ray;

• urinalysis for blood and protein. If abnormal a midstrean specimen of urine for cells, casts, proteinuria and evidence of infection, and 24-h urine collection to measure creatinine clearance and protein loss;

• blood, urea and electrolytes to assess renal function and look for hypokalaemic alkalosis of Conn's or Cushing's syndrome (or diuretic therapy);

• 24-h urine collection to measure vanilly mandelic acid (VMA) or 4-hydroxy-3-methoxymandelic acid (HMMA) output (phaeochromocytoma).

If renovascular disease (p. 380), Cushing's syndrome (p. 214), Conn's syndrome (p. 216), phaeochromocytoma (p. 218) or aortic coarctation (p. 394) are suspected, further investigation should be performed.

Treatment

Patients should attempt to achieve an ideal weight, avoid excessive alcohol or salt and take regular exercise.

Thiazide diuretics inhibit distal tubular sodium reabsorption. Low doses (e.g. bendrofluazide 2.5 mg daily) have maximal antihypertensive effect. Higher doses confer little additional antihypertensive effect, but cause more marked adverse metabolic effects, including hypokalaemia, hyponatraemia, hypochloraemic alkalosis, hyperuricaemia, hyperglycaemia and hyperlipidaemia.

β-Blockers reduce blood pressure and cardiac output, block peripheral adrenoceptors and alter baroreceptor reflex sensitivity. β-Blockers with intrinsic sympathomimetic activity (e.g. acebutalol, pindolol) stimulate as well as block adrenergic receptors, and may cause less bradycardia and coldness of the extremities. Water-soluble β-blockers (e.g. atenolol, nadolol) are less likely to cross the blood–brain barrier and cause sleep disturbance. Some β-blockers have less effect on β_2-(bronchial) receptors (e.g. atenolol, bisoprolol, metoprolol). They are

TRIALS

Most studies showing beneficial effects of antihypertensives have used diuretics or β-blockers. Recent trials studying the effect of antihypertensives on blood pressure (BP) control, morbidity and mortality are summarized below.

The **MAPHY (Metoprolol Atherosclerosis Prevention in Hypertension)** study compared propranolol and thiazide diuretics (hydrochlorothiazide or bendroflumethiazide) in 3234 men aged 40–64 with diastolic BP 100–130 mmHg. Additional hypertensives were allowed if BP did not respond.

The findings suggest that metoprolol produces greater 5-year survival benefits than thiazide diuretics, being associated with significant reductions in total mortality, cardiovascular mortality, cardiovascular events, coronary mortality and stroke mortality. *Hypertension* 1991; **17**: 579–588: *Am J Hypertens* 1991; **4**: 151–158.

The **IPPPSH (International Prospective Primary Prevention Study in Hypertension)** compared oxprenolol with placebo in 6357 patients with diastolic BP 100–125 mmHg. Additional hypertensives were allowed if BP did not respond.

BP was reduced more effectively in the group receiving oxprenolol, but there was no difference in the incidence of sudden death, cerebrovascular accidents or myocardial infarction between the two groups. *J Hypertens* 1985; **3**: 379–392.

The **HAPPHY (Heart Attack Primary Prevention in Hypertension)** trial compared β-blockers and diuretics in 6569 men aged 40–64 years with diastolic BP 100–130 mmHg. If monotherapy failed, additional drugs were used. After a mean follow-up of 45.1 months there were no significant differences in BP control or cardiovascular events between the two groups. *J Hypertens* 1987; **5**: 561–572.

The **MRC young hypertensives trial** compared bendrofluazide, propranolol and placebo in the treatment of 17 354 patients aged 35–64 with diastolic BP 90–109 mmHg. Additional hypertensives were allowed if BP did not respond.

Bendrofluazide and propranolol were equally effective at lowering BP. Active treatment did not significantly influence overall mortality, nor overall coronary events at 5 years. However, the incidence of cardiovascular events and the incidence of stroke were both reduced by active treatment. *Br Med J* 1985; **291**: 97–104.

continued

TRIALS (continued)

The **MRC elderly hypertensives trial** compared atenolol, amiloride plus hydrochlorothiazide and placebo in the treatment of 4396 patients aged 65–75 years with systolic BP 160–209 mmHg.

After a mean follow-up of 5.8 years both active treatments were effective in reducing BP compared to placebo. Active treatment reduced stroke, coronary artery events and all cardiovascular events, compared to placebo. These benefits were entirely attributable to the diuretic treatment group. *Br Med J* 1992; **304**: 405–412.

The **EWPHE (European Working Party on Hypertension in the Elderly)** compared active therapy (first-line: hydrochlorothiazide and triamterine; second-line: methyldopa) with placebo in the treatment of 840 patients aged over 60 years with diastolic BP 90–119 mmHg. Active treatment was associated with a reduction in cardiovascular mortality, deaths from myocardial infarction and non-fatal strokes, but total mortality was not reduced. *Am J Med* 1991; **90** (suppl 3A): 1S–64S.

SHEP (Systolic Hypertension in the Elderly Program) compared chlorthalidone (switching to atenolol or reserpine if necessary) with placebo in 4736 patients aged over 60 with systolic BP 160–219 mmHg and diastolic BP less than 90 mmHg. Treatment lowered both BP and the risk of stroke and myocardial infarction. *JAMA* 1991; **265**: 3255–3264.

STOP–Hypertension (Swedish Trial in Old Patients with Hypertension) used atenolol, or hydrochlorothiazide plus amiloride, or metoprolol, or pindolol, or placebo in 1627 patients aged 70–84 with systolic BP 180–230 mmHg and diastolic BP 90 mmHg or above. Active treatment reduced BP and the incidence of fatal and non-fatal strokes. *Lancet* 1991; **338**: 1281–1285.

STONE (Shanghai Trial of Nifedipine in the Elderly) compared nifedipine with placebo in 1632 elderly hypertensives (aged 60–79 years). Nifedpine reduced the risk of stroke and severe arrhythmia. *J Hypertens* 1996; **14**: 1237–1245.

therefore relatively cardioselective, and less likely to provoke bronchospasm. However, all β-blockers should be avoided in patients with asthma or chronic obstructive airways disease.

Calcium-channel blockers inhibit inward movement of calcium ions through slow channels in cell membranes. They influence the function of cardiac myocytes, the specialized conducting cells of the heart, and vascular smooth-muscle cells.

Three classes, which differ in their relative effects on the heart and blood vessels, are available:

- the phenylalkylamine, verapamil, slows conduction in the sinoatrial and atrioventricular nodes and depresses myocardial contraction, but is less potent as a vasodilator
- the benzothiazepine, diltiazem, slows conduction in the sinoatrial and atrioventricular nodes, but causes less myocardial depression and vasodilatation
- the dihydropyridines (nifedipine, nicardipine, amlodipine, felodipine, isradipine, lacidipine) have little effect on cardiac contraction or conduction, but are more potent arterial vasodilators. Dihydropyridines vary in their effects on different vascular beds. Nimodipine acts preferentially on cerebral arteries and is used to prevent vascular spasm following subarachnoid haemorrhage.

Although calcium-channel blockers are effective treatments for hypertension, evidence that they improve long-term outcome is awaited.

ACE inhibitors inhibit conversion of angiotensin I to II, which is a vasoconstrictor and stimulates aldosterone production. They should be considered for treatment of hypertension when β-blockers or thiazides are contraindicated or ineffective. They may cause excessive hypotension, particularly in the presence of sodium depletion. First doses are usually given at bedtime, and where possible diuretic therapy should be stopped for a few days before initiating treatment. Side effects include hyperkalaemia (particularly in the presence of renal disease), persistent dry cough, blood dyscrasias, rashes and angioedema. ACE inhibitors should be used with caution in renal disease (see below).

Vasodilator antihypertensives include hydralazine and minoxidil. Sodium nitroprusside and diazoxide may be given by intravenous injection in hypertensive emergencies. *α-Blockers* cause vasodilatation and their antihypertensive effect may be profound and associated with tachycardia. They are used in combination with β-blockers in suspected cases of phaeochromocytoma, when β-blockade alone may cause hypertensive crisis due to unopposed α-adrenoreceptor effects.

Severe hypertension

Very severe hypertension (diastolic >140 mmHg) or malignant hypertension (with papilloedema) should be treated in hospital. BP should be reduced gradually with an oral β-blocker (with α-blockade if phaeochromocytoma is suspected) or calcium-channel blocker. Rapid falls in BP can precipitate myocardial ischaemia, and reduce cerebral and renal perfusion, leading to stroke and deteriorating renal function.

HYPERTENSION IN RELATION TO OTHER CONDITIONS
Diabetes

Hypertension is commoner in diabetics than non-diabetics. Possible reasons include:

- obesity;
- increased sympathetic nervous stimulation and catecholamine production;

- diabetic nephropathy; and
- insulin resistance and the associated hyperinsulinaemia.

Treatment

Thiazide diuretics (which may provoke hyperglycaemia) and β-blockers (which reduce awareness of hypoglycaemia) have potential disadvantages in diabetics. ACE inhibitors and calcium antagonists are preferable. In patients with nephropathy, BP control slows the decline in renal function. ACE inhibitors appear to have a specific renal protective effect that is independent of their antihypertensive action.

Renal disease

Hypertension is an important cause and consequence of renal disease.

Hypertension as a cause of renal disease

Estimates of the prevalence of chronic renal failure due to hypertension vary widely from 0.002% to 20%. Renal failure due to hypertension is commoner in blacks than whites, and there appears to be familial clustering of hypertensive renal disease within the black population, raising the possibility of a genetic susceptibility to hypertensive renal damage.

Renal failure is an invariable feature of *accelerated hypertension* in which acute, severe hypertension is associated with gross intimal hyperplasia leading to occlusion of the lumen of small arteries and arterioles within the kidney. Renal failure is a rapid consequence if the BP is not controlled.

Renal disease as a cause of hypertension

Hypertension may occur in renal disease as a result of:
- activation of the renin–angiotensin–aldosterone system;
- retention of salt and water;
- altered production or excretion of vasoactive substances (e.g. endothelin); and
- alterations in the structure and function of resistance vessels.

Renovascular hypertension

Ischaemia of the kidney due to renal artery disease is an important treatable cause of hypertension, although renovascular hypertension occurs in less than 1% of the total hypertensive population. The diagnosis should be considered when the onset of hypertension is abrupt, or occurs before age 30 or after age 50. The presence of an abdominal bruit, atherosclerosis elsewhere, hypokalaemia, or deteriorating renal function following treatment with ACE inhibitors are also suggestive.

Atherosclerotic renal disease accounts for approximately 70% of cases, is bilateral in 25% of cases, is commonest in elderly men, and usually results from a plaque in the first part of the renal artery. Fibrous renal artery disease occurs predominantly in young women, is frequently bilateral, and often involves the distal portion of the artery, giving rise to a beaded appearance on arteriography.

Diagnosis

Renal arteriography remains the principal method, although duplex ultrasonography, magnetic resonance imaging scanning and differential isotope renography before and after captopril may also provide useful information.

Treatment

ACE inhibitors provide an attractive means of reducing BP, but should be used with caution as renal perfusion in the presence of renal artery stenosis is dependent on angiotensin II. Rarely, ACE inhibitors cause membranous glomerulonephritis. Angioplasty is the treatment of first choice in many centres. The procedure can be repeated if restenosis occurs, and does not preclude surgical revascularization, which may have a better success rate in atherosclerotic lesions.

Pregnancy

Stroke volume and heart rate increase during pregnancy, leading to increased cardiac output. BP usually falls during early pregnancy as a result of reduced peripheral resistance, but rises towards non-pregnant values by term.

Pregnancy-induced hypertension has been defined as diastolic BP 110 mmHg or above, or two readings of 90 mmHg or above after 20 weeks in previously normotensive women (International Society for the Study of Hypertension in Pregnancy). Diastolic BP above 90 mmHg before 20 weeks suggests chronic hypertension, which is confirmed if hypertension persists after delivery.

Pre-eclampsia is defined by pregnancy-induced hypertension and proteinuria greater than 300 mg/24 h. Serum uric acid is usually raised. It may lead, often rapidly, to haemolysis, epileptic seizures, abnormal liver function tests, and low platelet count (HELP syndrome). Pre-eclampsia affects about 5% of primiparae, but is less common in subsequent pregnancies by the same father.

Treatment

Methyldopa is safe and effective in reducing BP. β-Blockers and labetalol α- + β-blocker) are also effective, but may cause intrauterine growth retardation if started early. Calcium antagonists are as yet unlicensed for use in pregnancy, and ACE inhibitors may adversely affect the fetal kidney. Diuretics interfere with physiological plasma volume expansion and should be avoided. Pre-eclampsia warrants admission to hospital. Parenteral hydralazine may be used for control of severe hypertension. Delivery cures pre-eclampsia.

Valvular heart disease

AORTIC STENOSIS
Aetiology
Valvular stenosis
- Under 60 years: calcification of congenital bicuspid valve; rheumatic valve disease

- Over 60 years: the above + degenerative calcification of otherwise normal valve.

Subvalvar aortic stenosis (rare)

Fibromuscular hypertrophy, diffuse narrowing or hypertrophic obstructive cardiomyopathy.

Supravalvar stenosis (very rare)

Congenital abnormality associated with 'fish face' and infantile hypercalcaemia.

Symptoms

There may be no symptoms initially. Later angina, dyspnoea and syncope (which may be due to the low cardiac output) occur. Left ventricular failure may occur, and sudden death is relatively common, probably due to ventricular arrhythmia.

Signs

- Regular slow-rising, slow-falling (plateau) pulse.
- Small pulse pressure (e.g. blood pressure 105/90 mmHg).
- Left ventricular hypertrophy (sustained and heaving apex).
- There may be an aortic thrill in systole.

Auscultation. An aortic systolic ejection murmur maximal in the right second intercostal space radiating to the neck with a quiet delayed or absent second sound. An ejection click indicates valvar stenosis. The murmur becomes less marked when the stenosis is very tight because the flow falls as the pump fails.
NB   Neither supravalvar nor subvalvar stenosis has an ejection click, and post stenotic dilatation is uncommon in subvalvar stenosis (see below).

Investigations

- ECG: LVH and sometimes left atrial hypertrophy. Severe stenosis in adults is unlikely if LVH is not present.
- Chest X-ray: left ventricular enlargement may not be present, even in the presence of a prominent apex beat. The aorta is small and may be dilated distal to the valve (post stenotic dilatation). The aortic valve may be calcified (best seen on lateral chest X-ray).
- Echocardiography: defines the size of the orifice and degree of thickening and calcification of the valve, which may be bicuspid. Doppler can be used to assess the gradient across the valve.
- LVH and function can also be assessed.
- Cardiac catheterization: accurate assessment of the gradient across the valve can usually be obtained by Doppler. The pressure gradient can be measured during angiography by withdrawing a catheter across the valve. In addition, coronary arteriography should be performed as 25% of patients over 50 will have significant coronary artery disease.

Complications

- Left ventricular failure.
- Infective endocarditis.
- Syncope.
- Sudden death.

Management

Valve replacement is indicated for asymptomatic severe stenosis (e.g. gradient > 50 mmHg) or for symptomatic deterioration including syncope, a rapidly enlarging heart and strain on the ECG, as soon as heart failure has occurred. Catheter studies are performed to confirm the site of the obstruction and gradient, and assess the state of the coronary arteries. Operative mortality is about 3%. (Antibiotic prophylaxis—see p. 397.)

AORTIC REGURGITATION

Aetiology

Congenital bicuspid valve and infective endocarditis are the commonest identifiable causes. Rheumatic valve disease is now a rare cause. Less common associations include seronegative arthritis (ankylosing spondylitis, Reiter's syndrome, colitic and psoriatic arthropathy), congenital lesions (coarctation of the aorta, Marfan's syndrome), syphilis and traumatic rupture.

Atherosclerosis and hypertension are of disputed importance.

Symptoms

There are usually none until dyspnoea from pulmonary oedema occurs. Angina is not common.

Signs

The pulse has a sharp rise and fall ('waterhammer' or 'collapsing') and there is a wide pulse pressure. There may be marked carotid pulsation in the neck (Corrigan's sign). The left ventricle is enlarged and the apex displaced laterally.

There is an early blowing diastolic murmur at the left sternal edge maximal in the left third and fourth intercostal spaces, heard best with the patient leaning forward with the breath held in expiration. The second sound is quiet. There is usually a systolic flow murmur which does not necessarily indicate aortic stenosis. There may be a diastolic murmur at the apex as the regurgitant aortic jet strikes the mitral valve (Austin Flint murmur, which sounds like mitral stenosis).

Investigations

- ECG: LVH.
- Chest X-ray: shows cardiac enlargement.
- Echocardiography: will demonstrate dilatation of the aortic root and the separation of the cusps. Left ventricular functions and dimension can be assessed. The

mitral valve can be affected with fluttering of the anterior leaflet and premature closure, if the regurgitation is severe.

Management
- Medical: identify any underlying cause. Antibiotic prophylaxis (treat endocarditis if present). Treatment of heart failure.
- Surgical: valve replacement should be considered for symptomatic deterioration, if the heart size increases rapidly, or if the left ventricular internal diameter is >55 mm on echocardiography in a young patient, even when asymptomatic.

Dominance of lesion in combined rheumatic aortic stenosis/aortic regurgitation
Aortic regurgitation is present if the pulse volume is high and the pulse pressure collapsing. The left ventricle is enlarged and displaced. Aortic stenosis is dominant if the pulse is of small volume ('plateau pulse') and the pulse pressure low. The ventricular apex, though hypertrophied, is not necessarily displaced.

MITRAL STENOSIS
Aetiology
Almost invariably due to rheumatic fever. It is the commonest rheumatic valve lesion and is four times more common in women than men. It develops 2–20 years after the acute episode of rheumatic fever, and 30% of patients give no history of the illness (either very mild or forgotten).

Symptoms
- Dyspnoea—nocturnal and on exertion due to pulmonary oedema.
- Palpitations from atrial fibrillation (risk of embolization).
- Haemoptysis (pulmonary hypertension, pulmonary oedema, pulmonary embolism).
- Fatigue and cold extremities from a low cardiac output. Angina may occur rarely.

Signs
- Mitral facies (dusky purple flush of the cheeks with dilated capillaries — malar flush).
- Arterial pulse: small volume (obstruction to flow at mitral valve). May be irregular (atrial fibrillation).
- Apex: the apex beat is tapping (palpable first sound).
- If pulmonary hypertension has developed there is a left parasternal heave of right ventricular hypertrophy. A diastolic thrill can be present in severe disease.

Auscultation
The mitral first sound is loud because the mitral valve is held wide open by high atrial pressure until ventricular systole slams it shut.

The length of the murmur is proportional to the degree of stenosis. The murmur starts when blood starts to flow through the mitral valve, i.e. when atrial pressure exceeds ventricular pressure. The tighter the stenosis, the higher the atrial pressure and the longer the murmur. In mild cases, exercise tachycardia may bring out the murmur and the patient should lie on the left side. The presence of an opening snap and loud first sound denotes a pliable valve. If the valve is already rigid this cannot occur. Presystolic accentuation is due to the increased flow through the valve produced by atrial systole and it is therefore absent in atrial fibrillation.

NB   Some of the signs of mitral stenosis can be given by the Austin Flint murmur of aortic regurgitation, and very rarely by a left atrial myxoma.

Assessment

The *degree of stenosis* can be assessed from the severity of dyspnoea, the duration of the murmur, and evidence of the degree of left atrial enlargement on ECG and chest X-ray. The tighter the stenosis, the longer the murmur and the closer the opening snap to the second sound.

The *mobility of the valve* is denoted by the presence of an opening snap and a loud mitral first sound (and absence of valve calcification on the chest X-ray).

Pulmonary hypertension. Fatigue, symptoms of right heart failure and a reduction in dyspnoea indicate raised pulmonary vascular resistance. The development of pulmonary hypertension is indicated by a dominant 'a' wave in the jugular venous pulse (unless in atrial fibrillation), a loud pulmonary second sound, right ventricular hypertrophy, rarely pulmonary incompetence and low-volume peripheral arterial pulse (mnemonic: April).

Presence of other lesions. Mitral regurgitation and other valve lesions must be noted and assessed, particularly if symptoms indicate surgical intervention. Atrial fibrillation may suggest a greater degree of myocardial disease, which is always present to some extent.

ECG. Atrial fibrillation may be present; if not, the P mitrale of left atrial hypertrophy. Right ventricular hypertrophy may be present.

Chest X-ray. Left atrial enlargement. Upper lobe venous congestion with septal lines (Kerley B) just above the costophrenic angles may be present with enlargement of the pulmonary arteries. The mitral valve may be calcified. Absence of calcification in pure mitral stenosis suggests that closed valvotomy may be attempted. Haemosiderosis in the lung fields is rare.

Echocardiogram. Allows measurement of the reduced diastolic closure rate of the mitral valve. It also demonstrates valve thickening and calcification (a mitral valve area of <1.5 cm² indicates critical stenosis), and gives an assessment of ventricular function.

Complications

- Pulmonary oedema.
- Right heart failure.
- Atrial fibrillation.
- Systemic embolization.
- Infective endocarditis.

Management

Prophylactic antibiotics (p. 397). Anticoagulation is indicated when atrial fibrillation develops or there is left atrial enlargement. Some physicians anticoagulate all patients with mitral stenosis prophylactically. Ventricular rate is controlled by digitalis — attempts to restore sinus rhythm are not worthwhile.

No other treatment is indicated in the absence of respiratory symptoms, evidence of enlargement of the left atrium, pulmonary hypertension (normal 25/8 mmHg).

Valvotomy or balloon valvuloplasty is usually indicated for effort dyspnoea. The operative risk is 2–5%. Re-stenosis tends to occur in 5–10 years and may require re-valvotomy or mitral valve replacement. Mitral regurgitation may result from closed valvotomy.

Mitral stenosis in pregnancy. Fluid retention in pregnancy produces a 30% increase in blood volume during the last trimester and can precipitate heart failure in the presence of mitral stenosis. Valvotomy can be performed at any time during pregnancy if indicated by the above criteria. The cardiac output falls in the last 2 months of pregnancy and most patients who can manage at that time go to term. Antibiotics should be given through labour to cover organisms of the genital tract if there are obstetric complications.

MITRAL REGURGITATION
Aetiology

- Floppy (prolapsing) mitral valve leaflets.
- Ischaemic papillary muscle dysfunction, particularly after inferior myocardial infarction.
- Severe left ventricular failure with dilatation of the mitral ring.
- Rheumatic fever.
- Rarely, cardiomyopathy, congenital malformation (Marfan's syndrome), infective endocarditis and rupture of the chordae tendinae.

Symptoms

Progressive dyspnoea develops as a result of pulmonary congestion and this is followed by right heart failure. Angina and haemoptysis are common compared with mitral stenosis. Fatigue and palpitation are common.

Signs

LVH and systolic thrill. A left parasternal heave is present and due to systolic expansion of the left atrium (rather than from right ventricular hypertrophy).

Auscultation. There is an apical pansystolic murmur radiating to the left axilla. The mitral sound is soft. There may be a third sound (of rapid ventricular filling). A short mid diastolic murmur in severe mitral regurgitation does not necessarily indicate valve stenosis.

Mitral valve prolapse produces a late systolic click and murmur which is late because the posterior leaflet of the valve only starts to leak when the ventricular pressure is at its highest. It occurs in two clinical situations. In the middle-aged and elderly it is associated with disorder of the leaflet (wear and tear), chordae or papillary muscle (post myocardial infarction). A floppy valve can be detected in 5% of young people by echocardiography. The prognosis is usually excellent, although it has been associated with arrhythmias, syncope, atypical chest pain and bacterial endocarditis. Prophylactic antibiotics should be used (p. 397).

Investigations

- *ECG*: LVH. P mitrale of left atrial hypertrophy. Atrial fibrillation is less common than in mitral stenosis.
- *Chest X-ray*: the left atrium and ventricle are enlarged, the former sometimes being enormous.
- *Echocardiography*: helps to distinguish between the various causes, and assess left ventricular function.
- *Assessment*: dominance of lesions in combined mitral stenosis/mitral regurgitation. Mitral stenosis is more likely to be the dominant lesion if the pulse volume is small (in the absence of failure) and if there is no LVH.

Complications

As with mitral stenosis, except that infective endocarditis is more common and embolism less common.

Management

Prophylactic antibiotics. Valve replacement is indicated if symptoms are severe and uncontrolled by medical therapy, or pulmonary hypertension develops.

Indications for anticoagulation are atrial fibrillation (p. 73), systemic embolism and prosthetic valves.

TRICUSPID REGURGITATION
Aetiology

- *Dilatation of the tricuspid valve ring* in right ventricular failure from any cause.

- *Rheumatic* — invariably associated with disease of mitral and/or aortic valves (rare).
- *Endocarditis* in drug addicts.

Signs

Giant 'v' waves are present in the jugular venous pulse with systolic pulsation of an enlarged liver. Right ventricular enlargement causes marked pulsation at the lower left sternal edge, and a pansystolic murmur, loudest in inspiration, is heard at the lower end of the sternum.

There is often ankle and sacral oedema, ascites and jaundice from hepatic congestion.

PULMONARY STENOSIS
Aetiology

Congenital — may follow maternal rubella. Sometimes associated with Noonan's syndrome (Turner's phenotype with normal chromosomes). Rheumatic fever and carcinoid are extremely rare causes.

Symptoms

Fatigue and syncope if stenosis is severe.

Signs

Peripheral cyanosis, low-volume pulse and a large 'a' wave in the jugular venous pressure. Right ventricular hypertrophy causes a parasternal heave. There is a systolic thrill and murmur in the pulmonary area (second left intercostal space) and an ejection click. The pulmonary component of the second sound is quiet and late.

ATRIAL MYXOMA

Atrial myxoma is very rare. It usually occurs in the left atrium and presents with features of mitral stenosis, systemic emboli and constitutional upset with fever. It can mimic bacterial endocarditis. It is best diagnosed by echocardiography where the tumour produces characteristic echoes as it moves between the mitral valve leaflets in diastole and in the atrium in systole. It is fatal unless removed surgically.

Congenital heart disease

Congenital heart disease may present as an isolated cardiac abnormality or as part of a systemic syndrome.

Maternal rubella

It is dangerous in the first 3 months of pregnancy (particularly the first month — 50% of fetuses are affected). The cardiac lesions are in three groups:
- patent ductus arteriosus;

- septal defects: atrial septal defect (ASD), ventricular septal defect (VSD), Fallot's tetralogy; and
- right-sided outflow obstruction: pulmonary valve, artery or branch stenoses.

The systemic syndrome includes cataract, nerve deafness and mental retardation.

All children are offered rubella vaccine at the age of 12 years. Fertile women given vaccine must not become pregnant in the immediate future.

If a pregnant woman is in contact with rubella, serum should be taken for antibody levels to rubella if not known. If raised, this is evidence of previous infection and there is little or no risk to the fetus. If the titre is not raised, a repeat sample is measured 3–4 weeks later (or if symptoms appear in the mother) and if the titre has risen significantly, this is evidence of recent infection. The earlier the pregnancy, the greater the risk to the fetus. Some elect for termination of pregnancy. If termination would be unacceptable, normal immunoglobulin is sometimes given after exposure to reduce the risk of clinical attack.

Down's syndrome (usually 21-trisomy)
Associated with septal defects, particularly ventricular.

Turner's syndrome (XO)
Associated with coarctation of the aorta.

Marfan's syndrome (arachnodactyly)
An autosomal dominant connective tissue disorder which affects the aortic media, eyes and limb skeleton.

Incidence: 5000 in UK (5% of cases are a new mutation). Ten per cent are seriously affected.

It is characterized by disproportionate length of the long bones which results in span exceeding height and long fingers and toes. There is frequently a high arched palate, pectus excavatum, scoliosis, little subcutaneous fat and lens dislocation with myopia. The aortic media is weak with a tendency to dilatation of the ascending aorta and aortic valve ring, resulting in aortic valve regurgitation and dissection of the aorta. Mitral regurgitation may develop. Joints tend to be hyperextensible.

WORKING CLASSIFICATION
An asterisk denotes the most frequent.

Stenosis
- Semilunar valves: aortic stenosis (supra- and subvalvar and valve stenoses), pulmonary stenosis.
- Atrioventricular valves: mitral stenosis, tricuspid stenosis.
- Major arteries: coarctation of aorta,* pulmonary artery stenosis.

Regurgitation

- Semilunar valves: aortic regurgitation, pulmonary regurgitation (very rare).
- Atrioventricular valves: mitral regurgitation, tricuspid regurgitation, Ebstein's anomaly.

Shunts

- *left-to-right*: ASD,* VSD,* patent ductus arteriosus (PDA),* aortopulmonary window.
- *Right-to-left* (cyanotic: transposition of the great vessels (frequent but die at birth), Fallot's tetralogy,* Eisenmenger's syndrome.

ATRIAL SEPTAL DEFECT

Ten per cent of congenital heart disease. Occasionally in Marfan's syndrome.

Ostium secundum (70% of ASDs) is usually uncomplicated. Compared with congenital heart defects, there is a high (late) incidence of atrial fibrillation (20%) and an extremely low incidence of endocarditis.

Ostium primum (30% of ASDs) is often complicated because it tends to involve the atrioventricular valves and produces mitral and tricuspid regurgitation and even an associated VSD. In most respects (embryology, cardiodynamics, complications and prognosis) it is quite different from ostium secundum ASD.

Symptoms

In simple lesions there are usually no symptoms, though dyspnoea occurs in 10% of cases. Symptoms usually occur for the first time in middle age. It is usually detected at routine chest X-ray.

Signs

Characteristically there is fixed wide splitting of the second sound. Flow through the defect does not itself produce a murmur but increased right heart output gives a pulmonary flow murmur and large shunts may produce a tricuspid diastolic flow murmur. In ostium primum there may be signs of the associated lesions, and mitral regurgitation (tricuspid). The precordium may be deformed, the pulse volume small and a left parasternal lift of right ventricular hypertrophy may be present.

Assessment

ECG

- *Ostium secundum*: partial right bundle branch block with right axis deviation and right ventricular hypertrophy. Atrial fibrillation may occur.
- *Ostium primum*: there is usually left axis deviation with evidence of right ventricular hypertrophy. Conduction defects and junctional dysrhythmias occur.

Chest X-ray

Enlargement of the right atrium and ventricle with enlarged pulmonary arteries and plethoric lung fields (evidence of increased right-sided flow). The aorta appears small (evidence of decreased left-sided blood flow).

Cardiac catheterization: reveals a step up in oxygen saturation in the right atrium.

Complications

- Pulmonary hypertension may lead to flow reversal through the defect (Eisenmenger's syndrome).
- Atrial fibrillation.
- Tricuspid regurgitation (from right ventricular enlargement).
- Infective endocarditis occurs in ostium primum defects.

Management

- Ostium secundum: operate if pulmonary–systemic flow ratio is more than 2:1.
- Ostium primum: operate for symptoms or for cardiac enlargement with mitral regurgitation.

NB   Eisenmenger's syndrome precludes surgery.

PATENT DUCTUS ARTERIOSUS

Fifteen per cent of all congenital heart disease. It is associated with the rubella syndrome. It is commoner in females.

Symptoms

Usually there are none. Bronchitis and dyspnoea on exertion occur with severe lesions.

Signs

The pulse may be collapsing (water hammer) and the left ventricle hypertrophied. There is a continuous (machinery) murmur with systolic accentuation maximal in the second left intercostal space and posteriorly. This continuous murmur must be distinguished from other causes, i.e. jugular venous hum, mitral regurgitation plus aortic regurgitation, VSD plus aortic regurgitation, pulmonary arteriovenous fistulae.

Assessment

ECG: normal or there may be left ventricular hypertrophy.

Chest X-ray: aorta and left ventricle may be enlarged. The pulmonary artery is enlarged and there is pulmonary plethora.

Echocardiography: shows a dilated left atrium and left ventricle.

Complications

- Endocarditis (of the ductus).

- Heart failure (Eisenmenger's syndrome following pulmonary hypertension and shunt reversal).

Management

Indomethacin, if given within 1–3 weeks of birth and close the duct possibly by blocking prostaglandin E production in the duct muscle. If this is unsuccessful, surgical ligation (1–5 years) is required or possibly an umbrella occlusion device. Cyanosis contraindicates surgery. Antibiotic prophylaxis (p. 397).

VENTRICULAR SEPTAL DEFECT

Twenty-five per cent of congenital heart disease.

Small defect. Maladie de Roger, i.e. a loud murmur with a normal-sized heart, chest X-ray and ECG.

Large defect. The clinical importance depends on pulmonary vascular resistance which determines how much shunting is present and its direction of flow.

Symptoms

None unless the VSD is large, when there may be dyspnoea and bronchitis.

Signs

There may be a small-volume pulse and LVH may be present (and right ventricular hypertrophy if there is pulmonary hypertension). A pansystolic murmur (and thrill) is present in the fourth left intercostal space. A mitral diastolic flow murmur implies a large shunt.

Assessment

ECG: LVH.

Chest X-ray: enlargement of the left atrium and ventricle may be present. The pulmonary arteries are enlarged in pulmonary hypertension.

Complications

- Endocarditis in 20–30% with emboli into the pulmonary circulation.
- Eisenmenger's syndrome.

Management

- Chemoprophylaxis to prevent endocarditis (p. 397).
- Small VSD: these may close spontaneously. Surgery is not indicated for the endocarditis risk alone.
- Large VSD: surgery is indicated in most cases to prevent the development of irreversible pulmonary vascular damage developing. It is contraindicated once Eisenmenger's syndrome has developed.

FALLOT'S TETRALOGY

Ten per cent of congenital heart disease and 50% of cyanotic congenital heart disease.

The four features are:
- VSD in which the shunt is from right to left because of;
- pulmonary stenosis, infundibular or valvar;
- right ventricular hypertrophy due to the consequent load on the right ventricle;
- associated dextroposition of the aorta so that it sits over the defect in the septum.

Symptoms

- Syncope (20%).
- Squatting (this may help decrease the right-to-left shunt by increasing systemic resistance and reducing venous return).
- Dyspnoea.
- Retardation of growth.

Signs

Cyanosis and finger clubbing.

The typical murmur is of pulmonary stenosis. P2 is quiet or inaudible. There is no VSD murmur.

Assessment

ECG: usually moderate right atrial and ventricular hypertrophy.

Chest X-ray: there is a normal-sized, but boot-shaped heart and a large aorta with a small pulmonary artery and pulmonary oligaemia.

Polycythaemia is common.

Complications

- Cyanotic and syncopal attacks (sometimes fatal).
- Cerebral abscesses (10%).
- Endocarditis (10%).
- Paradoxical emboli.
- Strokes (thrombotic–polycythaemia).
- Epilepsy is commoner than in the general population.

NB   Only 1 in 10 reach 21 years if untreated.

Management

- Total correction on cardiopulmonary bypass.
- Blalock shunt (not performed now), i.e. anastomosis of the left subclavian to the left pulmonary artery to increase pulmonary blood flow.

PULMONARY STENOSIS

Five per cent of congenital heart disease. It is usually acyanotic unless it is part of a Fallot's tetralogy (central cyanosis) or is very severe (peripheral cyanosis). The stenosis is usually valvar but may be subvalvar (infundibular). It sometimes occurs late in the carcinoid syndrome (p. 239).

Symptoms

Even with considerable stenosis there may be no symptoms. Severe stenosis causes dyspnoea, fatigue, angina and syncope.

Signs

The characteristic sign is a pulmonary systolic murmur with or without a thrill. An ejection click implies a valvar stenosis. Classically its intensity increases with deep inspiration. Moderately severe stenosis produces a large 'a' wave in the jugular venous pulse, signs of right ventricular hypertropy and a wide split of the second sound (the delay in P2 is due to raised right ventricular pressure—the greater the delay, the tighter the stenosis). Severe stenosis results in a reduced cardiac output with a small-volume arterial pulse, peripheral vasoconstriction (with peripheral cyanosis) and P2 becomes soft or absent if very severe.

Chest X-ray: post stenotic dilatation of the pulmonary artery with pulmonary oligaemia when the stenosis is moderately severe or worse.

Assessment

ECG: degrees of right atrial hypertrophy (P pulmonale) and right ventricular hypertrophy (with 'strain pattern') corresponding to the degree of stenosis (a better guide than the symptoms).

Echocardiography: can show the stenosis and estimate the gradient across it.

Complications

- Endocarditis.
- Right heart failure.

Management

If mild or moderate (right ventricular systolic pressure <70 mmHg) observe: if more severe, balloon valvuloplasty or valvotomy (or infundibular resection) is indicated.

COARCTATION OF THE AORTA

Five per cent of congenital heart disease. It is associated with berry aneurysms, Marfan's and Turner's syndromes. Ninety-eight per cent are distal to the origin of the left subclavian artery.

Symptoms

Sixty per cent have none. Forty per cent have symptoms including stroke, endocarditis, occasionally intermittent claudication and those secondary to hypertension.

Signs

- Usually there is radiofemoral delay with a small-volume femoral pulse. Blood pressure may be raised in the arms, especially on exercise, different on the two sides and low in the legs. Asymmetry of radial pulses may be present.
- Visible and/or palpable scapular collaterals.
- LVH.
- The murmurs are:
  (a) a systolic murmur at front and back of the left upper thorax;
  (b) collateral murmurs over the scapulae; and
  (c) an aortic systolic murmur (of an associated bicuspid valve in 70% of cases) is usually obscured by the coarctation murmur.

Assessment

ECG: 50% have LVH.

Chest X-ray: double aortic knuckle due to stenosis and post stenotic dilatation, rib notching (and at the scapular margin), and normal or large cardiac shadow.

Associations

Bicuspid aortic valve, cerebral artery aneurysms (berry aneurysms) and PDA.

Prognosis

Ninety per cent die by the age of 40 years from endocarditis, heart failure or cerebrovascular haemorrhage.

Management

Surgical resection. The operative mortality is 5%. Antibiotic prophylaxis (p. 397).

EISENMENGER'S SYNDROME

This refers to the situation in which there is a reversal of a left-to-right shunt (e.g. VSD, ASD, PDA) due to pulmonary hypertension. With left-to-right shunts there is a pulmonary circulatory overload and an increase in pulmonary vascular resistance follows with the development of pulmonary hypertension. When the pressure on the right side of the shunt exceeds that on the left side, the shunt flow reverses. The patient becomes cyanosed and deteriorates rapidly with symptoms of dyspnoea, syncope and angina. The lesion must be surgically corrected before this stage is reached. Otherwise, heart–lung transplantation should be considered.

Infective endocarditis

Acute

This is a rare disease in which the heart valves are infected as part of an acute septicaemia, of which the features are swinging fever, rigors, delirium and shock. Healthy valves are affected in 50% of cases. It follows infection with staphylococcus, usually from primary infection of the lungs or skin. *Streptococcus pneumoniae*, *Haemophilus influenzae*, gonococcus and meningococcus may also be responsible.

The prognosis is that of the generalized septicaemia unless valve destruction leads in addition to acute intractable cardiac failure.

Subacute

This is usually bacterial and subacute in onset (subacute bacterial endocarditis).

Predisposing abnormalities
• *Congenital*: VSD, PDA, coarctation of the aorta and bicuspid aortic valves.
NB   ASD of the secundum (common) variety does not develop endocarditis, but the rare primum lesion, where the mitral valve is also involved, can.
• *Acquired*: any rheumatic valve may be affected, the mitral more than the aortic, and mitral regurgitation more frequently than mitral stenosis, but chronic rheumatic heart disease now accounts for less than a quarter of all UK cases. Mitral valve prolapse is present in 5–15% of young adults, particularly females. Calcified aortic stenosis and syphilitic aortitis (rare) predispose to endocarditis. It occurs postoperatively following cardiac catheterization or surgery and often on prosthetic valves which are at risk. The normal tricuspid valve is at special risk in drug addicts.

Organisms
• *Streptococcus viridans* (non-haemolytic) is the commonest (45%), and the usual source is teeth.
• *Staphylococcus aureus* and *albus* (25%).
• *Streptococcus faecalis* (7%) especially in young women (abortion) and old men (genitourinary catheterization). Other bacteria include gonococcus, *Brucella* and *Proteus*.
• *Coxiella burnetii* (Q fever).
• Fungi (*Candida, Aspergillus, Histoplasma*).
   The origin of infection varies with the infecting organisms and includes teeth and tonsils (*Streptococcus viridans*), urinary tract (*S. faecalis*), central venous catheterization (*Staphylococcus*) and the skin (*Staphylococcus*).

Clinical features

Classically the disease affects young adults (20–30 years) with rheumatic valve or congenital heart disease, although it is now commonly recognized in the over-60s (30%). The symptoms and signs may be considered in three groups:

I   *Signs of general infection*. Lethargy, malaise, anaemia and low-grade fever are frequent but not invariable (fever exists at presentation in 70%). Clubbing of the fingers (20%) and splenomegaly (40%) are fairly late signs (6–8 weeks). There may be transient myalgia or arthralgia (25%). The white cell count may be low, normal or high. *Café-au-lait* complexion is now exceedingly rare since it occurs only in the neglected late stage.

2   *Signs of underlying cardiac lesions* must be sought, though not present in 50% of patients. New lesions and changing murmurs are highly suggestive and the patient must be examined for these daily.

3   *Embolic phenomena.* Large emboli (30%) may travel to the brain (15%) and viscera or cause occlusion of peripheral arteries. Emboli from left-to-right shunts (VSD and PDA) and on right-sided heart valves go to the lungs, giving pleurisy and lung abscesses.

Vasculitic phenomena occur in up to 50% and cause splinter haemorrhages in the nail bed, and microscopic haematuria. Osler's nodes in the finger pulp are pathognomonic but rare. Roth spots in the eye also occur rarely.

The renal lesions in SBE are of two kinds:
• a diffuse proliferative glomerulonephritis (not specifically diagnostic of SBE); and
• a focal embolic glomerulonephritis. The tissue is sterile on culture.

Immune complexes are present in serum and complement levels reduced.

Diagnosis

The diagnosis should be considered in any patient with a predisposing cardiac lesion who becomes ill. It is made on the basis of the clinical picture alone, even if unconfirmed by the isolation of the organism from blood culture. The most efficient way to make the diagnosis is:
• repeated examination, particularly for changing murmurs;
• blood cultures (at least three sets);
• midstream urine examination for microscopic haematuria;
• immune complexes and low complement in serum;
• echocardiogram for vegetations; and
• positive rheumatoid factor.

NB   Endocarditis sometimes presents with atrial fibrillation in the elderly.

Prognosis

The mortality is 95% in untreated cases. It is still over 30%, even with modern therapy. Adverse features include the presence of congestive heart failure, advanced age or of peripheral emboli. Death is often from heart failure of valve destruction or from major (e.g. cerebral) emboli.

Management

Prophylaxis

When valves are abnormal antibiotics must be given during intercurrent infections and before any surgical procedures in the mouth, genitourinary tract or gastro-intestinal tract.

Dentistry. Under local or no anaesthesia oral amoxycillin 3 g 1 h before the procedure. For those who are penicillin-allergic, or have received a penicillin in the previous month give clindamycin 600 mg 1 h before. Under general anaesthesia intravenous or intramuscular amoxycillin 1 g at induction, then 500 mg 6 h later. Intravenous vancomycin and gentamicin can be used in those who have received a penicillin recently or are allergic. Good dental hygiene is essential.

Genitourinary, gastrointestinal or obstetric procedures. Amoxycillin 1 g and gentamicin at time of induction, followed by amoxycillin 500 mg 6 h later. (Vancomycin and gentamicin if penicillin allergy or recent exposure.)

Chemotherapy

It is essential to obtain blood culture before starting chemotherapy, but it should not be delayed in the presence of good clinical evidence even if cultures are negative. Penicillin G, 6–12 g/day intravenously in divided doses is the drug of first choice. Since 30% of organisms are now penicillin-resistant most physicians would add an aminoglycoside (e.g. gentamicin). When the results of bacterial sensitivities are available therapy is guided by this, an attempt being made to achieve serum levels of the antibiotic at least three times the minimal inhibitory concentration (MIC) of the organism. Therapy should be continued for at least 4 weeks (intravenously for the first 2 weeks), if effective blood concentrations can be achieved. The patient should be carefully followed for recurrence. Emboli may occur for up to 1–2 months after cure.

Indications for surgery

Surgery must be considered early for valve rupture, intractable heart failure, resistant infection particularly of a valve prosthesis, and if the organisms are drug-resistant.

Culture-negative endocarditis

This diagnosis is considered after six successive negative cultures when culture technique is known to be good. The following should be considered:
- unsuspected organisms—e.g. *Coxiella burnetii* (Q fever), especially if the aortic valve is diseased. The diagnosis depends on finding a rise in antibody titre. *Bacteroides* — anaerobic culture is required (and kept for up to 3 weeks). Fungi—*Candida, Aspergillus, Histoplasma*
- partly treated bacterial causes
- right-sided endocarditis
- systemic vasculitis, systemic lupus erythematosus (SLE), atrial myxoma
- non-bacterial thrombotic endocarditis associated with carcinoma.

Constrictive pericarditis

Aetiology

This is now rare. It may be due to tuberculosis following spread from the pleura or mediastinal lymph glands. It may follow acute viral or pyogenic pericarditis, but the cause is often unclear. Haemopericardium, irradiation and carcinoma account for a few. It never follows acute rheumatic fever. It may be stimulated by restrictive cardiomyopathy (p. 402).

Clinical features

Symptoms result from cardiac constriction with decreased filling and low cardiac output. Right heart failure predominates over left. Fatigue and ascites with little or no ankle swelling are characteristic, but dyspnoea and ankle swelling may occur later. Pulmonary oedema and paroxysmal nocturnal dyspnoea are rare.

Examination

The pulse is rapid and volume small and there may be arterial paradox (pulsus paradoxus, p. 399), as with acute pericarditis. Atrial fibrillation is present in 30% of cases. Ascites may be the presenting feature and the elevated JVP may be missed because it is so high. The classical JVP signs of diastolic collapse (steep 'y' descent), and a further rise on inspiration (Kussmaul's sign) are often not observed. The liver, and sometimes the spleen, is enlarged. Ventricular contraction may cause localized indrawing of the chest wall at the apex. The heart sounds may be normal, though quiet. A third sound due to an abrupt end to ventricular filling may be present. There in no rub.

Investigation

- ECG: there may be widespread ST changes with low-voltage complexes, and atrial fibrillation.
- Chest X-ray: there may be calcification of the pericardium (often seen only in the lateral film). Cardiomegaly, if present, is less than one would expect from the degree of right (and possibly left) heart failure.
- Echocardiography shows the rigid, thickened pericardium, particularly if calcified, large atria with normal (or small) ventricles, and ventricular filling predominantly in early diastole.
- CT scan demonstrates the thickened pericardium in almost all cases.

Management

No action is needed if the patient is symptom-free and the assessment confirms mild disease. Close follow-up is essential. Pericardiectomy should be performed if severe constriction is present.

Acute pericarditis

Aetiology

Pericarditis is common within the first week of acute myocardial infarction. Dressler's syndrome is uncommon and occurs 2 weeks–2 months after myocardial infarction or cardiac surgery. It is characterized by fever, pleurisy, pericarditis and the presence of antibodies to heart muscle.

Infective pericarditis is usually a complication of chest infection. Acute benign pericarditis affects young men, often follows a respiratory infection and is probably viral. A rising antibody titre to coxsackie B virus is sometimes found. Suppurative pericarditis is rare. It results from infection with the staphylococcus or occasionally haemolytic streptococcus. Tuberculous pericarditis is very rare and non-suppurative.

Pericarditis occurs as part of systemic syndromes: rheumatic fever, SLE, severe uraemia, local extension of carcinoma of the bronchus and following trauma.

Clinical features

There is central, poorly localized tightness in the chest which varies with movement, posture and respiration. There may be pain referred to the left shoulder if the diaphragm is affected. The pericardial rub varies with time, position and respiration.

The signs of pericardial effusion without tamponade are an absent apex beat, a silent heart and disappearance of the rub.

Tamponade, which is rare, produces:
- pulsus paradoxus. The pulse volume decreases in the normal person on inspiration. This is more marked with tamponade and is then known as pulsus paradoxus. The paradox which Kussmaul noted was that the heart continued to beat strongly whilst the peripheral arterial pulse virtually disappeared during inspiration.
- a rise in the JVP on inspiration (Kussmaul's sign).

Both pulsus paradoxus and Kussmaul's sign result from decreased cardiac filling on inspiration due to the descending diaphragm stretching the pericardium and increasing the intrapericardial pressure.

Assessment

ECG: there is raised concave elevation of the ST segment in most leads (especially II and V3–4) and T-wave inversion. The voltage is low in the presence of effusion.

Chest X-ray: it is unchanged in the absence of effusion. Effusion classically produces an enlarged pear-shaped cardiac shadow with loss of normal contours.

Echocardiography is the most sensitive way of detecting pericardial fluid with free space between the heart and percardium.

Management

Aspirate for tamponade (if the systolic arterial blood pressure falls below 90–100 mmHg). Treat the underlying condition. Steroids are used for systemic lupus erythematosus and in acute benign pericarditis if it is severe or prolonged. Recurrent effusion with tamponade is treated by insertion of a drain or creation of a pericardial window.

Syphilitic aortitis and carditis

It is now very rare in the UK. Acquired syphilis affects the aorta, the aortic ring to produce dilatation or aneurysm, and aortic regurgitation and the coronary artery orifices to cause angina.

NB   Congenital syphilis does not produce aortitis.

Pathology

Endarteritis and occlusion of the vasa vasorum of the aortic muscle wall which becomes degenerate and fibrotic. Atheromatous plaques form over the damaged areas.

Aortic regurgitation

The symptoms are similar to those of rheumatic aortic regurgitation (see p. 383 for differential diagnosis). It is often gross with no haemodynamic stenosis (though there may be a systolic murmur).

Syphilitic angina

Fifty per cent of patients with syphilitic aortitis are affected. The angina is severe, attacks are long, often nocturnal, and respond poorly to glyceryl trinitrate.

Syphilitic aneurysms

Ascending aorta. This is the 'aneurysm of signs' with evidence of gross aortic regurgitation, local pulsation and systolic bruit and thrill in the second or third right interspace, marked carotid pulsation in the neck, signs of superior vena cava obstruction if the aneurysm is sufficiently large, and dilatation and calcification of the ascending aorta.

Arch of aorta. This is the 'aneurysm of symptoms' as it compresses the trachea and recurrent laryngeal nerve to produce cough, the left bronchus to produce collapse of the left lower lobe, the vertebrae producing erosion and pain, and occasionally the oesophagus causing dysphagia. Horner's syndrome may result from compression of the sympathetic trunk, and the left radial pulse may be absent due to compression of the left subclavian artery.

Abdomen. These are usually atheromatous and rarely due to syphilis. They present as pulsating abdominal masses.

Cardiomyopathy

This word means disorder of heart muscle. It is usually restricted to cardiomyopathies of unknown cause or association. They are classified into three major groups depending upon the clinical effects of the abnormality of the function of the left ventricle, which may be: hypertrophied, dilated or restricted.

HYPERTROPHIC CARDIOMYOPATHY

Also known as HCM, it is usually familial. It results in asymmetrical LVH associated with:

• loss of left ventricular distensibility which leads to symptoms of dyspnoea, pulmonary oedema and syncope. Some patients develop angina;

• hypertrophy, particularly of the left ventricle and septum with mitral regurgitation. In some patients this disappears with progression of the disease as the heart muscle fails.

Signs

There is a steep-rising jerky pulse (unlike the slow-rising plateau pulse of aortic valve stenosis), cardiac hypertrophy, a palpable atrial beat followed by a late systolic aortic ejection murmur, usually heard best in the left third and fourth intercostal spaces. There may be associated signs of mitral regurgitation. Complications include atrial fibrillation (10%), systemic embolism, congestive heart failure and sudden death.

Investigation

Echocardiography shows asymmetrical septal hypertrophy, systolic anterior movement of the mitral valve and a narrow left ventricular cavity with hypertrophied trabeculae and papillary muscles. A 24-h ECG record identifies those most at risk from sudden death from dysrhythmias.

Management

β-Adrenergic blockade is given to increase left ventricular compliance and reduce the incidence of dysrhythmias and angina. The response is variable. If the patient develops atrial fibrillation, anticoagulants and digoxin or verapamil are added. Serious arrhythmias may need amiodarone. Patients are at risk from endocarditis. Treat for cardiac failure and if medical therapy fails, consider transplantation.

DILATED (CONGESTIVE) CARDIOMYOPATHY

This is very rarely familial.

The label 'congestive cardiomyopathy' covers a large group of aetiologically unrelated disorders which tend to present as low-output congestive heart failure. By convention the more common and more easily diagnosed myocardial disorders are excluded, i.e. ischaemic, hypertensive and rheumatic heart diseases.

Angina (10%), systemic and pulmonary infarcts, conduction defects and arrhythmias occur.

Aetiology

• Alcoholism and thiamine deficiency (beriberi).
• Infections: viruses, e.g. influenza A_2 Coxsackie B, *Toxoplasma*, diphtheria.
• Infiltrations: sarcoidosis, amyloidosis (primary and secondary to myeloma), haemochromatosis.
• Collagen disease: SLE, polyartertis nodosa, diffuse systemic sclerosis.
• Muscular dystrophies and Friedreich's ataxia.
• Endocrine: hyper- and hypothyroidism.
• Postpartum.

Management

Bed rest, diuretics and ACE inhibitors form the basis of treatment of the cardiac failure. Anticoagulants are given because of the risks of embolism. Any underlying pathology (e.g. thyroid disease, collagen disease) should be treated appropriately.

RESTRICTIVE CARDIOMYOPATHY

The efficiency of the ventricles as pumps are restricted by endocardial fibrosis or granulation tissue — respectively EMF (endomyocardial fibrosis of equatorial Africa) and Loeffler's eosinophilic endomyocardial disease. In the UK, amyloidosis is the commonest cause of this rare condition, and is best diagnosed by endomyocardial biopsy.

Peripheral arterial disease

There are four common clinical syndromes: intermittent claudication, acute obstruction, ischaemic foot and Raynaud's phenomenon.

INTERMITTENT CLAUDICATION

Ninety per cent are males over 50 years of age. The disorder is associated with smoking and diabetes mellitus, occasionally with hyperlipidaemia and occasionally precipitated by anaemia. Obstruction may be femoropopliteal (80%), aortoiliac (15%) or distal (5%).

Diagnosis

The history is of pain in the calf on effort with rapid relief by rest. The Leriche syndrome is buttock claudication with impotence. The major peripheral arterial pulses are reduced or absent. There may be arterial bruits over the aorta, iliac or femoral arteries. The tissues of the leg atrophy (muscle bulk is reduced) and hair loss is common. There may be cyanosis, pallor or redness, oedema, ulcers or gangrene.

Doppler ultrasound is useful to exclude obstruction in doubtful cases. Arteriography is required if surgery is contemplated.

Prognosis

The symptom indicates generalized vascular disease and 80% die from cardiovascular or cerebrovascular disease. Life expectancy is similar to a healthy population 10 years older. Diabetes mellitus and persistent smoking are associated with a worse prognosis. Age, cerebrovascular disease and ischaemic heart disease are poor prognostic features. Leg gangrene is uncommon.

Management

- Stop smoking.
- Exercise within the effort tolerance to help develop collateral vessels. Treat obesity, hypertension, hyperuricaemia and hyperlipidaemia, despite the lack of

firm evidence that this affects the prognosis: a positive attitude to therapy is itself reassuring.

• Check for diabetes, polycythaemia and anaemia and treat if necessary.
• Keep the body and arms warm, and the legs cool.
• Attend carefully to foot hygiene.
• Surgery. Endarterectomy is indicated if there is a high block with good distal blood flow on angiography. Bypass (prosthetic or vein graft) surgery may be indicated if angiography shows the vessels to be satisfactory distal to the block.
• Dilatation of narrowed arteries using balloon catheter angioplasty may be successful. Sympathectomy is rarely successful in relieving symptoms of muscle ischaemia.

ACUTE OBSTRUCTION

This may be due to thrombosis or to embolism (usually blood clot in atrial fibrillation). Ninety per cent are in the legs.

Diagnosis

Pain (usually severe) is associated with numbness, paraesthesiae and paresis. There is pallor and coldness of the limb below the obstruction followed by cyanosis. The limb becomes anaesthetic and the arterial pulses weak or absent.

Management

Maintain the limb at room temperature or below to decrease local cell metabolism and therefore its oxygen demand.

Assess early for disobliteration, which is the treatment of choice, even if shocked. The embolus is sent to the laboratory for histology and culture. The muscles are probably viable if firm and tender and resist movement. The skin is probably not viable if it is densely cyanosed and anaesthetic.

Hyperbaric oxygen, if available, may be helpful. Heparin and low-molecular-weight dextrans are used while awaiting surgery and, in addition, thrombolytic agents and vasodilators may be tried if surgery is contraindicated or delayed.

ISCHAEMIC FOOT

This is caused by chronic arterial obstruction distal to the knees. It is most commonly seen in diabetes, and is associated with neuropathy and local infection.

Symptoms

• Areas of necrosis and ulceration.
• Pain in the foot (often not present in diabetics because of associated peripheral neuropathy).
• Intermittent claudication.

Signs

If the large arteries are narrowed there is pallor and/or cyanosis, empty veins in the feet with trophic changes in nails and absence of hair. The feet are cold and pulses diminished or absent.

In diabetes, it is often chiefly the small vessels which are affected and the foot pulses are often present despite severe ischaemia of the toes.

Management

Foot hygiene is especially important in diabetes. Pain may be severe and require morphine. Sympathectomy may improve skin blood supply and reduce pain. Endarterectomy or vascular grafting are seldom technically feasible and angiography therefore seldom indicated. If amputation is required it is frequently above-knee. Conservative management includes stopping smoking and various drugs which are not fully evaluated. These include agents to reduce platelet stickiness (aspirin, dipyridamole), reduce blood viscosity (oxpentifylline), dilate arteries (isoxsuprine and naftidrofuryl) and alter tissue metabolism (nicofuranose). None is very effective.

RAYNAUD'S PHENOMENON

Definition

Intermittent, cold-precipitated, symmetrical attacks of pallor and/or cyanosis of the digits without evidence of arterial obstructive disease. The digits become white (arterial spasm), then blue (cyanosis) and finally red (reactive arterial dilatation).

Aetiology

- Idiopathic and familial, usually in young women (Raynaud's disease).
- Collagen disease, especially SLE and scleroderma.
- Arterial obstruction, e.g. cervical rib.
- Trauma, usually in occupations involving vibrating tools.
- Drugs including β-blockers, the contraceptive pill and ergot derivatives.

Management

Treatment is disappointing. The hands and feet should be kept warm and free from infection. The patient is reassured about the long-term prognosis (usually good) and advised to stop smoking. Electrically heated gloves can be very helpful. Calcium antagonists (e.g. nifedipine) or patches of glyceryl trinitrate can be tried. Sympathectomy is sometimes successful as a last resort, particularly in the presence of recurring skin sepsis. Intravenous prostacyclin (epoprostenol) has been used in severe cases.

Dermatology

The commonest dermatological diseases are dermatitis, psoriasis, acne vulgaris, drug eruptions, athlete's foot, warts and basal cell carcinoma.

Psoriasis

This affects about 1–2% of the population and may be inapparent, cosmetically debilitating or chronic. Rarely it may be acute and life-threatening. Partial remissions are characteristic.

Psoriasis may present acutely with multiple small round silver-scaly lesions on an erythematous base on the body, limbs and scalp (guttate psoriasis). Removal of the scales leaves small bleeding points. This tends to remit spontaneously over 2–4 months, but some patients subsequently develop chronic psoriasis.

Similar chronic skin lesions occur mainly on the extensor surfaces (back, elbows, knees) and scalp, but any area of skin may be affected and symmetry is a feature. Thimble-pitting of the nail-plate is common. In flexures it looks different with smooth, confluent red areas and pruritus is then fairly common, though not necessarily in the flexural parts.

Psoriatic arthropathy occurs in 5–10% and resembles seronegative rheumatoid arthritis and is associated with thimble-pitting in the nail-plate (p. 195).

Treatment

Topical treatments

Salicylic acid (2–6% ointment or lotion) reduces hyperkeratotic, scaling lesions. It is often used in combination with coal tar or dithranol.

Coal tar paste is effective but is unpleasant to use. Coal tar shampoo can be used for scalp lesions, and coal tar baths if lesions are extensive.

Dithranol is applied to lesions, covered with a dressing, and left for an hour or more. Skin irritation can occur (start with 0.1% and gradually build up to 5%). Stains skin, hair and clothes brown.

Calcipotriol and *tacalcitol* are vitamin D derivatives which can be used topically for mild to moderate psoriasis.

Systemic treatments

Psoralens and ultraviolet A phototherapy (PUVA) is successful in clearing and delaying recurrence in chronic psoriasis. There is a very slightly increased risk of skin cancer.

Eterinate, and its metabolite *acitretin*, are retinoids (vitamin A derivatives). They are used for severe resistant psoriasis. Side effects include dryness and cracking of skin and lips, transient hair loss, myalgia, hepatotoxicity and a rise in plasma lipids. They are teratogenic and must be avoided in pregnancy.

Methotrexate and cyclosporin A may also be useful for severe resistant psoriasis.

Lichen planus

An uncommon disorder, usually of the middle-aged, who present with an irritating rash affecting the flexures of the wrist and forearms, the trunk and the ankles. About 10% have nail involvement. The rash consists of discrete purple, shiny polygonal papules with fine white lines passing through them (Wickham's striae), often occurring in scratch marks and other sites of injury (Köbner's phenomenon). The lesions may be widespread or confined to one or two papules. Lesions may occur on the buccal mucosa with a white lacy network or in the nails without other lesions on the skin.

The disorder usually resolves within 6 months but recurrences may occur. The cause is unknown but many drugs may produce an identical eruption, e.g. gold, antimalarials and antituberculous drugs. The dermis is infiltrated with T cells. Only 50% resolve in 9 months (85% in 18 months).

Treatment

Topical steroids may be sufficient to suppress symptoms until resolution has occurred. Systemic steroids may be required to suppress the pruritus of widespread lichen planus, especially planta and palma lesions.

Pityriasis rosea

The rash is preceded by a *herald patch* — a solitary red, scaly oval lesion on the abdomen or over the scapular area. This is followed after 1–2 weeks by a mildly itching macular rash which may cover the entire trunk, the upper thighs and upper arms. The macules tend to be oval and aligned along the natural skin creases with peripheral scales. The disorder occurs in small outbreaks in schools and families and may be caused by a virus.

The disorder is self-limiting, usually within 6 weeks.

Treatment

Mild sedation can help. Mild to moderate topical steroids may be needed.

Dermatitis and eczema

Dermatitis is often used to refer only to skin inflammation due to an exogenous agent. The term is, however, synonymous with eczema, a term used colloquially for endogenous dermatitis, i.e. atopic dermatitis. It affects 10% of the population.

Clinical features

Clinically the term describes a patchy diffuse irritating and sometimes painful lesion, often with vesicles which rupture to leave a raw weeping surface. Itching may be the dominant symptom. Secondary infection is common. In chronic lesions scaling may be present and the skin may become thickened (lichenification). Healed lesions do not scar but may pigment.

Histologically, the initial abnormality is oedema of the epidermis and this finally results in vesicle formation. Vesicles or oedema dominate depending upon the thickness of the horny layer. In eczema of the face and genitalia oedema is marked, but on the palms and soles vesicles are more prominent.

Contact dermatitis

There are two groups, *irritant* and *allergic*.

1 *Irritant* contact dermatitis follows prolonged or repeated exposure to physical or chemical trauma (e.g. industrial solvents) and may occur in anyone exposed. It is a common problem in certain occupations such as hairdressers and engineers.

2 *Allergic* contact dermatitis requires previous sensitization and may subsequently be provoked by very small quantities of the allergen. The rash is usually confined to the sites of exposure. A careful history is often necessary to discover possible sensitizers. Patch tests should be performed on all suspected cases. Chromates, nickel, rubber, dyes, perfumes, antibiotics (topical), some plants and antiseptics are frequent sensitizers.

Seborrhoeic dermatitis

A red, itchy, inflamed and scaly remittent dermatitis which appears on oily areas of the skin, especially around the head, including the scalp, eyebrows and creases of the nose and ears. It also occurs in flexures (axillae, inframammary and perineal), as intertrigo and, with ammonia from urine, as nappy rash.

Atopic dermatitis

Atopy refers to a hereditary tendency to develop allergic responses to various allergens and is usually shown by asthma, rhinitis and conjunctivitis and well as dermatitis. About a quarter of the UK population is atopic. Atopic dermatitis usually presents in infancy in an individual (and from a family) with other atopic manifestations. Prick tests to common allergens are usually positive and serum immunoglobulin E (IgE) levels often raised, though this does not help management. There is itching and inflammation, usually flexural, and lichenification is common.

Treatment

The local irritant or sensitizer must be removed if possible and practicable. Dietary manipulation and hyposensitization have only a minor role in routine management. Commercial soaps may contain such irritants, and it is best, therefore, to wash with water only or use soap substitutes. If the lesion is weeping, local soaks (e.g. 1/8000 potassium permanganate) will aid healing, and then apply topical mild to moderate steroids. If dry, an emollient such as aqueous cream may be sufficient, but topical steroids may also be required. Sedative antihistamines by mouth may relieve pruritus and allow sleep. If secondary infection occurs in the skin, systemic antibiotics may be needed.

Acne vulgaris

A disease chiefly of puberty (but onset can be up to 40 years) in which androgens cause increased sebaceous gland activity. Plugging of hair follicles by keratin causes retention of sebum producing the characteristic comedo (blackhead). These may become secondarily infected with skin bacteria. The comedos are distributed on the face, the shoulders and upper thorax. The skin is usually greasy. It usually disappears in early adult life, often with residual scarring. Acne is seen in Cushing's syndrome (p. 214).

Treatment

Frequent washing with soap and water or local detergents (e.g. cetrimide) to degrease the skin.

Topical benzoyl peroxide cream or lotion (2.5–10%) or antibiotics (clindamycin or erythromycin) usually helps, often with oral antibiotics.

Oral antibiotics such as oxytetracyline (or erythromycin) 1 g daily are given for 6 months or longer and are usually effective for mild to moderate disease, though results may take 3 months to appear.

Isotretinoin (Roaccutane) is a vitamin A derivative taken orally for severe disease when topical therapy and oral antibiotics have failed. Side effects are common, including facial erythema, dry skin, myalgia and a rise in plasma lipids and abnormal liver function tests. It is teratogenic.

Rosacea

A disorder, more common in women, beginning usually after 30 years of age, with erythema, papules, pustules and telangiectasia over the cheeks, nose, chin and forehead.

Treatment

Avoid precipitating factors (e.g. hot drinks, sunlight, alcohol and topical steroid preparations).

Oxytetracycline (500 mg bd) may be effective when given long-term intermittently, 2 months at a time with or without topical metronidazole.

Fungus infections

CANDIDIASIS (*Monilia*, thrush)

In general medical practice this yeast infection, though common in fit people, should raise the suspicion of underlying diabetes mellitus (and the rare hypoparathyroidism), or other factors which suppress normal immune mechanisms, e.g. leukaemia, Hodgkin's disease, steroid therapy, AIDS when overwhelming systemic infection may occur.

The nail folds are commonly involved, sometimes producing obvious paronychia. Thrush occurs frequently in the vagina, on the penis, and on the oral mucosa, especially in users of inhaled steroids. It may spread to affect the entire gastrointestinal tract, especially after antibiotics.

NB   Oesophageal moniliasis has a characteristic radiological appearance with barium adhering to the patches of *Monilia*.

Treatment

Nystatin orally (500 000 units 6-hourly). Imidazole creams (e.g. clotrimazole) are the drugs of choice but may be ineffective if the underlying disorder does not respond to specific therapy. Itraconazole is used orally. Griseofulvin is ineffective.

PITYRIASIS VERSICOLOR

This is a yeast infection with *Pityrosporum orbiculare* (*Malassezia furfur*) usually of the trunk which causes brownish scaly lesions of varying size which may coalesce. Depigmentation, which may last many months after effective treatment, may resemble vitiligo because only the unaffected skin pigments in sunbathers. Diagnosis is made by skin scrapings. An application of 2.5% selenium sulphide repeated after a week may be sufficient. Topical imidazole for several weeks may be used. Griseofulvin is not effective.

RINGWORM (tinea)

The ringworm fungi are a group of related organisms (*Trichophyton*, *Microsporum*, *Epidermophyton*) which live in the keratin layer of the skin. The disorders produced are described after their site on the body — tinea pedis, tinea cruris and tinea capitis. Diagnosis is confirmed either by observing fungal hyphae in skin scrapings treated with potassium hydroxide or by culture. Ringworm is commonly misdiagnosed and treated inappropriately.

Tinea pedis (athlete's foot)

The most common of the group affecting the interdigital skin, usually between the fourth and fifth toes. The nails may be involved. The lesion is irritating and the skin appears white and macerated. It may provide an entry for bacterial infection (streptococcal cellulitis). The infection tends to be recurrent or chronic. The disorder must be distinguished from simple skin maceration, atopic dermatitis, psoriasis and footwear (contact) dermatitis.

Tinea cruris

This may result from spread of infection from the feet. The lesion affects the upper inner thighs and has a slightly raised, well-defined, spreading scaly margin. In contrast, *Monilia* is symmetrical, with ill-defined edges and small satellite lesions. Tinea gives pruritus.

Tinea capitis

A disease of prepubertal children who present with an area of baldness with scaly skin and stumps of broken hair. Some infections show characteristic fluorescence when viewed under Wood's light. The underlying scalp is scaly and may become secondarily infected.

Treatment of dermatophytes in general

Topical imidazole (e.g. clotrimazole, miconazole) treatment is usually effective for localized areas, but if the infection is severe, widespread or if there is nail and hair involvement, systemic therapy may be needed. Griseofulvin (0.5–1 g daily) is given for 6 weeks for simple scalp infections and for up to 2 years for toenail involvement. They should only be started after laboratory confirmation of the diagnosis.

Drug eruptions

Many drugs can produce eruptions which may be erythematous, maculopapular, urticarial or purpuric. The pattern for any one drug may not always be the same and most drugs may at times produce one or other type of reaction, i.e. virtually any drug can produce any eruption—an overstatement but necessary to consider in any patient with a rash. The commonest now are the thiazides, allopurinol, captopril and penicillamine. Topical antibiotics, particularly the penicillins and the neomycin group, frequently produce skin eruptions. The common drug rash of ampicillin is maculopapular and may be specific to it and not to all penicillins. (It is almost universal in patients with infectious mononucleosis.)

URTICARIAL REACTIONS

The penicillins are probably the most common group of drugs which produce urticaria. Of all patients receiving a penicillin, 1–2% have adverse reactions, and many of them (if asked) give a history of previous sensitivity. Reactions are more frequent in adults, probably a measure of previous exposure. Sensitivity to one penicillin may mean sensitivity to all, and cephalosporin sensitivity in about 1 in 10 patients. The urticarial eruption usually occurs 3–7 days after therapy is started. Rarely, an acute hypersensitivity reaction occurs within minutes and is associated with serum sickness-like features of fever, wheezing, arthralgia and hypotension. Chronic cases should avoid dairy produce as antibiotics are generously used in farming.

Other drugs which produce urticarial reactions include barbiturates, salicylates, streptomycin, sulphonamides, tetracyclines, phenothiazines and chloramphenicol.

PURPURA

This may be a feature of any severe drug reaction and results from capillary damage. Bone marrow suppression by gold, carbimazole or phenylbutazone may cause thrombocytopenic purpura (p. 106).

OTHER DISORDERS

- Light sensitivity (amiodarone, sulphonamides, tetracyclines, thiazides, chlorpropamide, tolbutamide, griseofulvin, chlorpromazine).
- Fixed drug eruption. This describes an eruption which has the same character and occurs in the same site when the causative drug is taken. Phenolphthalein, used in some laxatives, is frequently incriminated. Other drugs include penicillin, phenylbutazone, aspirin and sulphonamides.
- Lichen planus (gold, phenylbutazone, quinidine; p. 407).
- Exfoliative dermatitis (gold, barbiturates, phenytoin, chlorpropamide).
- Erythema multiforme (p. 417).
- Systemic lupus erythematosus (p. 178).

Management

- Stop all drugs.
- Oral antihistamines for urticaria.
- Mild topical steroids may help itching.
- Adrenaline may be life-saving in acute hypersensitivity reactions including shock and angioneurotic oedema (p. 337), and systemic steroids may be required in severe but less acute cases.

Skin manifestations of systemic disease

ERYTHEMA NODOSUM
Clinical presentation

Tender, red, raised lesions usually on the shins and less frequently the thighs and upper limbs. The lesions pass through the colour changes of a bruise. It is five times commoner in females and occurs usually between 20 and 50 years of age. Arthropathy, especially in the legs, occurs in 50% and bilateral hilar lymph gland enlargement is usually seen on chest X-ray in sarcoidosis.

Aetiology

- Sarcoidosis is probably the most common cause in this country (35%).
- Streptococcal infection and hence rheumatic fever.
- Tuberculosis.
- Drugs, particularly sulphonamides and including penicillin and salicylates.
- Other causes include ulcerative colitis, Crohn's disease, Behçet's disease and fungal infections (e.g. *Histoplasma*). Erythema nodosum occasionally occurs as an isolated, sometimes recurrent, disorder.

LYME DISEASE (erythema chronicum migrans—ECM)

Borrelia burgdorferi is a spirochaete spread by ioxdid ticks from deer and rodents to humans. The infection may produce clinical features in the skin (ECM), joints, central nervous system and heart.

- ECM begins as an indistinct red macule, from around the tick bite, which enlarges progressively.

There may be other features of infection with fever, malaise, myalgia and lymphadenopathy plus:
- migratory arthralgia, usually of large joints;
- neurological features including aseptic meningitis and cranial nerve lesions (especially seventh nerve);
- cardiac disease with atrioventricular block and myocarditis.

The diagnosis is confirmed serologically by the presence of a high titre of antibodies to *B. burgdorferi*, and treatment is with tetracycline, penicillin or a third-generaton cephalosporin (e.g. cefotaxime).

HAEMOLYTIC STREPTOCOCCAL INFECTION

Skin lesions frequently occur as a sign of streptococcal sensitivity and present as erythema nodosum, erythema marginatum (very rare but virtually diagnostic of rheumatic fever) and erythema multiforme (also occurs in rheumatic fever). Skin infections produce cellulitis or erysipelas (slightly raised, well-circumscribed, acutely painful bright red lesions of half to one hand's-breadth in diameter). The elderly are more commonly affected and the legs and face the most common sites. There may be generalized symptoms of headache, fever and vomiting. Response to parenteral penicillin is usually rapid. Transient skin rashes are common with streptococcal infection but the classical endotoxic rash of scarlet fever is now rarely seen.

Herpes zoster (shingles)

Although it usually occurs in isolation, herpes zoster may occur in any debilitating disease and particularly with Hodgkin's disease, the leukaemias and patients on steroids. The lesion consists of groups of vesicles on an inflamed base. Pain precedes the lesions in nerve root distributions. Postherpetic neuralgia may be severe and intractable. The virus (varicella-zoster) is identical with the virus of chickenpox and denotes earlier clinical or subclinical infection in childhood. The virus remains latent within dorsal root ganglia until diminished resistance allows reactivation. Patients should be isolated from the non-immune and immunocompromised population until the lesions are crusted, otherwise chickenpox may develop. Topical idoxuridine or acyclovir may help if given early, and parenteral acyclovir is usually required in the imunosuppressed (p. 455).

MALIGNANCY

Generalized pruritus is associated with tumours of the reticuloendothelial system such as Hodgkin's disease (also renal and hepatic failure, and old age).

Dermatomyositis (see p. 185)

Twenty per cent of adult cases occur in association with carcinoma, leukaemia or lymphoma.

Acanthosis nigricans

Brown pigmented warts or plaques most marked in the axilla are associated with underlying carcinoma, particularly of the bronchus, gastrointestinal tract, prostate, breast and uterus. It is very rare. Benign forms occur, especially in the obese.

Other manifestations

These include acquired ichthyosis (Hodgkin's disease), chronic myeloid leukaemia, skin infiltration, secondary skin metastases, migratory thrombophlebitis and exfoliative dermatitis.

XANTHOMATOSIS

Tendon xanthomata, usually most easily felt in the Achilles tendon and in the finger extensors on the dorsum of the hand, are characteristic of familial hypercholesterolaemia and associated with premature cardiac death. Xanthelasmata are dull yellow plaques commonly in the inner angles of the eyelids. They may, though not always, indicate hyperlipidaemia with raised serum cholesterol and are associated with myxoedema, diabetes and primary biliary cirrhosis. Eruptive xanthomata may occur with greatly elevated serum lipid levels.

OTHER RARE MANIFESTATIONS

The following conditions are well-recognized:

- necrobiosis lipoidica in diabetes mellitus;
- pretibial myxoedema in thyrotoxicosis;
- lupus pernio (a purple eruption) in sarcoid;
- lupus vulgaris and erythema induratum (Bazin's disease) in tuberculosis;
- *café-au-lait* spots and multiple neurofibromata of neurofibromatosis (von Recklinghausen's disease);
- light sensitivity and blistering in porphyria (p. 236); and
- ECM in Lyme disease.

Mucosal ulceration

This may be localized to the buccal mucosa or associated with generalized disease. Causes include aphthous ulcers, herpes simplex ulceration, herpangina (coxsackievirus type A), agranulocytic ulcers in aplastic anaemia, usually drug-induced or leukaemic, erythema multiforme and Stevens–Johnson syndrome, Behçet's syndrome, and under dental plates (often *Monilia*).

BEHÇET'S DISEASE

A disease of unknown aetiology characterized by a relapsing iritis associated with crops of oral and genital ulceration. It is twice as common in males and the peak age of onset is in the 20s. There may also be a migrating superficial thrombophlebitis which may occasionally present with deep vein thrombosis (and occasionally pulmonary involvement), arthralgia of large joints (50%), erythema nodosum (up to 80%) and neurological complications (10%). The diagnosis is chiefly clinical, though the erythrocyte sedimentation rate (ESR), is usually over 50 mm/h and there is a neutrophilia. It is treated with anti-inflammatory drugs (steroidal and non-steroidal) and with anticoagulants when indicated. Cytotoxic drugs (azathioprine or cyclophosphamide), colchicine and thalidomide have been used in the more severe cases.

Bullous lesions

Drugs may produce bullous eruptions. There are four other primary bullous skin disorders which are well-regconized. All are rare.

DERMATITIS HERPETIFORMIS

All patients have a gluten-sensitive enteropathy, though in 50% it is subclinical. The skin of the limbs and trunk is affected. In 80% histocompatibility locus antigen (HLA) B8 is present. Subepidermal IgA is usually present.

Clinical presentation

Symmetrical clusters of urticarial lesions on the occiput, interscapular and gluteal regions and extensor aspects of the elbows and knees. Vesicles follow and only rarely become bullous as skin trauma is provoked by the intolerable itching. There are seldom lesions in the mouth and there is no fever.

Prognosis and management

The disease starts acutely and may remit spontaneously, but tends to become chronic. Secondary bacterial infection is common. Dapsone is the drug of choice for the skin lesion.

PEMPHIGUS VULGARIS
Clinical presentation

A rare disease of middle age, some of the characteristics of which are explained by the very superficial site of the lesion: there is splitting in the epidermis above the basal layer. Degeneration of the cells of the epidermis (acantholysis) is seen on skin biopsy. IgG is present on the intercellular substance and patients have antibodies against desmoglein. Clinically it presents with widespread erosions and relatively few bullae (because they rupture so easily) spread over the limbs and trunk. Most (90%) patients have lesions in the mouth and these may be the only lesions at first. The surrounding skin is normal. The superficial skin layer can be moved over the deeper layers (Nikolsky's sign) and tends to disintegrate, allowing secondary infection. Lesions appear at sites of pressure and trauma and are then extremely painful. There is fever and severe constitutional disturbance. It may be precipitated by drugs, e.g. penicillamine.

Complications and management

Secondary bacterial infection is common and septicaemia may result. Protein loss from weeping skin may occur in widespread disease. Prednisolone (initially 60–100 mg, later reduced) may be required to control the eruptions. The prognosis is poor without treatment, but it can be no more than inconvenient in mild, treated cases.

PEMPHIGOID

A disease of the elderly in which the lesion is at the basement membrane between the dermis and epidermis—deeper in the skin than in pemphigus. IgG is deposited in the basement membrane zone and patients have antibodies against bullous pemphigoid antigens (BPAG1 and BPAG2). Acantholysis is not seen on histology. Clinically it presents after prodromal itch for a few weeks, with the sudden onset of bullae on the limbs and, to a lesser extent, on the trunk. The large, tense subepidermal bullae have less tendency to break than in pemphigus but can be provoked by trauma. Nikolsky's sign is negative. The surrounding skin shows erythematous patches. Mucosal ulceration is rare (10%). Secondary infection is common, and the patients are not usually ill.

Management

Steroids (prednisolone 40–60 mg daily) are required to control the eruption and may be required in low dose for years.

Pemphigoid gestationis (herpes gestationis) presents with vesicular and urticarial lesions during the second or third trimesters of pregnancy. It resolves after delivery and is associated with an IgG antibody against bullous pemphigoid antigens.

ERYTHEMA MULTIFORME

Clinical presentation

A generalized disease that may present in well people or sometimes with prodromal symptoms of fever, sore throat, headache, arthralgia and gastroenteritis. These are followed by a pleomorphic erythematous eruption which may become bullous. The forearms and legs are commonly affected first and the rash may spread centripetally to involve the entire body. The buccal mucosa may be involved. Target lesions — concentric rings of differing shades of erythema — are characteristic but late. The disease remits spontaneously in 5–6 weeks but may recur.

Stevens–Johnson syndrome is a severe form of erythema multiforme characterized by systemic illness with lesions in the mouth, conjunctiva, anal and genital regions.

Aetiology

The disease sometimes follows drug therapy (sulphonamides, penicillin, salicylates and barbiturates) and herpes simplex infection. The aetiology often remains unknown.

Management

- Withdraw drugs.
- Local treatment with mild-potency steroids for pruritus.
- Stevens–Johnson syndrome may require steroids to suppress the eruption but infection must be identified and specifically treated.

SKIN PIGMENTATION

This is usually racial or due to sun tanning. Other causes include pregnancy and the oral contraceptive (chloasma), Addison's disease, Nelson's syndrome (post-adrenalectomy), haemochromatosis, cirrhosis, uraemia, heavy-metal and chronic arsenic poisoning. In neurofibromatosis the patches are of varying size, discrete and associated with subcutaneous neurofibromata. In Peutz–Jeghers syndrome there are small discrete patches around the mouth and multiple small intestinal polyps. Other dermatological causes include the post-inflammatory changes which follow a number of dermatoses. Remember cosmetic preparations intended to simulate suntan. The *café-au-lait* pigmentation of bacterial endocarditis is now rarely seen because patients are treated early.

Haematology

Anaemia

The symptoms given by all anaemias are much the same, though the rate of onset of anaemia, age of the patient and symptoms from other aspects of an underlying disease process may alter the presenting symptomatology. These are tiredness, physical fatigue and dyspnoea, with angina, heart failure and confusion in older people.

Classification (pp. 97–102)
Deficiency
- Iron (including sideroblastic anaemia).
- B$_{12}$.
- Folic acid.

Haemolysis
Abnormal red cells (intrinsic disorders):
- *Membrane disorder*: hereditary spherocytosis; hereditary elliptocytosis
- *Haemoglobinopathy*: sickle-cell anaemia; thalassaemia
- *Enzyme deficiency*: glucose-6-phosphate dehydrogenate (G6PD); pyruvate kinase.

Normal red cells (extrinsic disorders):
- *Immune*: newborn, autoimmune (especially systemic lupus erythematosus); lymphomas (especially chronic lymphocytic leukaemia and Hodgkin's disease); cold haemoglobinuria, drug-induced (methyldopa, mefenamic acid).
- *Non-immune*:
  (a) *Mechanical haemolytic anaemias*: disseminated intravascular coagulation,

thrombotic thrombocytopenic purpura, haemolytic–uraemic syndrome, prosthetic heart valves and march haemoglobinuria

(b)   *Infections*: malaria, *Clostridium perfringens*, viral infections
(c)   *Paroxysmal nocturnal haemoglobinuria*
(d)   *Drugs*: e.g. oxidative damage, dapsone, salazopyrine.

Marrow failure

• *Aplasia*.
• *Suppression*: idiopathic or secondary to infiltration, drugs, infections or other disorders such as uraemia, hypothyroidism and chronic disease.
• *Dyserythropoeisis*: myelodysplastic syndrome.

IRON-DEFICIENCY ANAEMIA
Diagnosis

The peripheral blood count shows hypochromia (mean corpuscular haemoglobin (MCH) $<$ 27 pg) and microcytosis (mean corpuscular volume (MCV) $<$ 80 fl), possibly with poikilocytosis (variation in shape) and anisocytosis (variation in size). The serum iron is low and the transferrin (or total iron-binding capacity; TIBC) raised, with a low saturation. Serum ferritin reflects the state of the iron stores and is therefore low. There is a reduction in stainable iron in the marrow. The cause of the iron deficiency must be identified and corrected. In premenopausal women, excess menstrual loss is often the cause, though this should not be accepted uncritically because other important causes may be present as well. Slow gastrointestinal loss is a common cause, with peptic ulceration, gastric carcinoma and carcinoma of the descending colon commonest of the causes which usually give symptoms. Carcinoma of the ascending colon or caecum frequently produces no symptoms and its possible presence must be considered positively in all cases of iron-deficiency anaemia. Dietary deficiency remains an important cause, particularly in the elderly. (Other causes of hypochromic, microcytic anaemia include thalassaemia, and anaemia secondary to chronic disease where serum iron and TIBC are usually reduced and ferritin normal or even raised; since it is an acute-phase protein.) The bone marrow shows adequate iron in macrophages but reduced amounts in developing erythroblasts. Collagen disease such as rheumatoid arthritis, and renal failure are two of the commoner causes. *Examination* will include assessment of pallor (very imprecise), glossitis, angular stomatitis, koilonychia and rectal examination. Investigate the gastrointestinal tract if no other cause is identified.

Management

Ferrous sulphate, 200 mg bd before food is usually all that is required. The reticulocyte count rises first and then the haemoglobin (at about 1 g per week), but iron should be continued for another 3 months to replenish the stores.

B_{12} AND FOLIC ACID DEFICIENCY

Vitamin B_{12} is present in liver, and small amounts also in milk and dairy products, and requires intrinsic factor for absorption. Folic acid is found in green vegetables and liver.

B_{12} deficiency

This is usually caused by lack of intrinsic factor: B_{12} deficiency due to the presence of parietal cell and intrinsic factor antibodies is the most common cause in the UK. Rare causes of B_{12} deficiency include gastrectomy, intestinal blind loops (in which bacteria multiply using up B_{12}), a vegan diet, Crohn's disease involving the absorbing surface in the terminal ileum, other causes of malabsorption and *Diphyllobothrium latum*—a Finnish tapeworm which consumes B_{12}.

Folate deficiency

• *Dietary deficiency*. In the UK this is most commonly seen in chronic alcoholics, the poor and the elderly who get no green vegetables. In the tropics it is often seen in association with multiple deficiencies and with gut infection and infestation.
• *Malabsorption* (p. 316).
• *Increased requirement*. Haemolysis (increased red cell formation) requires folate more than B_{12}; pregnancy and infancy.
• Therapy with phenytoin interferes with folate metabolism.

PERNICIOUS ANAEMIA

This is due to the inability to produce intrinsic factor leading to deficient B_{12} absorption. Stores of B_{12} last 3–4 years. Achlorhydria is invariably present. It is associated with other organ-specific autoimmune disorders.

Clinical features

Pernicious anaemia occurs in the middle-aged and elderly and is more common in women. Exhaustion and lethargy are the commonest presenting complaints, though the anaemia may be noticed incidentally. Classically, the skin has a pale lemon tint, the hair is snow white and the sclera may be slightly jaundiced due to mild haemolysis which is a typical feature. Cardiac failure is common if the anaemia is marked. The tongue may be tender, smooth and red due to atrophy of the mucosa. Peripheral neuropathy may be the presenting feature with pain, soreness or numbness of the feet on walking. Later, features of subacute combined degeneration of the cord may develop (p. 164). The spleen is sometimes palpable. There is an increased incidence of gastric carcinoma.

Diagnosis

The haemoglobin may be very low, i.e. 3–4 g or less. The blood film shows macrocytes usually with anisocytosis and poikilocytosis, and the MCV is usually >100 fl. The total white blood cell (WBC) count may fall due to reduced numbers of both lymphocytes and neutrophils. Some neutrophils may show hypersegmentation of the nuclei (>5 lobes). There may also be a moderate fall in the platelet count. Reticulocytes are generally not increased until treatment is started. Giant metamyelocytes and megaloblasts are present in the marrow which is hypercellular, evidence that anaemia is in part due to suppression of cell release. Serum bilirubin is raised, haptoglobins reduced, and urobilinogen is present in the urine as a result of reduced red cell survival and ineffective erythropoiesis. Antibodies to parietal cells are present in >90% of patients and to intrinsic factor in approximately 55%. Not all individuals who have parietal cell antibodies have pernicious anaemia.

Treatment

Vitamin B_{12} as hydroxocobalamin 1 mg (1000 µg) is given five times at 2 day intervals and then every 3 months for life.

The response of the marrow to therapy is very rapid with an early reticulocyte response maximal on the fourth to sixth day. The haemoglobin follows this and rises about 1 g/dl every 1–2 weeks. The WBC and platelets will be normal in about 7 days.

The rapid production of cells with therapy may reveal an associated deficiency of, and demand for, iron, potassium or folic acid and supplements should be given where necessary.

Neurological features of B_{12} deficiency usually improve to some degree: sensory abnormalities more completely than motor, and peripheral neuropathy more than myelopathy. However, neurological features may remain static and occasionally even deteriorate.

NB   If folic acid is given alone to patients with pernicious anaemia the neurological features may become worse.

Blood transfusion contains enough B_{12} to correct the marrow and to make interpretation of serum B_{12} levels difficult. It may precipitate heart failure and death — some authorities believe that transfusion must *never* be given to patients with pernicious anaemia. A poor response to B_{12} therapy suggests that the diagnosis is wrong.

HAEMOLYTIC ANAEMIA   (Table 21.1)

Haemolysisis is characterized by jaundice with a raised unconjugated serum bilirubin, increased urobilinogen in urine and stools, decreased haptoglobins and reticulocytosis. The blood film may show polychromasia, spherocytes, crenated and fragmented red cells. There may be features of:

• rapid red cell destruction — increased plasma haemoglobin, methaemalbuminaemia, decreased haptoglobins, haemoglobinuria and haemosiderinuria; and

• excess red cell formation — reticulocytosis and erythroid hyperplasia and increased folate requirements.

Hereditary spherocytosis

An autosomal dominant disorder which causes increased osmotic fragility and produces spherocytes in the peripheral blood. Patients present with intermittent

HAEMOLYTIC ANAEMIAS

Intrinsic red cell disorders	Extrinsic red cell disorders

Membrane disorder
Hereditary spherocytosis*; hereditary elliptocytosis
	Immune
	Isoimmune
	Mismatched transfusion, haemolytic disease of the newborn
	
	Autoimmune
	Warm antibodies
	  Idiopathic
	  Secondary (CLL, SLE, lymphoma, carcinoma, drug)
	Cold—agglutinins
	  Idiopathic
	  Secondary (*Mycoplasma*, glandular fever, lymphoma)
	  Lysis

Enzyme deficiency G6PD*; pyruvate kinase	
Haemoglobinopathy Sickle-cell anaemia; thalassaemia	
	Non-immune March haemoglobinuria; postcardiotomy; microangiopathic haemolytic anaemia (thrombotic thrombocytopenic purpura); paroxysmal nocturnal haemoglobulinuria (p. 425)

*Most frequent.

Table 21.1 Classification of haemolytic anaemias. G6PD, Glucose-6-phosphate dehydrogenate; CLL, chronic lymphoid leukaemia; SLE, systemic lupus erythematosus.

jaundice which may be confused with Gilbert's syndrome or recurrent hepatitis. Gallstones, leg ulcers, splenomegaly and haemolytic or aplastic crises during intercurrent infections may occur.

Splenectomy relieves the symptoms but does not cure the underlying defect.

Hereditary elliptocytosis

This is also inherited as an autosomal dominant and produces elliptical red blood cells (RBCs), variable degrees of haemolysis and, rarely, splenomegaly.

Glucose-6-phosphate dehydrogenase deficiency

A disease found in Africa, the Mediterranean, the Middle and Far East. Inheritance is sex-linked on the X chromosome (i.e. affected males always show clinical manifestations but females will have variable degrees of haemolysis). Because of the phenomenon of random inactivation of the X chromosome, females will have two populations of RBCs, one normal and one G6PD-deficient: the susceptibility to haemolysis will be greater, the greater the size of the deficient population. In the UK, acute haemolytic episodes are usually drug-induced (sulphonamides, primaquine) or occur during acute infections. Other features are neonatal jaundice and favism.

The diagnosis is confirmed by reduced or absent enzyme activity in the red cells.

HAEMOGLOBINOPATHIES
Clinical features

Normal adult haemoglobin is made up of two polypeptide chains, the α- and β-chains, which are folded such that each chain can hold an oxygen-binding haem molecule. The haemoglobinopathies are a diverse group of autosomal recessive disorders of haemoglobin synthesis which include sickle-cell anaemia (abnormal β-chain synthesis) and the thalassaemias (deficient or absent α- or β-chain synthesis). Together they form the commonest group of single-gene disorders in the world population.

Genetic basis of haemoglobinopathies

Genes encoding five different β-globin chains and three different α-globin chains are expressed in a precisely regulated manner during different stages of development. During fetal life the two β-globin variants called γ-globin combine with two α-globin chains to give rise to fetal haemoglobin (HbF). During adult life the β-globin variants themselves combine with α-globin chains to form adult haemoglobin (HbA). HbA_2 is $<3\%$ of haemoglobin in adults and possesses two α- and two δ-chains.

The five β-globin chain genes are clustered on chromosome 11, whereas the α-globin chain genes occur together on chromosome 16. Numerous different mutations in the α-globin and β-globin genes have been described, which give rise to α- or β-thalassaemia respectively. Sickle-cell anaemia is caused by a point mutation, which involves substitution of T for A in the second nucleotide of the sixth codon changing the sixth amino acid from glutamine to valine.

NB   HbA is 95% of haemoglobin in adults and possesses two α- and two β-chains $(\alpha_2\beta_2)$.

HbF is $<0.5\%$ of haemoglobin in adults and possesses two α- and two γ-chains $(\alpha_2\gamma_2)$.

Sickle-cell haemoglobin (HbS) possesses two α- and two abnormal β-chains.

Haemoglobin A_2 (HbA_2) is $<3\%$ of haemoglobin in adults and possesses two α- and two δ-chains $(\alpha_2\delta_2)$.

Sickle-cell disease

A disease found in Africa, the Middle East, the Mediterranean and India, transmitted as an autosomal dominant. Sickle-cell trait occurs in heterozygotes (HbA–HbS) whose haemoglobin contains characteristically 60% HbA and 40% HbS. Patients with the trait are usually symptom-free except when the oxygen tension is very low, e.g. through altitude and anoxic anaesthesia. The outlook is excellent. The prevalence of the gene is probably because the HbS protects against the serious and occasionally lethal effects of falciparum malaria.

Sickle-cell anaemia occurs in homozygotes (HbS–HbS) and the abnormal haemoglobin renders the RBCs susceptible to very small reductions in oxygen tension leading to the sickling phenomenon and abnormal sequestration with thrombosis in small arterioles with subsequent infarction which may affect any part of the body.

Clinical features

Anaemia occurs within the first months of life as levels of HbF fall. Acute haemolytic crises begin after 6 months, causing bone infarcts which are common, and children may present with pain and swelling in the fingers and toes (dactylitis). Infarcts may cause abdominal pain, haematuria or cerebrovascular accidents. Splenic infarction is common and by the age of 1 most children are functionally asplenic. Repeated renal infarction causes tubular damage and failure to concentrate urine compounding sickle-cell crises.

Prognosis

The disease carries a high infant and child mortality from thrombosis to a vital organ or infection, with pneumococcus the most common as a result of hyposplenism. Children who survive beyond 4–5 years continue to have chronic ill health with anaemia, haemolytic and thrombotic crises, leg ulcers and infections (which may precipitate crises), and rarely survive beyond 35–40 years. Folate supplements are required throughout life. Pneumococcal vaccine should be given and penicillin prescribed to reduce mortality from pneumococcus.

Thalassaemia

Thalassaemia is found in the Middle and Far East and the Mediterranean, and is due to deficient α- or β-chain synthesis.

The deficiency is genetically determined and results in α-thalassaemia or β-thalassaemia. In the latter, γ-chains continue to be produced in excess into adult life and excess HbF is present.

β-Thalassaemia minor trait (heterozygote)

This often produces no symptoms or a mild microcytic hypochromic anaemia which may be confused with iron deficiency. It is diagnosed by finding a raised HbA_2 level generally (4–7%). HbF levels may also be slightly raised (1–3%).

β-Thalassaemia major (homozygote)

Both parents possess the trait. Patients are relatively normal at birth (little β-chain anyway) but develop severe anaemia later with failure to thrive and are prone to infection. The anaemia is hypochromic and the film contains target cells (Mexican hat cells) and stippling. Erythroid hyperplasia occurs in the marrow and chain precipitation appears as inclusion bodies on supravital staining.

Infants who survive develop hepatosplenomegaly, bossing of the skull, brittle and overgrown long bones, gallstones and leg ulcers.

Treatment consists of transfusion to maintain the Hb at 10 g/dl but this, combined with increased iron absorption, results in iron overload. Desferrioxamine is given to reduce haemosiderosis (p. 303) with folic acid replacement, and splenectomy may be indicated if hypersplenism supervenes. Bone marrow transplantation has been used successfully.

HAEMOPHILIA

Haemophilia A (classical haemophilia) or haemophilia B (Christmas disease) results from defects in the clotting factor VIII (on chromosome Xq28) or factor IX (on chromosome Xq27) respectively. They are sex-linked recessive clotting disorder in which patients suffer mainly from spontaneous bleeding into joints and soft tissues, and excessive bleeding in response to trauma or surgery. Treatment is by replacement of the deficient clotting factor.

PAROXYSMAL NOCTURNAL HAEMOGLOBINURIA

An acquired clonal disorder of haematopoiesis in which cells have deficient production of the phospholipid glycosylphosphatidylinositol which anchors certain proteins to the cell surface. These include CD59 which protects cells from complement-mediated lysis. This accounts for the increased sensitivity of red cells to complement, which forms the basis of Ham's acid lysis test.

The clinical features usually occur in the over-30s who develop paroxysmal haemolysis (with anaemia, macrocytosis, reticulocytosis, haemoglobinuria and haemosiderinuria) and life-threatening venous thromboses. Patients may develop aplastic anaemia. Spontaneous remission occurs in about 15% of cases. Long-term anticoagulation should be considered.

ANAEMIA SECONDARY TO CHRONIC DISEASE

There is an anaemia down to about 10 g/dl, usually normocytic (though sometimes slightly microcytic), associated in particular with chronic infection, malignant disease, chronic renal failure and the collagen diseases. The serum iron is characteristically reduced, and so is the transferrin (iron-binding capacity), unlike the findings in iron-deficiency anaemia. The marrow iron stores are increased, but the iron is not incorporated fully into red cell precursors. The erythrocyte sedimentation rate (ESR) is usually raised (and also ferritin and other acute-phase proteins). Haematinics have no significant effect. This condition can be complicated by true iron-deficiency anaemia, for instance when rheumatoid arthritis is treated with non-steroidal anti-inflammatory drugs (NSAIDs), or collagen disease with steroids, because blood loss may occur from gastric erosions or an ulcer.

MARROW APLASIA

Patients present with anaemia and/or spontaneous bleeding due to lack of platelets and/or infection due to lack of polymorphonuclear granulocytes. A peripheral blood film reveals a pancytopenia, though one cell line may be affected more than the others. A bone marrow aspiration is performed. If it is difficult to aspirate (possible myelofibrosis or malignancy), a trephine biopsy may be necessary to obtain a diagnostic specimen of marrow. The drugs which most commonly cause marrow suppression include phenylbutazone (now only on hospital prescription), gold, indomethacin, chloramphenicol and cytotoxic drugs. Half are idiopathic. Remember ionizing radiation.

Some marrow suppression is associated with uraemia, rheumatoid arthritis and hypothyroidism.

Myelodysplastic syndrome

This refers to peripheral cytopenia with cellular marrow. It presents mostly as a serendipitous finding on a routine peripheral blood film, usually as macrocytosis (with normal B_{12}, folates, liver and thyroid function tests, and γ-glutamyl transferase). Less commonly, it may present as a refractory anaemia, pancytopenia, neutropenia or thrombocytopenia. Marrow examination shows a dysmyelopoietic picture with excess blasts, with normal or increased cellularity.

There are six major subgroups with decreasingly satisfactory prognoses:
1 refractory anaemia with sideroblasts, with >15% ringed sideroblasts, but none in the periphery;
2 refractory anaemia: less than 5% blasts in a dyserythropoietic marrow, but no blasts in the peripheral blood;
3 refractory anaemia with excess blasts, amounting to 5–20% nucleated marrow cells;
4 refractory anaemia in transformation, with 20–30% sideroblasts or >5% in the periphery or of Auer's rods in the blast cells, regardless of the marrow blast count;
5 chronic myelomonocytic leukaemia, with a peripheral monocyte count >1 × 10^9 and monocytic precursors in the marrow. Philadelphia chromosome-negative; and
6 acute myeloblastic leukaemia.

Treatment

Haematinics have usually been tried and found to be ineffective. Blood transfusion is necessary and has to be repeated regularly.

Prognosis depends on the occasional transformation to blasts and is then that of the leukaemia, with bone marrow failure.

Complications

Anaemia (requiring the transfusion of about 1 unit of blood per week), infection, haemorrhage and blast transformation.

Leukaemias

Malignant proliferation of blood-forming cells. Broadly classified according to whether lymphocytic or myeloid (marrow-related) cell lines are involved, and whether the disease untreated is likely to follow an acute, rapidly fatal, or more prolonged chronic course.

ACUTE LYMPHATIC LEUKAEMIA

Commonest form of childhood leukaemia (accounts for 75–80% of all childhood leukaemias). Infiltration of bone marrow with lymphoblastic cells causes anaemia, bruising (thrombocytopenia) and infections (neutropenia). Lymphoblasts are usually present in the peripheral blood and always in the marrow. Lymphadenopathy, splenomegaly and hepatomegaly occur. Seventy per cent of children with acute lymphatic leukaemia can now be 'cured'.

CHRONIC LYMPHATIC LEUKAEMIA

Occurs in the elderly. Generalized lymphadenopathy. Raised white cell count with lymphocytosis. Usually follows a benign course—treatment only indicated if symptoms develop.

ACUTE MYELOID LEUKAEMIA

All ages but less common in childhood. Myeloblasts infiltrate the marrow and are found in the blood. Anaemia, bleeding or infections are common. Involvement of other organs is unusual.

CHRONIC MYELOID LEUKAEMIA

Usually presents in middle age, often insidiously with anaemia, weight loss and fever. White cell count is markedly raised with myeloid precursors in the marrow and peripheral blood. The spleen, and in later stages the liver, are markedly enlarged. In over 90% of patients leukocytes contain the Philadelphia chromosome, a translocation of the breakpoint cluster region (*bcr*) gene on the long arm of chromosome 22 to a position adjacent to the *c-abl* gene on chromosome 9. This results in formation of a *bcr-abl* fusion gene, and the subsequent expression of the BCR-ABL fusion protein is involved in the malignant transformation of myeloid cells.

Lymphoma

Solid tumour of the lymphoreticular system. Divided histologically into two main types — Hodgkin's disease characterized by the presence of multinucleated giant cells (Reed–Sternberg cells) and non-Hodgkin's lymphoma.

Clinical features

Patients may present with painless lymphadenopathy. Symptoms, if present,

TRIALS

The **International Lymphoma Study Group** (*Blood* 1994; **84**: 1361–1392) has agreed a classification for non-Hodgkin's lymphoma, and lymphoid neoplasms have been broadly classified into:

B-cell neoplasms
• Precursor B-cell neoplasm (most present as acute leukaemia but a few present as solid tumours).
• Peripheral B-cell neoplasms (includes B-cell chronic lymphocytic leukaemia, mantle cell lymphoma, follicular lymphoma, mucosa-associated lymphoid tissue (MALT) lymphoma, hairy-cell leukaemia, plasmacytoma, Burkitt's lymphoma).

T-cell and putative natural killer-cell neoplasms
• Precursor T-cell neoplasm (precursor T-lymphoblastic lymphoma).
• Peripheral T-cell and natural killer-cell neoplasms (includes T-cell chronic lymphocytic leukaemia, large granular lymphocyte leukaemia (LGL), mycosis fungoides/Sézary syndrome.

Hodgkin's disease
• Stage I: lymphocyte predominance
• Stage II: nodular sclerosis
• Stage III: mixed cellularity
• Stage IV: lymphocyte depletion.

include lethargy, anorexia, weight loss, fever, night sweats, pruritus. Hepatomegaly and splenomegaly may occur.

Lymphomas are staged according to the extent of disease:
• Stage I: involvement of a single lymph node region
• Stage II: two regions involved on the same side of the diaphragm
• Stage III: disease on both sides of the diaphragm, but limited to nodes, spleen or a single extralymphatic organ or site
• Stage IV: diffuse involvement of one or more extralymphatic sites, with or without lymph node involvement.

In Hodgkin's disease the suffix A (e.g. stage IIA) denotes the absence of symptoms, whereas the suffix B denotes the presence of weight loss (>10%), fever or night sweats.

The diagnosis is usually made on lymph node biopsy. Staging requires careful examination for superficial nodes and chest X-ray for mediastinal involvement computed tomographic (CT) scanning above and below the diaphragm can avoid the need for laparotomy.

Treatment is with combination chemotherapy, radiotherapy or a combination of the two depending on clinical, radiological and histological staging.

Burkitt's lymphoma was first described as a tumour of the jaw in African children who had been exposed to Epstein–Barr virus (EBV). It also occurs in a non-endemic form in the absence of EBV exposure. In the majority of patients with this lymphoid tumour there is a translocation between chromosomes 8 and 14. This results in the *c-myc* gene, which is an important regulator of cell growth and cell death on chromosome 8, being juxtaposed with the immunoglobulin heavy chain locus on chromosome 14. Overexpression of *c-myc* in its new position has been implicated in the pathogenesis of the lymphoma.

Myeloma

Malignant proliferation of a specific clone of plasma cells resulting in the production of a monoclonal immunoglobulin known as a paraprotein.

Clinical features

Eighty per cent of cases occur after the age of 50. Non-specific symptoms include malaise, lethargy and weight loss. Bone destruction from the expanding plasma cell clone causes pain, fractures and hypercalcaemia. Normochromic anaemia, thrombocytopenia and leukopenia (infections are common) occur as the normal bone marrow is replaced. Renal failure may result from hypercalcaemia or the presence of light chains which may be nephrotoxic or become precipitated in tubules.

Investigation

There is usually anaemia with a markedly raised ESR. The monoclonal antibody is detected as a discrete M band on plasma protein electrophoresis. Free immunoglobulin light chains may be detectable in the urine as Bence-Jones protein (precipitate on heating to 56°C, redissolve on boiling). There may be hypercalcaemia and renal failure. Osteolytic lesions are seen on X-ray. Alkaline phosphatase is usually normal (lesions are destructive without osteoclastic activity).

Diagnosis

Diagnosis depends on the presence of one major and one minor criteria, or three minor criteria, one of which must be increased plasma cells in bone marrow.

Major criteria
- Tissue plasmacytoma.
- Excess (>30% plasma cells in bone marrow).
- Monoclonal M band on plasma protein electrophoresis (>3.5g/dl immunoglobulin G (IgG) or >2g/dl IgA); or >1g/24h of κ or λ light chains in urine.

Minor criteria
* 10–30% plasma cells in bone marrow.
* presence of M band or urinary light chains at lower levels.
* osteolytic lesions on X-ray.
* evidence of immunosuppression with reduced normal (polyclonal) immunoglobulins.

In *Waldenström's macroglobulinaemia* a monoclonal IgM paraprotein is produced. Radiological involvement of bone is rare, but anaemia and a bleeding tendency occur. Plasmapheresis is indicated if symptoms related to hyperviscosity are present.

Cryoglobulinaemia
Cryoglobulins are immunoglobulin proteins that precipitate in the cold. They may be idiopathic or associated with connective tissue disease or haematological malignancies. They may occlude small peripheral vessels (causing digital gangrene) in cold weather.

Detection of cryoglobulins
Samples are collected into prewarmed (37°C) tubes and transferred to the laboratory at body temperature, where aliquots are incubated at 4, 20 and 37°C and visually inspected after 24, 48 and 72 h for precipitation in the 4 or 20°C samples. Any precipitate should redissolve at 37°C.

Amyloidosis
Amyloidosis is characterized by the tissue deposition of fibrillar proteins which stain with Congo red. Excess κ and λ light chains, associated with abnormal plasma cell proliferation, can form AL-type amyloid. In reactive (secondary or AA-type) amyloidosis, amyloid A protein is deposited, usually after many years of an inflammatory response induced by chronic infection or rheumatic disease. Amyloid A is a 76-amino-acid polypeptide fragment of an acute-phase protein termed serum amyloid A.

Although any organ can be involved, proteinuria is the commonest presenting feature. Other sites commonly involved are the gastrointestinal tract, heart and liver.

In long-term dialysis patients β_2-microglobulin is deposited as amyloid in musculoskeletal tissue and the carpal tunnel. In Alzheimer's disease and Down's syndrome amyloid plaques are found in the cerebral cortex.

Management
Management of haematological malignancies is under continuous review, and many patients are entered into multicentre trials. Patients should be treated in units with specialist experience of the drug regimes, and supportive treatment, including transfusions and antibiotics.

Cytotoxics (to destroy rapidly dividing cells) are used alone or in combination with radiotherapy. In some cases induction of remission by intensive chemotherapy is followed by bone marrow transplantation. The following drugs are commonly used.

Alkylating agents

Alkylating agents transfer alkyl groups to DNA, interfering with its replication. They reduce fertility in males (consider sperm storage) and may be associated with premature menopause in females. They are teratogenic, but there does not appear to be an increase in fetal abnormalities in patients who are fertile after treatment. Bone marrow depression is common and prolonged use is associated with an increased incidence of acute non-lymphocytic leukaemia.

Cyclophosphamide is used as a cytotoxic for chronic lymphocytic leukaemia and lymphomas, and as an immunosuppressant in autoimmune diseases. Haemorrhagic cystitis, caused by the metabolite acrolein, can be prevented by adequate hydration and mesna.

Chlorambucil is used for chronic lymphatic leukaemias and lymphomas.

Melphalan is predominantly used for myeloma.

Busulphan is used for chronic myeloid leukaemia. It can cause pulmonary fibrosis.

Lomustine (CCNU) is a nitrosourea which is used mostly for Hodgkin's disease. Nausea and vomiting are particular problems.

Antimetabolites

Antimetabolites are usually competitive analogues of normal metabolites. They cause gastrointestinal upsets and bone marrow depression.

Mercaptopurine and its derivative *azathioprine* are purine analogues. Mercaptopurine is used as maintenance therapy in acute leukaemias, whereas azathioprine is primarily used as an immunosuppressant in autoimmune disorders and transplantation.

NB Reduce dose if given with allopurinol, which interferes with metabolism of mercaptopurine and azathioprine.

Cytarabine, *fludarabine* and *fluorouracil* interfere with pyrimidine synthesis. Cytarabine is used in acute myeloblastic leukaemia, whereas fludarabine is used for chronic lymphocytic leukaemia.

Methotrexate inhibits dihydrofolate reductase, preventing synthesis of tetrahydrofolic acid which is needed as a coenzyme for synthesis of nucleic acids. It is used for treatment of lymphoma and childhood acute lymphoblastic leukaemia. Folinic acid can be given as rescue therapy to terminate the effects of high-dose methotrexate.

Vinca alkaloids

The *vinca alkaloids* arrest the cell cycle in mitosis. They cause peripheral and autonomic neuropathy and alopecia. Nausea is common.

Vincristine, *vinblastine* and *vindesine* are used for lymphomas and acute leukaemias. *Etoposide* may be given orally or intravenously.

Cytotoxic antibiotics

Cytotoxic antibiotics interfere with DNA or RNA synthesis through various mechanisms.

Doxorubicin is used to treat lymphomas and acute leukaemias. It causes nausea, myelosuppression and alopecia. Cardiomyopathy can occur with prolonged use. *Daunorubicin* has similar effects and is used for treatment of human immunodeficiency virus-related Kaposi's sarcoma.

Bleomycin is used to treat lymphomas. Mucositis and skin pigmentation occur. Dose-related pulmonary fibrosis limits prolonged use.

Other agents

Pentostatin is useful in treatment of hairy cell leukaemia; hydroxyurea is used for chronic myeloid leukaemia. Procarbazine is often used in combination with other agents for Hodgkin's disease. Nausea is a common side effect which can be aggravated by alcohol.

Drug Overdoses

Self-administered drug poisoning accounts for 10% of all acute medical admissions to hospital. Accidental poisoning is common in children and drugs are best kept in child-proof containers out of their reach. In adults the common drugs taken are: the tricyclic antidepressants (e.g. amitriptyline, nortriptyline, protriptyline), the benzodiazepines (e.g. diazepam, nitrazepam, chlordiazepoxide), household substances (e.g. bleach, detergents), paracetamol, co-proxamol and aspirin. Barbiturates are now less commonly abused. The weedkiller paraquat and insecticides (e.g. organophosphates) are occasionally taken accidentally. Carbon monoxide poisoning from domestic gas no longer occurs in areas where North Sea gas is used and carbon monoxide poisoning is usually now due to incomplete combustion from blocked flues and car exhausts.

Clinical presentation (Table 22.1, pp. 434–435)

Most patients who take overdoses are still conscious when seen and will usually state which tablets they have taken and/or bring the bottle. If unconscious, the other causes of coma must be considered even if a bottle is found in the pockets (p. 133). It is well worth searching for a diabetic (to exclude hypoglycaemia) or steroid card, or a hospital outpatient card. Relatives or friends may know whether the patient is currently under treatment. Patients often take more than one drug and very often alcohol in addition.

Management

1 Maintain the airways and ventilation.

2 Remove the drug with emetics if fully conscious or by gastric lavage with tracheal intubation if not (except with corrosives), and diuresis or dialysis if indicated.

3 General care of the unconscious patient — nursing, physiotherapy, fluid balance maintenance of renal function and treatment of shock.

4 Psychiatric assessment.

5 Poisons centres.

433

Ventilation

After ensuring that the airway is clear the patient should be admitted to hospital. It may be necessary to insert an endotracheal tube and give oxygen. Artificial ventilation is rarely necessary but spontaneous ventilation should be assessed regu-

COMMON DRUG OVERDOSE

Drug	Clinical features	Notes	Diuresis or dialysis	Specific antidotes
Aspirin	Hyperventilation, visual disturbance, tinnitus, nausea, vomiting, acidosis	May be well on admission and later very ill Bicarbonate intravenously for severe acidosis	Alkaline diuresis successful Start if initial blood level over 2,8 mmol/l (500 mg/l) or if condition deteriorares	Nil
Barbiturates	Drowsiness and coma, hypotension, hypoventilation, red wheals on pressure points of limbs, wide dilated pupils, absent reflexes	Most patients require supportive therapy only. Ventilation rarely required	Rarely required	Nil
Digoxin	Nausea and vomiting arrhythmias	Common if potassium levels are reduced (diuretic therapy)	Not indicated	Fab digoxin-specific antibody fragments
Benzodiazepines	Drowsiness to coma	Rarely fatal and very rarely requires ventilation (potentiated by alcohol)	No value	Flumazenil
Phenothiazines (e.g. chlorpromazine)	Hypotension, hypothermia, arrhythmias and dystonic movements; respiratory and cerebral depression	May require: 1 Diazepam for fits 2 Antiarrhythmics 3 Orphenadrine for dystonia	No value	Nil
β-Blockers	Bradycardia and shock	Glucagon for severe reduced blood pressure 10 mg intravenous infusion 3 mg/h	No value	
Lithium	Nausea, vomiting, muscle tremor, rigidity and twitching with or without nystagmus and dysarthria Apathy proceeding to coma		Forced diuresis or haemodialysis if concentration is 5 mmol/l acutely	Nil
Tricyclic antidepressants	Dry mouth, convulsions, arrhythmias, fits, respiratory depression, coma, dilated pupils	1 Diazepam for hyperexcitability 2 Physostigmine to block anticholinergic effects	No value	Nil
Paracetamol	Hepatotoxicity is usually apparent at 48 h (LFTs + INR)	Monitor liver function for up to 2 weeks if INR initially abnormal		N-acetylcysteine intravenously
Paraquat	Respiratory failure 10–14 days later	Oral Fuller's earth, followed by oral $MgSO_4$	Haemodialysis early (about 6 h) if more than minimal quantities	

Table 22.1 Clinical features of common drug overdose.

COMMON DRUG OVERDOSE (continued)

Drug	Clinical features	Notes	Diuresis or dialysis	Specific antidotes
Iron	Nausea and vomiting, agitation, liver damage	Usually seen in children. Chelate gastric iron with desferrioxamine solution for gastric lavage. Chelate absorbed iron with desferrioxamine intramuscularly	No value	Desferrioxamine
Methanol and ethylene glycol	Blurred vision, acidosis	Gastric lavage with 3% HCO_3^- and give ethanol to block methanol acetaldehyde	With heavier intoxication	Ethanol

LFTs, Liver function tests; INR, international normalized ratio.

larly and the decision to ventilate decided on the basis of a falling minute ventilation (e.g. <4 l/min).

NB   Severe respiratory depression from morphine or dextropropoxyphene is reversed with naloxone.

Remove poison from stomach and blood

The object is to remove drugs before they are absorbed. Gastric lavage is used in most centres. Forced vomiting is less efficient in removing tablets, though more commonly used in paediatric practice, and should only be performed in the conscious. It is very important to explain what is happening to the patient and friends and relatives because the procedure is frightening and unpleasant.

The head of the bed should be lowered and, in unconscious patients, the trachea intubated and the cuff inflated to prevent inhalation.

Specimens should be saved from gastric lavage for identification, and blood levels of likely poisons determined if these may be useful guides to determining the need for intensive therapy, e.g. forced alkaline diuresis.

Alkaline diuresis and dialysis. The alkalinity is more important than the quantity of urine and a normal urine output is adequate for effect (1.5–2 l/24 h), though it seems reasonable to load the circulation at the onset if the cardiovascular system is stable and can cope. Salicylates in severe overdose may be removed by alkaline diuresis, and also by peritoneal dialysis or haemodialysis: amitriptyline, diazepam, nitrazepam and paracetamol cannot. The decision to use these techniques depends upon the patient's general condition, particularly if this is deteriorating. It is useful to know the initial blood level of salicylate because an initially high level in a deteriorating patient is an indication for diuresis or dialysis. Contraindications are renal failure, shock and heart failure. The value of these techniques for other specific poisons may be obtained by contacting specialist poisons centres.

In paracetamol overdose, the use of oral methionine or intravenous *N*-acetylcysteine is determined by the initial blood level and the time after ingestion using standard charts that are available for reference (usually pinned to casualty department notice boards).

Care of the unconscious patient and shock

Expert nursing is essential and aimed at care of the airway and prevention of chest infection and bed sores. Fluid intake and output and assessment of renal function may be critical, particularly if the patient is hypotensive. This is commonly seen with barbiturate and phenothiazine poisoning. Most young patients will maintain good renal function at a systolic blood pressure of 80 mmHg and sometimes less. In the elderly or if there is doubt about renal perfusion, monitor the central venous pressure to detect hypovolaemia (maintain at 2–5 cm of water) and continuously monitor the urine output.

Chest infections due to inhalation or recumbency should be treated energetically with physiotherapy and antibiotics.

Psychiatric assessment

When the patient has recovered a careful assessment is required with the object of aiding the acute problem and preventing further attempts. About 10% of patients who take overdoses seriously intend suicide and 10–20% take a further overdose. It is useful to interview family and friends about the immediate background and their willingness to help in care after discharge. The patient may admit to planning a future suicidal attempt and a lack of plans for the future may be evidence of depression. The patient should be asked about:
- previous depression and suicide attempts;
- personal instability with a history of many jobs and different personal relationships;
- evidence of schizophrenic personality and schizophrenic thoughts;
- family history of depression, schizophrenia, alcohol abuse; and
- social history, especially living alone.

NB
- Both aspirin poisoning and hypoglycaemia produce sweating.
- Both aspirin poisoning and diabetic ketoacidosis produce confusion, hyperventilation and glycosuria.
- Most patients with drug overdose rarely require more than active supportive therapy.
- Keep drugs away from children.

Specialist centres

If in doubt, or the poison is unusual, specialist poisons centres provide advice and maintain a central database.

Imported Diseases and Infections

Within the community virus infections of the upper respiratory and gastrointestinal tract are the most common, followed by common virus infections usually of children such as measles, German measles, chickenpox and mumps, and the venereal diseases. Infections seen more frequently in hospitals usually relate easily to a single body system and are dealt with there (pneumonia p. 338, endocarditis p. 395, gastroenteritis p. 53, hepatitis p. 292, pyelonephritis p. 264, and meningitis p. 153, and see Table 11.2, p. 154).

Less frequent, but in diagnostic and management terms more difficult, are the imported diseases, septicaemia, pyrexia of unknown origin and infections of the immune-suppressed. The common infections, likely organisms and antibiotics of choice are shown in Table 23.1 (pp. 438–440).

Imported diseases

The common diseases of travellers (Table 23.2) returning to temperate climates are malaria, acute gastroenteritis including typhoid, infectious hepatitis and worm infestation. Diarrhoea in returning travellers requires investigation for worms and parasites (especially *Giardia* and amoeba) but usually no organism is found and the symptoms settle spontaneously or with simple therapy. Other diseases common in the tropics but rarely seen in returning travellers include tuberculosis, schistosomiasis, hydatid disease, poliomyelitis, tetanus, cholera, leprosy and trypanosomiasis.

Malaria

A disease of the subtropics and where the anopheline mosquito is found. Transmission is via the mosquito which carries infected blood from infected to uninfected humans. The mosquito lives chiefly between latitude 15° north and south and not more than 1500 m (5000 feet) above sea level.

Clinical features

The patient presents with fever and rigors usually within 4 weeks of returning from or travelling through a malarial zone. Occasionally symptoms may not

INFECTIONS AND ANTIBIOTICS

Infection	Likely organism	Antibacterial of choice (adult doses whilst awaiting microbiology)
Ear, nose and throat*†		
Sore throat	Viral	Nil
	Haemolytic streptococcus (*Streptococcus pyogenes*)	Pencillin V oral 250 mg qds (i.m. × 1 or 2 doses initially if severe) or erythromycin 250 mg qds if allergic to penicillin
Sinusitis	*Streptococcus pneumoniae* (pneumococcus) *Haemophilus influenzae*	Amoxycillin 250–500 mg tds, co-trimoxazole 2 bd or trimethoprim 200 mg bd
Otitis media	As above plus haemolytic streptococcus *Haemophilus influenzae* in under 5s	Amoxycllin under 5 years old: 200 mg/kg per 24 h
Acute epiglottitis	*Haemophilus influenzae*	Maintain airway plus cefotaxime or chloramphenicol
Urinary tract		
Acute cystitis	*Escherichia coli* (85%)	Trimethoprim 200 mg bd or
Acute pyelonephritis	*Proteus vulgaris* (5%)	co-trimoxazole 2 bd
Bone and soft tissue‡		
Cellulitis	Haemolytic streptococcus *Staphylococcus aureus*	Cloxacillin 500 mg qds flucloxacillin 250–500 mg qds orally (by injection initially if severe) for 7–10 days
Drip sites	*Staphylococcus aureus*	
Erysipelas	Haemolytic streptococcus	Penicillin (by injection initially for 24–48 h)
Osteomyelitis	*Staphylococcus aureus* *Haemophilus influenzae* in under 5s	Flucloxacillin or cloxacillin by injection plus amoxycillin in under 5s
Gastrointestinal infections§		
Acute gastroenteritis	Viral	Nil
	Campylobacter	Erythromycin 250–500 mg qds for 7 days

continued

Table 23.1 Common infections and antibiotics of first choice.

INFECTIONS AND ANTIBIOTICS (continued)

Infection	Likely organism	Antibacterial of choice (adult doses whilst awaiting microbiology)
Dysentery	Bacillary (*Shigella* species)	Ciprofloxacin (or chloramphenicol or ampicillin or co-trimoxazole) If septicaemic, doses as for typhoid
	Amoebic—*Entamoeba histolytica*	Metronidazole 800 mg 8-hourly for 5 days
Typhoid	*Salmonella typhi*	If septicaemic, ciprofloxacin 200 mg bd i.v. for 24 h, then 500 mg bd to complete 10–14 days (chloramphenicol, ampicillin or co-trimoxazole are alternatives)
Salmonella food poisoning	*Salmonella* species (>1000)	Nil (usually) unless septicaemic
Pseudomembranous colitis	*Clostridium difficile*	Metronidazole 400 tds or vancomycin 500 mg qds orally for 7 days
Acute cholangitis	*Escherichia coli*	Penicillin plus gentamicin or cefotaxime (one-third of biliary coliform-resistant to ampicillin/amoxycillin)

Chest infections—in hospital practice Gram-stain of sputum may identify the organism

Acute bronchitis	Viral	Nil
Acute on chronic bronchitis	Bacterial (*H. influenzae*) (*Streptococcus pneumoniae*)	Amoxycillin 250–500 mg qds Co-trimoxazole 2 bd Trimethoprin 200 g bd
Bronchopneumonia (off the streets)	*S. pneumoniae* *Mycoplasma pneumoniae* *Legionella pneumoniae* (rare *H. influenzae* 5% psittacosis)	Erythromycin 500 mg–1 g qds
In very unwell or immunosuppressed	Consider Coliforms *Klebsiella* Staphylococci during flu epidemics Pneumocystis in AIDS	Erythromycin plus third-generation cephalosporin (cefotaxime, cefoxitime) Pentamidine by inhalation Septrin by mouth or i.v.

*Meningitis (adult)–
  most are viral (90%)*
Viral
  Herpes simplex .... Acyclovir

continued

INFECTIONS AND ANTIBIOTICS (continued)

Infection	Likely organism	Antibacterial of choice (adult doses whilst awaiting microbiology)
Bacterial Pneumococcal Meningococcal Haemophilus (more common in children)	Streptococcus pneumoniae Neisseria meningitidis Haemophilus influenzae	Penicillin by injection in large doses 12–20 g/24 h for 5–10 days Cefotaxime 4–8 g daily (adult) (chloramphenicol by injection 1 g 6–8-hourly in adults 50–100 mg/kg per 24 h in hourly doses (children) is an alternative)

---

* Recurrent infection or 'odd' organisms, e.g. Klebsiella, Pseudomonas, suggest an underlying abnormality such as stone or tumour and further investigation is required. It is rarely possible to clear infection if there is an indwelling catheter (only treat if systematically ill). It is best to remove it if possible, and if not, try instilling an antiseptic, e.g. chlorhexidine 0.2%. Antibiotic use encourages the development of resistant organisms.

† Persistent bacteriuria is difficult to eradicate but patients can be kept relatively symptom-free with regular daily ampicillin 500 mg or nitrofurantoin 100 mg nocte or co-trimoxazole 1 tablet nocte.

‡ Treatment of osteomyelitis may be started by injection for 5–7 days depending upon response and may need to continue for about 6 weeks.

§ Patients with mild gastroenteritis without systemic illness or suspected systemic infection and who are excreting Shigella or Salmonella (including S. typhi) do not require antibiotics. The major problem is usually dehydration which may lead to deep venous thrombosis and pulmonary embolism in adults. Children need fluid and electrolyte replacement. Dioralyte sachets or electrosol tablets (which contain no dextrose) dissolved in water are satisfactory except in severe depletion.

develop for 12 months or more. The patient has usually failed to take antimalarials regularly, not slept under mosquito nets or failed to continue prophylaxis for 6 weeks after returning. The fever may be tertian (a 3-day pattern with fever peaking every other day (Plasmodium vivax and P. ovale)), quartan (a 4-day pattern with fever peaking every third day), or subtertian (a non-specific febrile pattern: P. falciparum). Diagnosis depends upon clinical awareness and then seeing the parasite in a blood film. The species of parasite may be differentiated by an experienced observer. In the UK, P. falciparum and P. vivax are most frequently seen in travellers from Africa and Asia. Malignant tertian malaria refers to P. falciparum which very occasionally produces high levels of parasitaemia (only P. falciparum gives red blood cell parasitaemia of >1–2%), serious complications of cerebral malaria or acute haemolysis and renal failure (blackwater fever).

Prophylaxis

Prophylaxis is by a combination of mosquito control, sleeping under mosquito

DISEASES OF THE RETURNING TRAVELLER

Common	Malaria
	Typhoid
	Diarrhoea often viral as pathogens rarely found but consider:
	Giardia lamblia and worms
	Amoebic colitis ⎤ which must be distinguished from
	Salmonella and ⎥ ulcerative colitis and Crohn's disease
	Shigella infection ⎦
	Tropical sprue
	Infectious hepatitis
Rare	Tuberculosis—usually not acute and more likely in Asian immigrants
	Amoebic liver abscess
	Hydatid liver cyst
Exceedingly rare	Rabies
	Cholera
	Exotic viruses
	Lassa fever
	Marburg
	Ebola

Table 23.2 Infections imported by returning travellers.

nets and specific prevention with proguanil (Paludrine) 200 mg daily, with chloroquine 300 mg twice weekly. For regions known to have chloroquine-resistant malaria, Maloprim (pyrimethamine with dapsone) and mefloquine have been used. Prophylaxis should be continued for 6 weeks after returning home.

NB   Before advising travellers, check whether they are entering a malarial zone, and seek advice from the nearest centre for tropical diseases about the current recommended prophylaxis because drug resistance, particularly of *P. falciparum* malaria, is continually changing.

Treatment

See Table 23.3.

Acute attacks

Patients with malaria should be given oral quinine. Intravenous quinine is potentially dangerous because it may produce cardiac asystole but is used in those who are vomiting or too ill to take oral therapy. Exchange transfusion may be required in very ill patients with high parasitaemia — consider levels above 10%. Some require full intensive care, including treatment of cerebral oedema, renal and liver failure and shock. Hypoglycaemia from a combination of liver failure and quinine-induced insulin secretion is easily overlooked; and pulmonary oedema from fluid overload is common in those treated for shock.

ANTIMALARIAL DRUGS

Drug	Important side effects	Comments
Chloroquine	Gl upset, headache, retinal damage and cataracts, rarely myelotoxicity, psychosis. Contraindicated in epilepsy.* Reduce dose in renal failure	Resistance is widespread, but confined to *Plasmodium falciparum*. Not active against dormant hepatic forms (hypnozoites) of *P. vivax* and *P. ovale*
Proguanil	Gl upset, rarely mouth ulcers. Reduce dose in renal failure	Prophylaxis only
Fansidar (pyrimethamine and sulfadoxine)	Skin rash, myelotoxicity	For eradication of *Plasmodium falciparum* infection
Maloprim (pyrimethamine and dapsone)	Skin rash, myelotoxicity	Prophylaxis only
Halofantrine	Contraindicated in pregnancy. Gl upset, pruritus, transient elevation of serum transaminases, cardiotoxicity	Treatment of uncomplicated *Plasmodium falciparum* infection
Primaquine	Gl upset, haemolysis, particularly in G6PD deficiency	Eradication of dormant hepatic forms (hypnozoites) of *Plasmodium vivax* and *P. ovale*
Mefloquine	Contraindicated in first trimester, breast-feeding, neurological disease, epilepsy* (including family history), liver disease, concurrent β-blocker therapy. Causes neuropsychiatric effects and Gl upset. Avoid pregnancy for 3 months after stopping treatment. Treatment duration should not exceed 1 year	Prophylaxis and treatment of chloroquine-resistant. *Plasmodium falciparum* malaria
Quinine	Tinnitus, hypoglycaemia, headaches, flushing, Gl upset, rash, myelotoxicity	Agent of choice for treatment of chloroquine-resistant or severe *Plasmodium falciparum* malaria

* Doxycycline is an alternative in epileptic patients.
Gl, Gastrointestinal; G6PD, glucose-6-phosphate dehydrogenase.

Table 23.3 Antimalarial drugs. (From *The Infectious Diseases Manual*, Wilks, Farrington & Rubenstein, Blackwell Science 1995; with permission.)

After treatment of the acute attack, falciparum malaria is cleared with Fansidar or tetracycline, and vivax with primaquine (check the glucose-6-phosphate dehydrogenase status first).

Typhoid

Clinical features

Symptoms begin with malaise, headache, dry cough and vague abdominal pain, up to 21 days after returning from a typhoid area. Travellers to any area with poor sanitation are at risk and typhoid occasionally occurs in non-travellers. In the first week fever is marked with cough and constipation which are typical features. In the second week, the fever persists, the abdomen distends, diarrhoea may or may not occur and rose spots develop as crops of pale pink macules on the sides of the abdomen. Delirium and death (10%) may occur in the third week in untreated cases.

NB   Symptoms of dry cough, constipation and fever should be sufficient to alert the clinician, particularly in returning holiday-makers.

Investigation

Leukopenia and neutropenia may or may not be present. Blood culture is mandatory if typhoid is suspected and culture of urine and stool should also be performed.

Treatment

Salmonella typhi responds to ciprofloxacin. Chloramphenicol, ampicillin and co-trimoxazole (Septrin) are also effective.

NB

• It is unnecessary to give antibiotics to patients who are clinically well, but from whom *S. typhi* is grown from the stools. If these patients are given antibiotics, they are more likely to become chronic excretors of resistant *S. typhi* (antibiotic-induced resistance).

• Typhoid must be reported to the public health authorities.

• Excretors of *S. typhi* are not allowed to work in the food industry.

Dysentery

BACILLARY DYSENTERY

Bacillary dysentery is caused by the genus *Shigella*. *S. sonnei* is the most common and occurs in outbreaks in children's homes. It produces the most serious clinical form of the disease, including septicaemia.

It is transmitted by faecal contamination of food and water and 2–4 days after ingestion produces acute diarrhoea, sometimes accompanied by abdominal colic, vomiting and tenesmus. If severe, there is rectal blood, mucus and pus.

Asymptomatic carriage can occur.

The disease is prevented by good sanitation and clean water supplies and good personal hygiene.

Infected patients should be isolated and rehydrated. Antibiotics (ampicillin, co-trimoxazole, ciprofloxacin or chloramphenicol) are required if the patient is septicaemic.

The public health service must be informed and patients and close contacts should not handle food until the stool cultures are negative.

Shigella dysentery can be confused with *Salmonella* food poisoning, amoebic and ulcerative colitis (p. 309).

AMOEBIC DYSENTERY

An infection of the colon by the protozoon *Entamoeba histolytica*. In the acute dysenteric form, the illness begins suddenly with fever, abdominal pain, nausea, vomiting and diarrhoea containing mucus and blood. More commonly, amoebic colitis presents less acutely with intermittent diarrhoea with or without abdominal pain, mucus and blood.

The major complications are hepatic abscesses and pericolic amoebomas which can be confused with colonic carcinoma. The diagnosis is made by finding trophozoites or cysts in fresh faeces, rectal mucus or rectal biopsy and supported by a positive complement fixation test.

Metronidazole is the treatment of choice for all invasive forms of amoebiasis, but abscesses may have to be drained if they do not resolve on drug therapy. Diloxanide is used to eradicate chronic amoebic cysts.

Cyst excretors should not handle food, and the contacts should be screened. Acute amoebiasis can be confused with bacillary dysentery, *Salmonella* food poisoning and ulcerative colitis, and chronic infection with *Giardia lamblia*, tropical sprue, ulcerative colitis and diverticular disease (p. 321).

Giardiasis

G. lamblia is a flagellate protozoon which infects the small intestinal wall but not the blood. Viable cysts are ingested with contaminated food and may be excreted asymptomatically, or produce diarrhoea and steatorrhoea.

The diagnosis is confirmed by the presence of trophozoites or cysts in stools or duodenal aspirates.

Tinidazole or metronidazole are the drugs of choice.

Pyrexia of unknown origin

There are many definitions of pyrexia of unknown origin. In practice, the difficulty arises when the cause is unidentified after the clear clinical possibilities have been excluded, and a basic set of tests performed. It is usually a hospital problem. A broad-spectrum antibiotic has usually been given. The causes are listed in Table 23.4 (p. 445).

MNEMONIC — IMAGINE

Infections	*Bacterial.* Bacillary endocarditis and septicaemia (including culture-negative) *Collections of pus
	Subphrenic
	Intrahepatic
	Perirenal
	Pelvic
	Pleura
	Bone (osteomyelitis)
	Viral/rickettsial
	(including hepatitis B)
	Protozoal
	Malaria, amoeba, spirochaetes
	Specific
	Tuberculosis* (all sites), typhoid, *Brucella*, Lyme disease (*Borrelia burgdorferi*)
Malignancy	Kidney and liver (primary and secondary)
	Pancreas, micrometastases, lymphoma (Hodgkin's and non-Hodgkin's), leukaemia
Autoimmune diseases	*Systemic lupus erythematosus, polyarteritis nodosa
	Chronic active hepatitis
	Rheumatoid disease, Still's disease (including adult Still's disease, p. 194)
Granulomata	Sarcoid
	Crohn's disease
Iatrogenic	Drug fever
Nurses and doctors and all paramedicals	Factitious fever
Etcetera	Consult exhaustive lists in big books, but remember that the cause is more often a rare manifestation of a common disease than a common manifestation of a rare disease

* Denotes a more likely cause of pyrexia of unknown origin—all are treatable and potentially curable.

Table 23.4 Mnemonic list (Imagine).

Special points in the history

• Exposure to infection (meals away from home, febrile illness in household contacts, unpasturized milk or cheese, undercooked eggs and poultry).

• Occupation, especially if a doctor or nurse (factitious fever). Farmer, veterinary surgeon, sewer worker, forester (for *Brucella*, *Leptospira*, anthrax, cat-bite fever, Lyme disease).

• Drug history, e.g. antibiotics, methyldopa, hydralazine, phenytoin, including non-prescribed preparations.

- Travel (malaria, amoebiasis) and sexual history.
- Pets, including dogs, cats and birds.

Special points in examination

NB   Repeat regularly, e.g. on alternate days, if the fever persists.
- *Cardiovascular.* Murmurs, especially if changing, suggest infective endocarditis. Tender temporal arteries. Dressler's syndrome.
- *Respiratory.* Crackles (crepitations or rales) for early pneumonia (e.g. legionnaire's). Sinuses. Consider recurrent pulmonary thromboembolic disease.
- Abdomen. Palpable liver, gall bladder or spleen (with or without tenderness).
- Musculoskeletal. Muscle stiffness and tenderness of collagen diseases, e.g. polymyalgia rheumatica.
- Skin rashes (drugs, rose spots of typhoid). Splinter haemorrhages. Osler's nodes.
- Lymphatic. Glands (all group).
- Check all orifices: mouth (teeth for apical abscesses), ears, perineum (anus and genitourinary tract).

Basic screening tests already performed (check)

Most will need to be repeated until a diagnosis has been achieved.
- Haemoglobin. If anaemia is present and considerable, it is usually relevant. If iron-deficient and there is no overt blood loss, exclude gut malignancy.
- White blood cell (WBC) count. Neutrophilia is associated with pyogenic infection and neoplasia, and neutropenia with viral infection. Lymphocytosis may suggest tubercle. Leukaemia and infectious mononucleosis are usually associated with abnormal peripheral counts and cell types (remember direct tests for infectious mononucleosis). Eosinophilia may suggest parasites or polyarteritis nodosa.
- Erythrocyte sedimentation rate. If over 100 mm/h, check for myeloma, polymyalgia rheumatica, and secondaries from carcinoma in bone or liver (also see p. 102).
- Midstream urine. Haematuria, possibly microscopic, occurs with bacterial endocarditis, renal carcinoma, polyarteritis nodosa and leptospirosis. WBCs in infection. Early-morning urine for acid-fast bacillus (AFB). NB   Glycosuria suggests infection somewhere.
- Chest X-ray. Carcinoma (primary or secondary) in lungs, and bone metastases. Miliary shadowing in miliary tuberculosis and sarcoid. Hilar nodes in tuberculosis, lymphoma, sarcoid and carcinoma.
- Sputum for microorganisms, including AFB.
- Liver function tests (LFTs) for secondary or primary malignancy, abscess, biliary disease, hepatitis (p. 49).
- Infectious mononucleosis screening test, e.g. Monospot.
- Blood culture (×3).

Further tests commonly required as determined by clinical leads

- Agglutination enzyme-linked immunosorbent assay (ELISA) tests for *Salmonella*, *Brucella* and *Coxiella*.
- Viral, mycoplasma and human immunodeficiency virus (HIV) antibody titres immediately and 2 weeks later.
- ASO titre and rheumatoid factors.
- Autoimmune screen (etc.).
- Ultrasound or computed tomographic (CT) scan of abdomen for liver abscesses, and for secondaries, for renal tumours and abscesses, and for splenic enlargement, and of the pelvis for pelvic lesions.
- Echocardiography for vegetations.
- CT scanning of chest and abdomen for lymphadenopathy.

Invasive procedures as indicated

- Temporal artery biopsy.
- Liver needle biopsy (tuberculosis, granulomata, neoplasm).
- Muscle biopsy.
- Laparoscopy and laparotomy are seldom necessary since the advent of modern scanning.

Go back again and again to take a new history, to re-examine the relevant areas, and to repeat selected investigations, especially those which might have been performed too early, i.e. before they could have become abnormal.

Other imported pathogens: nematodes, schistosomes

The worms listed in Table 23.5 are found worldwide and not uncommonly in travellers who live rough or enter areas of poor sanitation.

Septicaemia (bacteraemia)

Traditionally this is classified as Gram-positive, Gram-negative or unknown. In practice bacteraemia occurs most often postoperatively. Less commonly patients are admitted from home with suspected bacteraemia, often without an obvious source or site of infection (Table 23.6).

POSTOPERATIVE BACTERAEMIA

The clinical features are of fever, often swinging and with rigors, and later hypotension and oliguria. The major differential diagnosis of postoperative shock is pulmonary embolism.

Management

General measures include good nursing care and fluid and electrolyte balance, and in severe cases intensive therapy, including treatment of shock and renal failure.

COMMON WORMS

Worm	Major clinical features	Treatment
Threadworm (*Enterobius vermicularis*)	Anal itch Worm on stool	Piperazine Thiabendazole (treat all household members to prevent reinfection)
Roundworm (*Ascaris lumbricoides*)	Worm on stool	Piperazine
Hookworm (*Necator americanus: Ancylostoma duodenale*)	Nil. If severe infection, iron-deficient anaemia; malnutrition in children Eggs or worms in stools	Bephenium (Alcopar) Pyrantel Tetrachloroethylene
Schistosoma 1 *S. mansoni* (spur on side) 2 *S. haematobium* (spur on tail)	Fever and eosinophilia Initially diarrhoea Haematuria	Oxamniquine Metriphonate Praziquantel (for both)

Table 23.5 Worms commonly found in areas of poor sanitation.

Special measures

A wound abscess is often the site of infection and obvious pus must be drained. This may result in a rapid fall in temperature and obviate the need for antibiotics.

The choice of antibiotic depends upon the organism grown from the wound or blood. If the patient's condition demands that treatment must be started before microbiological cultures are available, the type of operation allows a best guess at the likely organism. The choice of antibiotic depends in turn upon the likely organism and local knowledge of antibiotic sensitivities (see Table 23.1, pp. 438–440).

The key management points are:

1 Drain pus.

2 Antibiotics (see Table 23.1 for appropriate choice).

3 Expert nursing care.

4 Fluid balance and monitor renal function.

If the patient is shocked:

5 Treat hypovolaemia with plasma or equivalent.

6 Give expert intensive care monitoring;

   (a) renal function and fluid balance

   (b) right atrial pressure

   (c) left atrial pressure (pulmonary artery flow catheter).

7 Inotropes — dopamine to increase pumping efficiency for hypotension and increased renal blood flow. Dopamine will also cause arteriole relaxation to reduce afterload if systemic vascular resistance is high.

SEPTICAEMIA — THERAPY

Postoperative

1 Drain pus
2 Expert supportive or intensive care:
   - Fluids
   - Electrolytes
   - Urine output and renal failure
   - Shock
   - DIC
3 Treat infection with antibiotics

Operation site	Likely organism	Antibiotics of choice ('blind therapy' while awaiting cultures)
Gastrointestinal	Coliforms and anaerobes	Gentamicin, metronidazole plus ampicillin (ampicillin plus gentamicin for *Streptococcus faecalis*)
Hepatobiliary	Coliforms and *Streptococcus faecalis*	Gentamicin plus ampicillin
Urinary	Coliforms	Ampicillin and gentamicin or cefotaxime
Gynaecological	Staphylococci (skin) and anaerobes (vagina)	Flucloxacillin and metronidazole (Augmentin for minor infection)
Cardiothoracic/CNS	Staphylococci (skin)	Flucloxacillin

Off the streets (differential diagnosis influenza, or malaria in travellers)

1 Observe for site of infection:
   - Throat
   - Leg ulcer
   - Wound
   - History of urinary or chest infection
   - Rash—drugs, virus, staphylococcus/streptococcus
   - Hidden infection—ear, nose and throat, teeth, pelvis, liver, kidney
2 Urgent investigation:
   - White blood cells
   - Chest X-ray
   - Urine examination and culture
   - Blood cultures (± stool)
   - Ultrasound of liver and kidney for abscesses
3 Management:
   - Drain pus if present
   - General expert supportive or intensive care
   - Antibiotic therapy

continued

Table 23.6 Septicaemia: guidelines to therapy.

SEPTICAEMIA — THERAPY (continued)

Site of infection	Likely organism	Antibiotics of choice
Skin	Staphylococci (± toxic shock syndrome) β-Haemolytic streptococcus	Flucloxacillin
Gynaecological (vaginitis, abortion)	Escherichia coli anaerobes Streptococcus faecalis, Clostridium, Staphylococcus, Streptococcus (coliforms and Streptococcus faecalis)	Penicillin and gentamicin and metronidazole (anaerobes)
Nil obvious	Probably Staphylococcus or Streptococcus	Flucloxacillin
	Abscess:	
	Liver (Streptococcus milleri, amoebae)	Drain plus penicillin Drain plus metronidazole
	Biliary (Escherichia coli and Streptococcus faecalis)	Gentamicin plus ampicillin
	Renal (Escherichia coli and Streptococcus faecalis)	Gentamicin plus ampicillin

NB   *Shocked patients:*
- Monitor right atrial pressure (+8–10 cmH$_2$O) and maintain circulating volume.
- Monitor left atrial pressure (pulmonary artery flow catheter).
- Inotropes (dopamine, dobutamine).
- Monitor urine output and renal function—dialysis may be required.
- Treat DIC.

NB   Antibiotic choice:
- Always seek expert microbiological advice as choice and dosage alters with changing character of organisms.
- Use intravenous therapy initially to guarantee adequate blood levels.

DIC, Disseminated intravascular coagulation; CNS, central nervous system;

8   Treat disseminated intravascular coagulation (DIC) by replacing deficient blood factors as measured. The presence of DIC indicates a poor prognosis, and the best means of treatment remains uncertain. Endotoxin triggers both extrinsic and intrinsic coagulation systems leading to consumption of coagulation factors and in turn to the widespread bleeding of DIC.

NB   Steroids are not of proven value in septicaemic shock unless there is associated adrenal damage (short Synacthen test).

Human immunodeficiency virus infection

HIV-1 and HIV-2 are members of the Lentivirus family of retroviruses. The virus preferentially infects CD4+ helper T lymphocytes, leading to a decline in CD4 cell counts with impaired cell-mediated immunity. Eventually the immune system becomes clinically compromised and the patient develops the infectious, neurological and neoplastic complications characteristic of acquired immunodeficiency syndrome (AIDS).

HIV-2 shares 45% sequence homology with HIV-1, and is found mainly in west Africa. It is less pathogenic *in vitro*, and transmission rates appear to be lower.

Viral transmission is through sexual contact (homo- and heterosexual) or blood-borne (intravenous drug abuse or transfusion of blood or blood products). In the UK blood for transfusion is now screened. Approximately 20% of children born to HIV-positive mothers are infected, some through breast-feeding, which should be avoided.

Clinical features

Half of cases develop a febrile illness with malaise, headache, pharyngitis, lymphadenopathy, and maculopapular rash 2–4 weeks after infection. Antibody tests for HIV become positive 2–6 weeks after this illness. Patients then remain free from serious illness for a number of years. They may then develop symptoms of malaise, fever, weight loss with features of mild immunodeficiency (e.g. oral *Candida*, cutaneous herpes zoster or herpes simplex) or immune dysfunction (immune thrombocytopenia, drug allergies). There may be generalized lymphadenopathy.

Progression to AIDS is defined in the UK by the development of one of the AIDS-defining illnesses listed in Table 23.7. In the USA a CD4 count less than $200/mm^3$ is diagnostic of AIDS. The rate of progression to AIDS varies considerably—maintenance of normal CD4 counts and low levels of viral RNA in plasma are markers of slower progression.

Opportunistic infections

These remain the most important complications of HIV infection.

Candidiasis

Oral *Candida albicans* infection is common, presenting with typical white plaques or mucosal erythema or candidiasis. Topical treatments (nystatin or amphotericin lozenges) may be effective, but oesophageal or genital candidiasis are indications for systemic therapy with fluconazole.

Pneumocystis carinii pneumonia (PCP)

Pneumocystic carinii has recently been classified as a fungus. Exposure is common in the general population, but clinical disease only occurs in severe immunodeficiency. Cough and progressive dyspnoea are accompanied by fever,

AIDS—INDICATOR DISEASES

AIDS indicator disease	Comments and qualifications
Bacterial infections, recurrent or multiple	In a child less than 13 years
Candidiasis	Affecting oesophagus, trachea, bronchus or lungs
Cervical carcinoma	Invasive
Coccidioidomycosis	Disseminated or extrapulmonary
Cryptococcosis	Extrapulmonary
Cryptosporidiosis	With diarrhoea for greater than 1 month
Cytomegalovirus disease	Onset after age 1 month, not confined to liver, spleen and lymph nodes
Cytomegalovirus retinitis	
Encephalopathy (dementia) due to HIV	HIV infection and disabling cognitive and/or motor dysfunction, or milestone loss in a child, with no other causes by CSF examination, brain imaging or post-mortem
Herpes simplex	Ulcers for longer than 1 month or bronchitis, pneumonitis or oesophagitis
Histoplasmosis	Disseminated or extrapulmonary
Isosporiasis	With diarrhoea for greater than 1 month
Kaposi's sarcoma	
Lymphoid interstitial pneumonia and/or pulmonary lymphoid hyperplasia	In a child less than 13 years
Lymphoma	Burkitt's or immunoblastic or primary in brain
Mycobacteriosis	Disseminated, extrapulmonary or pulmonary
Pneumocystis carinii pneumonia	
Progressive multifocal leukoencephalopathy	
Recurrent non-typhoidal *Salmonella* bacteraemia	
Recurrent pneumonia	Two episodes within 12 months
Toxoplasmosis of brain	Onset after age 1 month
Wasting syndrome due to HIV	Weight loss (over 10% of baseline) with no other cause, and 30 days or more of either diarrhoea or weakness with fever

Table 23.7 AIDS—indicator diseases. (From *The Infectious Diseases Manual*, Wilks, Farrington & Rubenstein, Blackwell Science 1995; with permission.)

cyanosis, tachycardia, tachypnoea and confusion. Auscultation of the chest may be normal.

Chest X-ray is normal early in the disease, but widespread, diffuse interstitial shadowing develops. Twenty per cent of cases have atypical features of lobar consolidation, upper zone shadowing or hilar lymphadenopathy. Pneumothorax is a recognized complication. Patients are usually hypoxic.

Diagnosis depends on identification of the organism by microscopy in sputum, bronchoalveolar lavage or transbronchial biopsy, although treatment is often commenced on clinical grounds.

Treatment is high-dose co-trimoxazole (100 mg/kg per day sulphamethoxazole and 20 mg/kg per day trimethoprim) in divided doses orally or intravenously for 21 days. Adverse reactions are common, and intravenous pentamidine 4 mg/kg per day is an alternative. High-dose oxygen and mechanical ventilation may be required in severe disease. Steroids improve survival in patients with hypoxia (Pao_2 less than 9.3 kPa).

Prophylaxis is continued with co-trimoxazole 960 mg daily three times per week, or monthly inhaled pentamidine.

Mycobacterial infections

Mycobacterium tuberculosis infection may occur as a result of reactivation or primary infection at any stage of HIV infection. Pulmonary presentation may be with typical apical cavitation and fibrosis, or more generalized lung infiltrates. Extrapulmonary tuberculosis (lymph nodes, bone, bone marrow, genitourinary tract, liver, spleen, skin, peritoneum, central nervous system) occurs in 50% of patients. Standard treatment regimes (e.g. isoniazid with pyridoxine, rifampicin, pyrazinamide and ethambutol) are used, although the duration is usually prolonged. Multi-drug-resistant tuberculosis is a particular problem in the USA.

Disseminated *Mycobacterium avium* complex infection is the commonest systemic bacterial infection in HIV-infected adults. It causes fever, night sweats, weight loss, abdominal pain and diarrhoea, and is associated with shortened survival. Clarithromycin monotherapy is effective treatment, but relapses associated with bacterial resistance are common. Combination treatment with rifabutin, ethambutol and clarithromycin may improve long-term survival. A number of studies have highlighted the advantages of prophylaxis.

Cytomegalovirus (CMV)

CMV retinitis occurs in 10% of AIDS patients, usually presenting as unilateral visual loss. Asymptomatic lesions may be detected as fluffy white areas of necrosis and haemorrhage on fundoscopy. Untreated progression to bilateral blindness occurs. Initial treatment is with intravenous ganciclovir. Maintenance therapy with oral or intravenous ganciclovir is continued, although ultimately progression occurs.

CMV encephalitis presents with cognitive loss, motor and behavioural abnormalities. It can be difficult to distinguish from other causes of AIDS dementia complex (direct effect of HIV infection, herpes simplex encephalitis, *Toxoplasma gondii*), although diagnosis can be established by brain biopsy. Response to ganciclovir is limited.

TRIALS

The **Canadian HIV Trials Network Protocol 010 Study Group** compared rifabutin, ethambutol and clarithromycin (three-drug group) with rifampicin, ethambutol, clofazimine and ciprofloxacin (four-drug group) in 229 patients with AIDS and *Mycobacterium avium*-complex bacteraemia. The three-drug regime led to more frequent and more rapid resolution, with better survival rates. *N Engl J Med* 1996; **335**: 377–383.

Pierce et al. compared clarithromycin with placebo as prophylaxis against *M. avium*-complex infection in 333 patients with advanced AIDS. Clarithromycin was well-tolerated, prevented *M. avium*-complex infection, and reduced mortality. *N Engl J Med* 1996; **335**: 381–391.

The **California Collaborative Treatment Group** compared prophylaxis with weekly azithromycin, daily rifabutin, or both in 693 HIV-infected patients with CD4 counts less than 100/mm^3. Combination therapy was most effective but poorly tolerated. Weekly azithromycin was more effective than daily rifabutin, and infrequently selected for resistant isolates. *N Engl J Med* 1996; **335**: 392–398.

Cryptococcal infection

Cryptococcus neoformans is a capsulate yeast, widely present in bird droppings. Infection occurs by inhalation. Meningitis is the commonest manifestation in AIDS, although pneumonia and skin sepsis also occur.

Presentation of cryptococcal meningitis is usually non-specific, with prolonged fever, headache, malaise, nausea and vomiting. Diagnosis is confirmed by identification of capsulate yeasts or cryptococcal antigen in cerebrospinal fluid. Treatment is with intravenous amphotericin followed by oral fluconazole, continued as life long maintenance therapy.

Toxoplasma

Primary infection with the protozoan *Toxoplasma gondii* is usually acquired during childhood by eating infected cat faeces or undercooked meat. An infectious mononucleosis-type illness is followed by persistence of *Toxoplasma* cysts in the central nervous system and elsewhere. Vertical transmission from mother to child also occurs and causes fetal abnormalities, including central nervous system abnormalities.

Reactivation of *T. gondii* in AIDS usually manifests with neurological features, including fever, confusion, fits and focal neurological deficit. Choroidoretinitis may precede encephalitis. Patients are seropositive for *T. gondii* are cranial CT reveals multiple hypodense lesions. Treatment is with pyrimethamine and folinic acid (to reduce haematological toxicity of pyrimethamine) and sulphadiazine or clindamycin.

Diarrhoea

Abdominal pain, diarrhoea and weight loss are common, and usually indicate infection, although no specific pathogen is identified in 25–50% of cases. Bacterial pathogens such as *Salmonella*, *Shigella*, *Campylobacter jejuni*, *Giardia lamblia* and *Entamoeba histolytica* should be excluded by stool microscopy and culture. *Cryptosporidium parvum* usually causes a self-limiting illness in normal individuals, but causes severe, prolonged diarrhoea in AIDS patients who may also develop cholangitis and cholecystitis. It may respond to paromycin.

Herpes simplex

Recurrent oral, genital or perianal ulceration is common and usually responds to systemic (oral or intravenous) acyclovir. Herpes simplex encephalitis typically presents with headache, fever, confusion and temporal lobe abnormalities. Culture of cerebrospinal fluid is usually negative for herpes simplex. Diagnosis can be established by brain biopsy, but treatment with intravenous acyclovir is usually started on clinical grounds.

Herpes zoster

Cutaneous dissemination of typical herpes zoster (p. 414) can occur. Treatment is with intravenous acyclovir.

Progressive multifocal leukoencephalopathy (PML)

This condition is caused by reactivation of the Polyomavirus JC which is a common asymptomatic infection in childhood. Two per cent of AIDS patients develop PML with development of multiple, progressive neurological defects. CT scan shows multiple non-enhancing lesions. Brain biopsy may be required to exclude other treatable lesions. There is no specific treatment for PML.

Malignancy

Kaposi's sarcoma, non-Hodgkin's lymphoma and cervical carcinoma are all AIDS-defining illnesses.

Kaposi's sarcoma occurs almost exclusively in homosexual males, suggesting that an additional sexually transmitted agent is important. Palpable, violaceous cutaneous nodules occur most commonly on the head and neck. Lesions also occur in other organs, including lungs and gastrointestinal tract. Radiotherapy can cause regression of local disease.

Non-Hodgkin's lymphoma often presents with widespread extranodal disease. Differentiation of central nervous system lymphoma from *Toxoplasma gondii* infection can be difficult and require brain biopsy.

Cervical carcinoma, abnormal cervical cytology and human papillomavirus infection are all more common in HIV-infected women, who should have cervical smears at least annually.

Primary treatment of HIV

The development of therapies for AIDS requires an understanding of how the HIV-1 virus integrates into the human genome, and how viral replication and viral gene expression are regulated.

The proviral genome of HIV-1 is 9–10 kb long, and has three main structural genes:
- The *gag* (group-specific antigen) gene encodes the core protein antigens of the virion (intact virus particle). These are formed as the cleaved products of a larger precursor protein.
- The *pol* (polymerase) gene encodes the viral reverse transcriptase, and also the IN protein required for integration of viral DNA into the host genome.
- The *env* gene encodes the two envelope glycoproteins, which are cleaved from a larger precursor.

When the HIV virion binds to a CD4 molecule on the cell surface, a conformational change occurs in the envelope glycoprotein, and the virus enters the cell via fusion of lipid bilayers at the cell surface. The uncoated core of the virion then uses its viral reverse transcriptase to transcribe one of the two identical strands of positive-sense RNA into DNA. This DNA is duplicated by a host cell DNA polymerase, and migrates to the nucleus where it is integrated at a random site into the genome. Transcription of the integrated viral DNA is regulated by both host factors (such as the DNA-binding protein NFκB), and viral regulatory proteins such as the tat and rev proteins. Virally encoded proteins are processed and assembled in the cytoplasm, and then bud from the cell surface as new infectious virions.

Therapy for AIDS

Despite increased understanding of the molecular biology of HIV infection, therapies remain elusive and AIDS remains a progressive, fatal disease. Several sites in the viral life cycle have been targeted, and effective treatment will probably require combination therapy (see Trials):

Inhibition of reverse transcriptase. This remains the mainstay of treatment. Zidovudine (AZT), and the newer agents didanosine (ddI) and dideoxycytosine (ddC; zalcitabine) are nucleoside analogues which bind preferentially to viral reverse transcriptase compared to human DNA polymerase.

Protease inhibitors. Ritonavir, indinavir and saquinavir prevent viral maturation. Gastrointestinal side effects are common (nausea, diarrhoea, abdominal pain, vomiting).

TRIALS

The **Aids Clinical Trials Group** compared zidovudine with didanosine in 617 patients with advanced HIV-1 infection with little or no previous treatment with zidovudine. Zidovudine appeared more effective as initial therapy, but after 8–16 weeks' exposure to zidovudine some patients may benefit from changing to didanosine. *Arch Intern Med* 1995; **155**: 961–974.

The **North American HIV Working Party** compared treatment with lamividine, zidovudine, or both in 366 HIV-positive patients with 200–500 CD4+ cells/mm^3. Treatment with lamividine and zidovudine in combination was well-tolerated and more effective than either agent alone in increasing CD4+ counts and reducing plasma HIV-1 RNA. *N Engl J Med* 1995; **333**: 1662–1669.

The **Delta trial** compared combinations of zidovudine (AZT) plus didanosine (ddI) or zalcitabine (ddC) with zidovudine alone in 3207 HIV-infected individuals. Treatment with combinations of AZT plus ddI or ddC prolonged life and delayed disease progression compared with AZT alone. The addition of ddI to patients already receiving AZT also improved survival. *Lancet* 1996; **348**: 283–291.

The **AIDS Clinical Trials Group** compared the effect of the HIV protease inhibitor saquinavir, in combination with nucleoside antiretroviral agents, with nucleoside agents alone in patients with HIV infection. Treatment with saquinavir, zalcitabine, and zidovudine was most effective in reducing HIV replication and increasing CD4+ counts. *N Engl J Med* 1996; **334**: 1011–1017.

The **AIDS Clinical Trials Group Study 175 Study Team** compared nucleoside monotherapy with combination therapy in 2467 HIV-infected adults with CD4 cell counts from 200 to 500/mm^3. Treatment with zidovudine plus didanosine, zidovudine plus zalcitabine, or didanosine alone slowed the progression of HIV disease, and was superior to treatment with zidovudine alone. *N Engl J Med* 1996; **335**: 1081–1090.

The **Terry Beirn Community Programs for Clinical Research on AIDS** compared zidovudine alone or in combination with didanosine or zalcitabine in 1102 HIV-infected patients with AIDS or CD4 cell counts less than 200/mm^3. In patients with advanced HIV infection combination therapy was not superior to zidovudine alone, although combination therapy may be more effective in patients with little or no exposure to zidovudine. *N Engl J Med* 1996; **335**: 1099–1106.

Prevention of new virion formation. A number of treatments aimed at inhibiting the production of new virus particles are under evaluation. These include agents which bind to and inhibit viral proteins such as tat, and the pro gene product.

HIV entry. Soluble truncated forms of the CD4 molecule are effective at neutralizing HIV *in vitro*. However, clinical trials of *soluble recombinant CD4* failed to show any benefit in HIV-infected patients. Several factors may have accounted for this lack of efficacy. Recombinant CD4 has a short half-life *in vivo*, and administration leads to the development of anti-CD4 antibodies. In addition, viruses present in the community may be less susceptible to neutralization by CD4 than their laboratory counterparts.

HIV vaccines

Emphasis is currently being placed on the development of vaccines against HIV. In addition to their importance in prevention, vaccines may also induce additional immunity to any immunity generated as a consequence of natural infection in patients.

A number of therapeutic trials using either modified whole virus particles or recombinant HIV proteins are currently in progress. The majority of current vaccines are based on the extracellular envelope protein gp120, or the envelope precursor protein gp160. One factor which may limit the success of these vaccines is the high variability of the envelope proteins between different strains of HIV.

Gene therapy for AIDS

• The gene encoding an HIV protein, such as the gp120 envelope protein, is introduced into the patient, either directly into muscle cells or *ex vivo* into cells that are harvested and reimplanted. Expression of the protein could then stimulate an immune response against the virus.

• Cells could be genetically engineered to secrete a potential therapy into the circulation. For example, lymphocytes could be transfected with a soluble CD4-IgG chimeric protein in the hope that continued secretion of soluble CD4 may be more effective at neutralizing HIV than injection of the recombinant molecule (see p. 456).

• Genes could be targeted directly to infected CD4 cells using retroviral vectors. For example, expression of a mutant *rev* gene could inhibit the production of structural HIV proteins. Alternatively, the expression of high levels of sequences that will bind HIV transcription factors (such as the *trans*-activation response region TAR), could sequester the viral transcription factors.

Infectious mononucleosis (glandular fever)

A common disease of the young with an excellent prognosis, usually transmitted by saliva. It is caused by the Epstein–Barr virus (a herpesvirus). Seroprevalence is >90% in adults.

Clinical presentation

Malaise, fever, sore throat, muscle and joint aches. Examination reveals a tonsillar exudate and palatal petechiae with generalized lymphadenopathy and splenomegaly. A macular–papular rash is common, and more frequent if ampicillin is given for the sore throat. Mesenteric adenitis with appendicitis may occur.

Investigation

The disease is confirmed by a leukocytosis ($10–50 \times 10^9$/l), with an absolute ($>4 \times 10^9$/l) and relative ($>50\%$ of total white cells) increase in mononuclear cells. Patients with infectious mononucleosis produce IgM antibodies which bind to and agglutinate red cells from other species. The Paul Bunnell test measures agglutination of sheep red cells with the patient's serum. In the Monospot test the patient's serum is used to agglutinate horse red cells.

Thrombocytopenia and abnormal liver function tests are common but rarely severe.

Complications

Tonsillar enlargement may be severe and prevent swallowing of saliva and even threaten airway obstruction. Rare complications include splenic rupture, autoimmune haemolytic anaemia, encephalitis, transverse myelitis, Bell's palsy and Guillain–Barré syndrome. Lethargy may last for several months.

Differential diagnosis

The disease may be confused with:

- acute tonsillitis;
- infections which produce a similar rash, e.g. measles, rubella;
- infections which produce similar malaise and lymphadenopathy (e.g. toxoplasmosis, brucellosis and tuberculosis);
- lymphomas and leukaemias;
- AIDS;
- drug hypersensitivity; and
- acute appendicitis.

NB   Diphtheria should not be forgotten.

Treatment

Usually rest, aspirin gargles and anaesthetic lozenges for the sore throat are sufficient. If the tonsillar enlargement is great and swallowing is difficult or the airway threatened (anginose glandular fever — usually with severe general symptoms), a short course of steroids (prednisolone 40 mg daily for 5–10 days) rapidly reduces the symptoms.

Tuberculosis

Tuberculosis (TB) most commonly causes pulmonary disease (p. 346) but can

BTS RECOMMENDATIONS

	Initial phase	Months	Continuation phase	Months
Adults				
Pulmonary TB	I, R, P, (E)*	2	I, R	4
Meningitis	I, R, P	2	I, R	10
TB lymphadenitis	I, R, P	2	I, R	4
Bone and joint	I, R, P	2	I, R	7
Pericarditis	I, R, P, E	2	I, R	4
Other extrapulmonary TB	I, R, P, E	2	I, R	4
Children				
Pulmonary TB	I, R, P	2	I, R	4
	or I, R	9		
Non-pulmonary	As above			

I, isoniazid; R, rifampicin; P, pyrazinamide; E, ethambutol.
*Ethambutol is added if there is reason to suspect drug-resistant organisms. Liver function tests (LFTs) should be checked before starting therapy. Transient asymptomatic increases in serum transaminases are very common after starting treatment. Discontinuation is not indicated unless there are symptoms of hepatitis (anorexia, vomiting, hepatomegaly) or jaundice. It is not necessary to monitor LFTs except in patients known to have pre-existing liver disease. Steroids are used in life-threatening or widespread TB in an attempt to reduce acute inflammation and allow time for drugs to work. They are usually indicated for pericarditis, extensive pulmonary disease, moderate or severe meningitis, ureteric TB and pleural effusion.

Table 23.8 BTS recommendations for treatment of TB. From *Thorax* 1990; **45**: 403–8.

affect any site, including central nervous system (p. 156). British Thoracic Society (BTS) recommendations for treatment are shown in Table 23.8.

Chronic fatigue syndrome

A report of the joint working group of the Royal Colleges of Physicians, Psychiatrists and General Practitioners used this term to describe the syndrome characterized by a minimum of 6 months of severe physical and mental fatigue and fatigability, made worse by minor exertion. The term myalgic encephalomyelitis (ME) was first used in 1955 to describe an unexplained illness in the staff of the Royal Free Hospital. Although ME has been linked to chronic fatigue syndrome, it describes a specific pathological process which is not found in these patients.

Apart from profound fatigue, there are no other features or physical signs which distinguish chronic fatigue syndrome. Associated psychiatric disorders, particularly anxiety and depression, are common. There is no convincing evidence that common viral infections are a risk factor for chronic fatigue syndrome, with the exception of the fatigue that follows less than 10% of Epstein–Barr virus infections.

Investigation

No laboratory tests can confirm the diagnosis. The following should be performed to exclude other causes of fatigue:

- full blood count, erythrocyte sedimentation rate;
- urea and electrolytes, liver function test, C-reactive protein;
- thyroid function;
- creatine kinase;
- urinalysis for protein and sugar.

Management

A gradual planned increase in exercise is the main objective. Cognitive behaviour therapy may help achieve this. Antidepressants should be given if there is evidence of an associated depressive disorder.

TRIALS

The Centers for Disease Control in Atlanta produced the CDC-1994 criteria for chronic fatigue syndrome (*Ann Intern Med* 1994; **121**: 953–959):

1 Clinically evaluated unexplained persistent or relapsing fatigue that is not:

- of new onset
- the result of ongoing exertion
- substantially alleviated by rest

and results in substantial reduction in previous levels of occupational, educational, social or personal activities

2 With four or more of the following symptoms, concurrently present for ≥6 months:

- impaired memory or concentration
- sore throat
- tender cervical or axillary lymph nodes
- muscle pain
- multijoint pain
- new headaches
- unrefreshing sleep
- post-exertion malaise

Appendices

Guide to UK medical standards of fitness to drive

EPILEPSY
Group 1 entitlement

First epileptic seizure/solitary fit. One year off driving with medical review before restarting.

Patients suffering from epilepsy
To be granted a licence patients should have been free from epileptic attacks for 2 years, or have had an epileptic attack whilst asleep more than 3 years previously and no epileptic attacks whilst awake but only whilst asleep since that attack.

If epileptic medication is withdrawn, the DVLA advises patients not to drive during withdrawal, and for 6 months after cessation of therapy. If an epileptic attack occurs the above criteria then apply.

Provoked seizures are dealt with by the DVLA on an individual basis.

A single loss of consciousness for which no cause is found requires cessation of driving for 1 year. Multiple episodes are treated as for epilepsy (i.e. at least 2 years off driving).

Group 2 entitlement

Patients with a history of epilepsy should:
- have been free of epileptic attack for at least the past 10 years;
- have not taken epileptic medication during this 10-year period;
- not have a continuing liability to epileptic seizure.

OTHER NEUROLOGICAL DISORDERS
Group 1 entitlement
Stroke
At least 1 month off driving after the event. When clinical recovery is fully satisfactory, driving may restart.

Subarachnoid haemorrhage due to intracranial aneurysm
If treated surgically, I year off driving for middle cerebral artery aneurysm, 6 months off driving for all other sites. Other treatment (e.g. embolization): cease driving until full clinical recovery. If no treatment, I year off driving.

Subarachnoid haemorrhage due to intracranial arteriovenous malformation
If treated surgically, I year off driving. Other treatment: cease driving until full recovery.

Cerebral abscess
Two years off driving (high risk of developing epilepsy).

Surgical treatment of benign supratentorial tumour
(e.g. meningioma, cyst)
One year off driving.

Surgical treatment of benign infratentorial tumour
(posterior fossa, e.g. acoustic neuroma)
Resume driving following recovery.

Malignant intracranial tumour
Grade I and II glioma — at least 2 years off driving; grade III and IV glioma or intracranial secondary deposits—at least 4 years off driving.

Serious head injury
One year off driving if craniotomy performed or if dural tear or intracerebral haematoma.

Group 2 entitlement
Refusal or revocation is recommended for all of the above with the exception of benign infratentorial tumour.

CARDIOVASCULAR DISORDERS
Group I entitlement
Angina
If angina occurs at wheel, driving must cease.

Myocardial infarction
At least I month off driving.

Successful coronary angioplasty
At least I week off driving.

Pacemaker insertion
One month off driving.

Arrhythmia
Off driving until satisfactory control of symptoms.

Group 2 entitlement
Refusal or revocation recommended for all of above. Relicensing may be permitted in some cases.

DIABETES MELLITUS
Group 1 entitlement
Insulin-treated
Must demonstrate satisfactory control, recognize warning symptoms of hypoglycaemia and meet visual standards.

Diet and tablet-treated
No restriction unless relevant disability (e.g. visual disturbance).

Diet alone
Need not notify DVLA unless relevant disability.

Group 2 entitlement
New applicants from 1/4/1991 are barred in law if on insulin. Patients on tablets or diet will be licensed unless relevant disability.

Glossary of useful pharmacological terms

First-pass metabolism
Metabolism of drugs after absorption from the gut lumen and before entry to the systemic circulation. This usually (but not exclusively) occurs in the liver. For example, GTN given sublingually bypasses the liver.

Pharmacodynamics
The study of the action of drugs at their sites of action, or 'the action of drugs on the body'.

Pharmacogenetics
The study of the different reactions to drugs based on hereditary differences, e.g. acetylation—'fast' and 'slow' of isoniazid and hydralazine.

Pharmacokinetics
The study of drug absorption, distribution, metabolism and excretion, or 'the action of the body on drugs'.

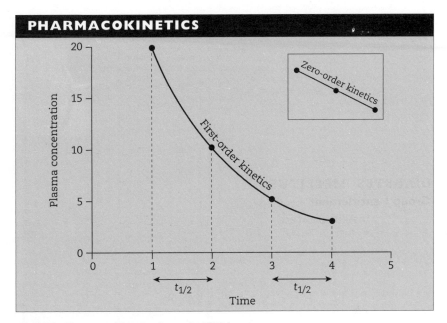

Fig. 24.1 Pharmacokinetics ($t_{1/2}$ = half life).

Receptors

Molecules with which drugs interact to produce pharmacological effects. The following terms describe this interaction:

- *Affinity*—a measure of how avidly the drug binds to its receptor.
- *Agonist*—a molecule that interacts with a receptor to produce a response.
- *Antagonist*—a molecule that binds to a receptor but does not activate it. They block the action of agonists.
- *Competitive antagonists* bind reversibly to the receptor—high doses of agonist can overcome the effect.
- *Irreversible antagonists* cannot be overcome by increasing concentrations of agonist.
- *Partial agonists* do not elicit the same response as full agonists, and antagonize the effect of full agonists.

Therapeutic ratio

The *toxic therapeutic ratio* is better termed the non-toxic therapeutic range. It is the plasma concentration range sufficient to produce a desired effect but below the toxic dose. The greater the ratio (e.g. penicillin when enormous doses are required to cause toxicity), the better.

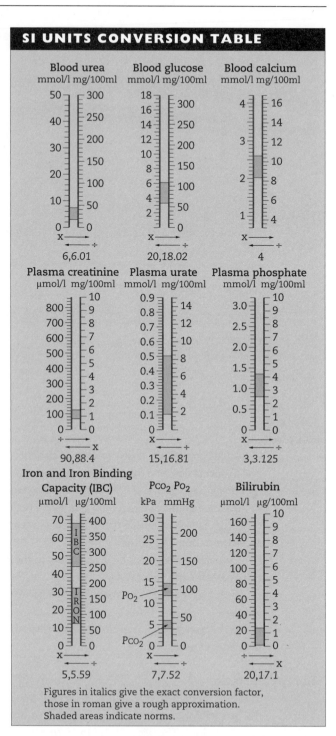

Fig. 24.2 SI units conversion table.

Trials
Phase I

Small studies in normal volunteers to determine the effective dose range and to detect and monitor side effects and toxicity.

Phase II

Studies on patients which include dose-ranging studies and small clinical trials.

Phase III

Clinical trials comparing the drug with other agents or placebo.

Half-life $(t_{1/2})$

The time for the plasma concentration of a drug to fall by half.

Zero-order kinetics

The rate of fall of plasma concentration is independent of concentration (e.g. ethanol).

First-order kinetics

The rate of fall of plasma concentration is related to the concentration, i.e. the more present, the faster the fall in plasma concentration (most drugs).

Index

abdominal carcinoma 46, 47, 48, 52, 55, 98

abdominal examination 42–6, 47, 48

abdominal mass 42, 43–4
  right subcostal region 45–6
  suprapubic region 46

absence seizures (petit mal) 134, 136

acanthosis nigricans 414

acetylcholine 122

achalasia 52, 53, 341

achondroplasia 220

acid alcohol-fast bacillus (AAFB) 346, 347, 348

acne vulgaris 39, 116, 409

acoustic neuroma 12, 28, 150

acromegaly 26, 110, 209, 210–12
  hypertension 211, 373
  secondary diabetes 108, 221

acyclovir 157, 414, 455

Addison's disease (adrenal insufficiency) 217–18, 288, 417
  acute (adrenal crisis) 217, 218
  chronic 217
  hypercalcaemia 252, 290
  hypoglycaemic coma 228
  hypoparathyroidism 255
  hypopituitarism 209

adenosine 364

adenovirus meningitis 157

adrenal adenoma 214, 219

adrenal carcinoma 214

adrenal cortex 213
  glucocorticoids 213–14
  mineralocorticoids 214
  sex hormones 214

adrenal crisis 217, 218

adrenal disorders 213–19

adrenal function tests 217–18

basal function 217
  Synacthen (tetracosactrin) tests 218

adrenal glands 213–14

adrenal insufficiency see Addison's disease

adrenal medulla 213

adrenaline 120, 121, 213, 218, 337, 365, 368, 412

adrenocorticotrophic hormone (ACTH) 208, 213
  deficiency 209
  ectopic secretion 214, 215, 287, 343

adrenogenital syndrome 216

adult respiratory distress syndrome (ARDS) 355–6

affective disorders 177

afterload 369

agnosia 16

agranulocytic ulcers 415

AIDS see human immunodeficiency virus (HIV)

AIDS dementia 172

albumin serum level 49

alcohol intake 172, 242, 323, 402
  coronary atherosclerosis 358
  epilepsy 135, 137
  hypertension 373

alcoholic hepatitis 48, 292, 296, 297
  cirrhosis 298
  hepatocellular failure 299

aldolase serum level 168

aldosterone 213, 214

alfacalcidol (1α-hydroxycholecalciferol) 248, 251, 256

alkaline diuresis 435

alkaline phosphatase serum level 49

alkylating agents 431

allergens 333

allergic contact dermatitis 408

allopurinol 257, 258

α$_1$-antitrypsin deficiency 298, 329

alphafetoprotein 50, 303

Alport's syndrome 267, 270, 275

Alzheimer's disease 135, 171, 173–4
  extrapyramidal component 147
  trials 174

amantadine 146

amiloride 288

5-amino salicylic acid 312

aminoglutethimide 215

aminoglycosides 12, 272

aminophylline 335

aminosalicylates 312

aminotransferase (transaminase) serum level 49

amiodarone 74, 76, 364, 412
  thyroid function effects 207

amitriptyline overdose 433, 435

amlodipine 379

amoebic cyst 45

amoebic dysentery 54, 55, 437, 444

amoebic hepatitis 292

amoebic liver abscess 292, 444

amoebomas 444

amoxycillin 307, 330, 339, 397

amphetamines 140
  overdose 135

amphotericin 272, 451, 454

ampicillin 265, 321, 443, 444

amyloidosis 44, 45, 151, 318, 430

amyotonia congenita 170

amyotrophic lateral sclerosis 144

anaemia 97–8, 418–26
  bronchial carcinoma 342
  cardiac failure 370

469